**diagnostic imaging** in cri

# diagnostic imaging
# in critical care

## A PROBLEM BASED APPROACH

Chris Joyce
Nivene Saad
Peter Kruger
Carole Foot
Nikki Blackwell

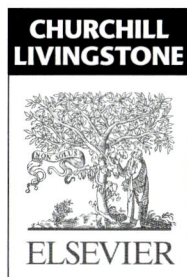

**CHURCHILL LIVINGSTONE**

ELSEVIER

Sydney  Edinburgh  London  New York  Philadelphia  St Louis  Toronto

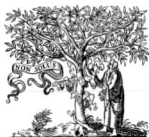

ELSEVIER

Churchill Livingstone
is an imprint of Elsevier

Elsevier Australia. ACN 001 002 357
(a division of Reed International Books Australia Pty Ltd)
Tower 1, 475 Victoria Avenue, Chatswood, NSW 2067

National Library of Australia Cataloguing-in-Publication Data

Diagnostic imaging in critical care : a problem based approach / Chris Joyce ... [et al.].

ISBN: 978 0 7295 3878 7 (pbk.)

Includes index.
Bibliography.

Diagnostic imaging.
Clinical medicine.

Joyce, Chris.

616.0754

Publisher: Sophie Kaliniecki
Developmental Editor: Sabrina Chew
Publishing Services Manager: Helena Klijn
Editorial Coordinator: Eleanor Cant
Edited by Mark Snape
Proofread by Kerry Brown
Design and typesetting by Pindar NZ, Auckland, New Zealand
Index by Max McMaster
Printed by 1010 Printing International Limited

# CONTENTS

# About the authors

**Chris Joyce**
MB ChB, PhD, FJFICM, FANZCA
Associate Professor, Department of Anaesthesiology and Critical Care, University of Queensland, Brisbane, Australia
Director of Intensive Care, Princess Alexandra Hospital, Brisbane, Australia

**Nivene Saad**
MB BCh, MS, MD, FRANZCR
Staff Radiologist, Princess Alexandra Hospital, Brisbane, Australia

**Peter Kruger**
MBBS, BSc(Hons), FJFICM, FANZCA
Senior Lecturer, Department of Anaesthesiology and Critical Care, University of Queensland, Brisbane, Australia
Deputy Director of Intensive Care, Princess Alexandra Hospital, Brisbane, Australia

**Carole Foot**
MBBS(Hons), FACEM, FJFICM, MSc(International Health Management)
Staff Specialist Intensive Care, Royal North Shore Hospital, Sydney, Australia

**Nikki Blackwell**
MBBS, BSc (Hons), FRCP, FRACP, FAChPM, DTMH, FJFICM
Senior Staff Specialist, The Prince Charles Hospital, Brisbane, Australia
Consultant Critical Care, Médecins Sans Frontières, Paris, France
Senior Lecturer, University of Queensland, Brisbane, Australia

# Reviewers

**Gerard Ahern**
MBBS
Prosector & Postgraduate Anatomy Coordinator, Monash University, Melbourne, Australia
Honorary Senior Fellow in Anatomy, University of Melbourne, Australia
Honorary Associate Professor, Oceania University, Apia, Samoa
Lecturer & Tutor, Royal Australasian College of Surgeons
Examination Contributor, Australian Medical Council

**Nicholas Barnes**
MB ChB, FJFICM
Clinical Director, Critical Care, Waikato Hospital, Hamilton, New Zealand

**Benjamin Harris**
MBBS, BSc(Med), PhD, FRACP
Respiratory Physician, Royal North Shore Hospital, Sydney, Australia
Research Fellow, The Woolcock Institute of Medical Research, Sydney, Australia

**Tim Harris**
FACEM, FCEM, DipImmCare, Dip O&G, BM, BS, BMedSci
Consultant, Emergency Medicine and Prehospital Care, Royal London Hospital and London HEMS, UK
Head of Research, School of Emergency Medicine and Department of Emergency Medicine, Royal London Hospital, London, UK

**Morry Silberstein**
MBBS, MD, DRACR, FRANZCR
Associate Professor, Radiology, Monash University, Melbourne, Australia

# Acknowledgements

Dr Daniel Mullany contributed images, critiqued the problems and helped with the annotations on the DVD. Dr Judith Bellapart contributed images for the problems on transcranial Doppler and provided advice on these problems. Our thanks to the radiographers, sonographers and PACS support personnel of Princess Alexandra hospital who helped with image acquisition and optimisation, and to Wendy Schipper who assisted with the preparation of the manuscript.

# Introduction: including how to use this book and DVD

This book is based on a series of problems about critically ill patients. Plain X-ray, CT, MRI, and ultrasound images from the full spectrum of disease processes seen in the critically ill patient are included. The problems are arranged in five chapters based on the region of the body being imaged (Chest, Abdomen and Pelvis, Head, Neck and Back, and Limbs). Each chapter starts with a section of applied anatomy related to imaging that region, except for the Limbs chapter. The final chapter is basic information about the imaging modalities presented in this book. Whether this is read first, last or when questions about the imaging modality are raised by the problems is up to the reader.

For each problem, there are two sets of radiological images. One set is in the book as part of the problem and, because of space, is limited to only those images necessary to solve the problem. The second set is contained on the DVD and comprises a full set of high-quality images such as a reporting radiologist would review. Each problem consists of a brief clinical scenario, the two sets of images and a series of questions. Answers to the questions (including our interpretation of the images) are provided in the book, along with a set of learning points.

While the book can be used independently of the DVD, the learning experience will be enhanced by reviewing the full set of images on the DVD when the problem is done. The DVD images are the same images seen on the digital X-ray system used in our clinical practice. This provides high-quality images on a computer screen that could never be achieved with printed reproductions. It also allows the user to scroll through MRI or CT images, which gives an appreciation of the three-dimensional anatomy that cannot be obtained from images in a book or on film printouts. Annotations on the DVD images illustrate the findings that we have made in our interpretation of the images. The DVD images can be viewed with these annotations switched on or off.

We hope that you find learning from this book as fulfilling as we have found the challenges of caring for the patients whose images are presented in this book.

# Acronyms

| | |
|---|---|
| **AP** | Anteroposterior |
| **ARDS** | Acute respiratory distress syndrome |
| **CXR** | Chest X-ray |
| **DISH** | Diffuse idiopathic skeletal hyperostosis |
| **GCS** | Glasgow coma scale |
| **Gd** | Gadolinium |
| **HIDA** | Hepatobiliary iminodiacetic acid (scan) |
| **HRCT** | High resolution computerised tomography |
| **ICU** | Intensive care unit |
| **IV** | Intravenous |
| **IVC** | Inferior vena cava |
| **NG** | Nasogastric |
| **PA** | Posteroanterior |
| **PCP** | Pneumocystis pneumonia |
| **TB** | Tuberculosis |
| **TPN** | Total parenteral nutrition |

# CHAPTER 1

# CHEST

# APPLIED ANATOMY

## Lobes and fissures of the lung

(Figures 1.1, 1.2 and 1.3)

In the right lung, there are two fissures. The greater or oblique fissure runs obliquely forwards and downwards from approximately the T4 vertebra posteriorly, then passes through the hilum to contact the front of the diaphragm 0–3 cm behind the anterior costophrenic recess. This greater fissure separates the lower lobe from the upper and middle lobes. The horizontal fissure runs horizontally and laterally at the level of the hilum and separates the upper from the middle lobe. The lower lobe lies against the diaphragm, the middle lobe lies against the heart, while the upper lobe lies against the superior mediastinum.

In the left lung, there is only one fissure, the oblique fissure. This fissure separates the lower lobe from the upper lobe. The part of the left upper lobe analogous to the right middle lobe is the lingula, but there is no fissure separating it from the rest of the upper lobe. The lower lobe lies against the diaphragm. The lingula lies against the heart and the remainder of the upper lobe lies against the upper mediastinum.

This explains the X-ray appearances when individual lobes are opacified. The normal borders between an affected lobe and adjacent soft tissue density mediastinal structures are lost (silhouette sign), while new borders are created where the opacified lobe lies against normal lung at fissures.

With a right upper lobe process there is loss of

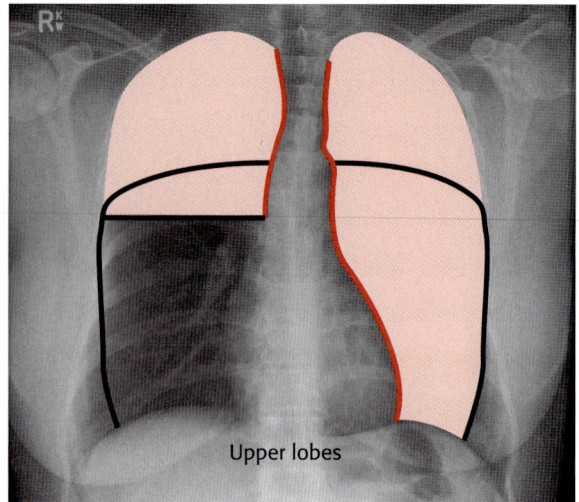

**FIGURE 1.2** Upper lobes.

the right upper mediastinal border and the creation of a border at the horizontal fissure.

With a left upper lobe process there is a loss of both the left upper mediastinal border and the left cardiac border. If the process is constrained to the lingula, only the left cardiac border is lost.

With a right middle lobe process, there is loss of the right cardiac border and creation of a new border at the horizontal fissure.

With a lower lobe process on either the right or left, there is loss of the diaphragmatic border. Note that the opacification can extend well above the level of the horizontal fissure, up to T4.

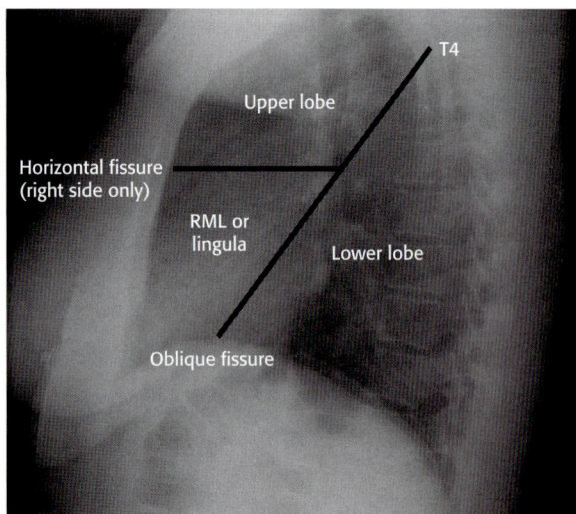

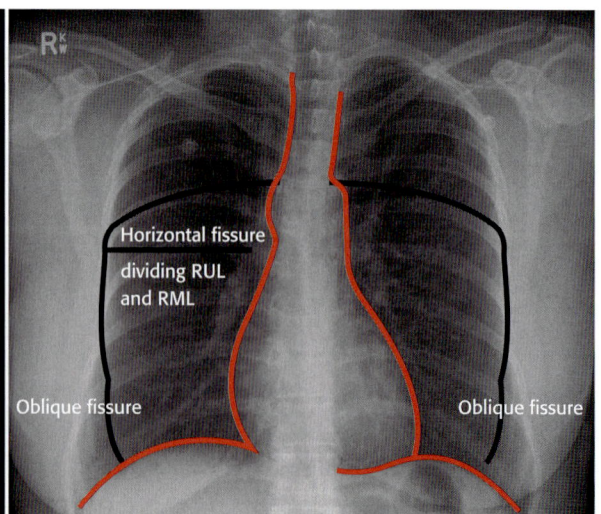

**FIGURE 1.1** The normal fissures and borders of the lung. RML = Right middle lobe; RUL = Right upper lobe.

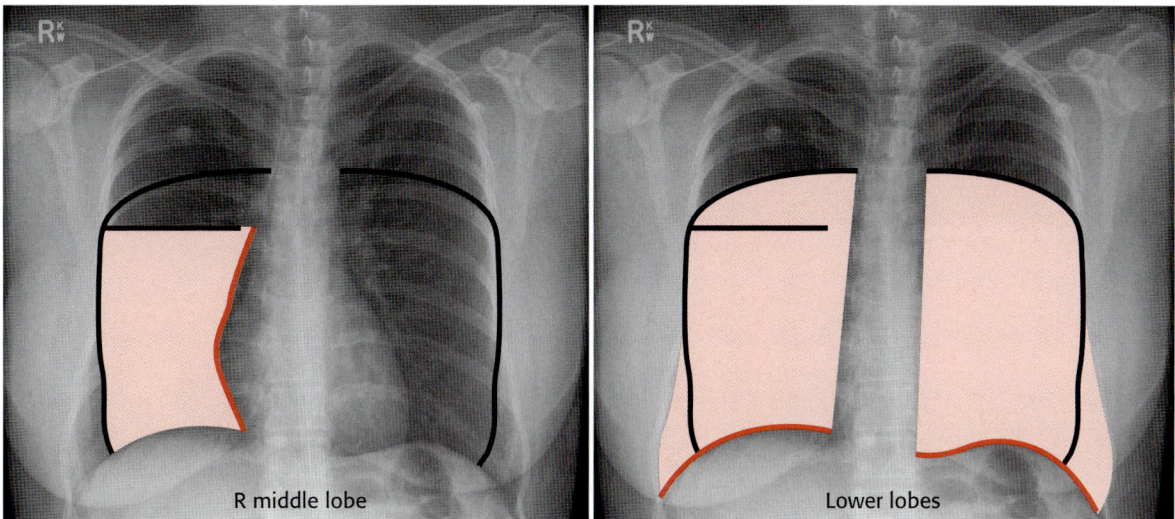

**FIGURE 1.3** Middle and lower lobes.

## Mediastinal borders (Figure 1.4)

The right side of the mediastinum is the "venous" side and, from above down, is formed by the brachiocephalic vein, the superior vena cava (SVC), the azygous vein, the SVC and the right atrium. The left or "arterial" side of the mediastinum is formed by the subclavian artery, the aortic knuckle, the pulmonary artery, the left atrium and the left ventricle. Understanding this anatomy facilitates determining which is the abnormal structure when there is an abnormal mediastinal or cardiac outline on the chest X-ray.

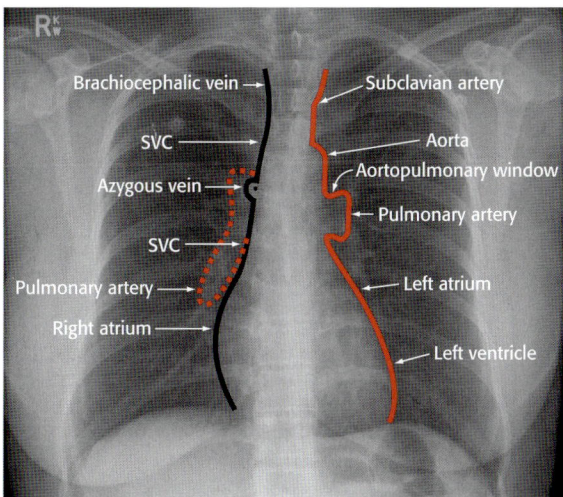

**FIGURE 1.4** Mediastinal borders and position of venous and arterial anatomical structures.

## PROBLEM 1.01

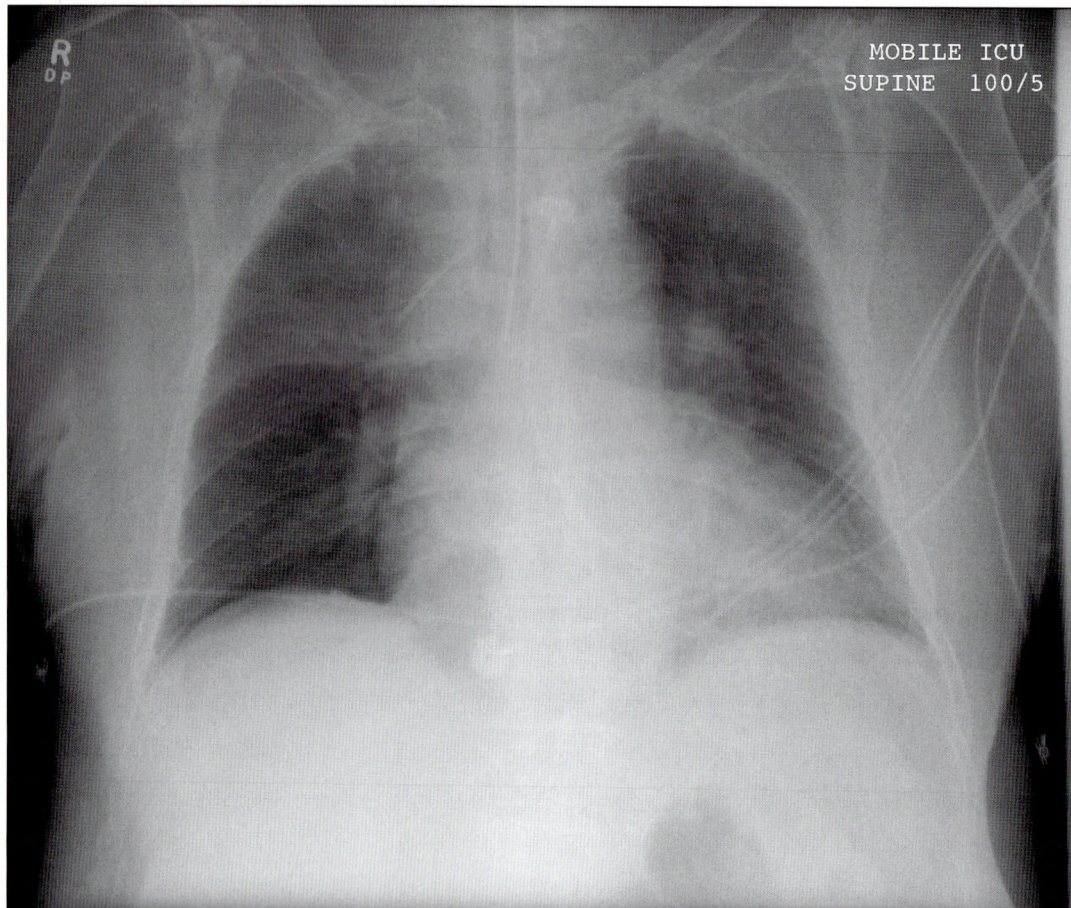

This 64-year-old man presented with shortness of breath for 24 hours. On admission to hospital, he had hypoxaemic respiratory failure.

## Q

1. Which lobe is abnormal?
2. What findings support this?
3. What is the likely process in the affected lobe?
4. What evidence supports this being the process?

# A

1. Right upper lobe.

2. Findings that support involvement of the right upper lobe are:
   • opacification in right upper zone
   • loss of right upper mediastinal border
   • creation of a new border at horizontal fissure

3. Consolidation.

4. Opacification without any evidence of shift of structures supports consolidation. An alternative process is collapse, which would be supported by the presence of the tip of the endotracheal tube at the carina. The lack of shift of structures argues against collapse unless it is incomplete.

## LEARNING POINT

Each lobe of the lung has a characteristic pattern of opacification. Loss/creation of borders allows identification of the site of a pathological process.

## PROBLEM 1.02

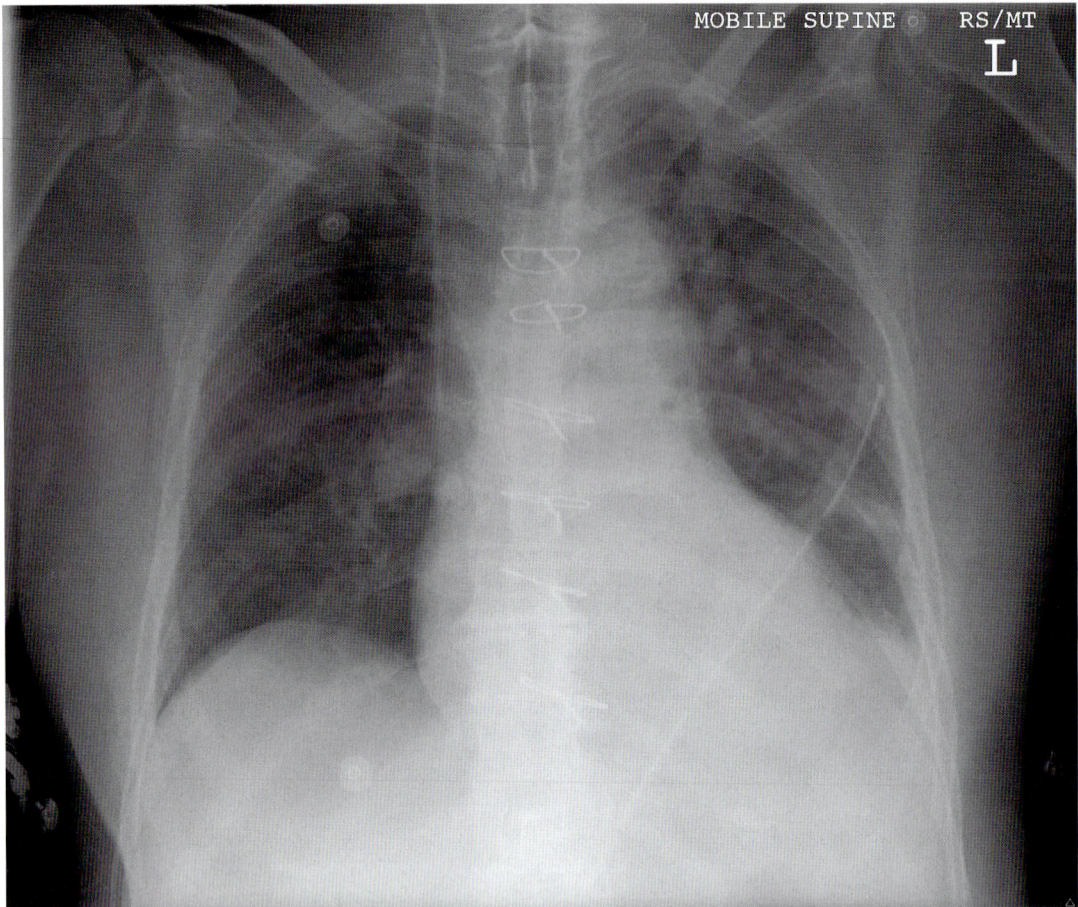

This 61-year-old man presented with unstable angina. He was found to have critical stenosis of the left main coronary artery and had emergency coronary artery bypass grafting yesterday.

## Q

1. Which lobe is predominantly abnormal?
2. What is the likely process affecting that lobe?
3. What findings support this?

# A

1. The left lower lobe. There is also patchy opacification elsewhere in both lungs, likely to be atelectasis.

2. Collapse, with some additional element of pleural effusion.

3. Findings which support this are:
   - increased cardiac density
   - loss of diaphragmatic border

   With complete collapse of the left lower lobe, the bronchus is typically shifted downwards, a sign that is not present on this image.

## LEARNING POINT

Left lower lobe collapse is very common following cardiac surgery.

## PROBLEM 1.03

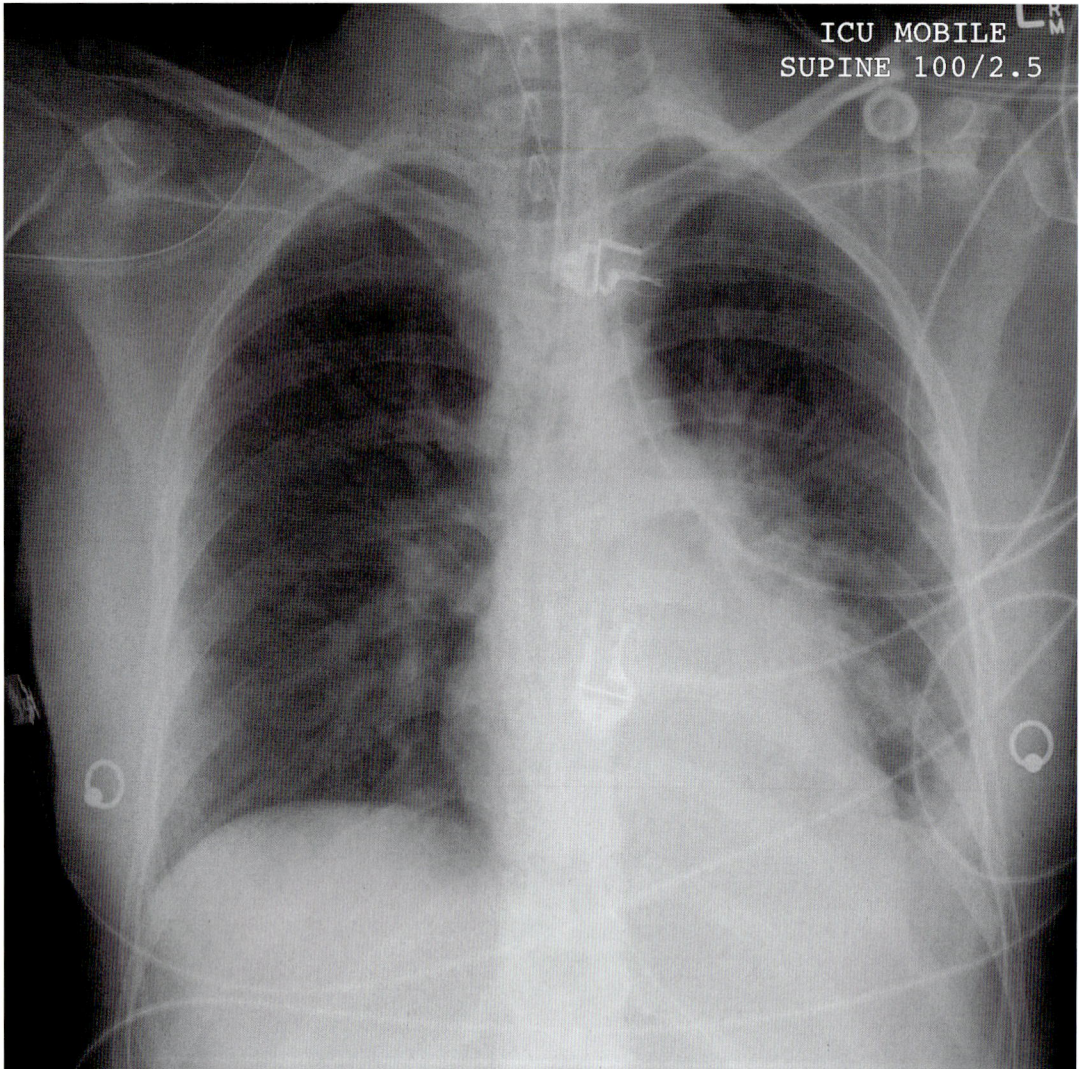

```
ICU MOBILE
SUPINE 100/2.5
```

This 25-year-old woman was an unrestrained front seat passenger during a high-speed motor vehicle collision. She sustained a severe head injury, with a GCS of 3 at the scene. She is thought to have aspirated prior to intubation.

**Q**

1. Which lobes are involved in the process?
2. What is the likely process?

## A

1. Lobes that are involved in the process are:
   - Lingula and left lower lobe are involved in the process.
   - Lingular involvement is evidenced by loss of the left cardiac border, with adjacent perihilar opacification.
   - Left lower lobe involvement is evidenced by patchy density behind the heart and partial loss of the left hemidiaphragm.

2. The likely process is consolidation, which, in this context, is probably due to aspiration. Collapse needs to be considered, but there is no obvious shift of structures.

## LEARNING POINT

Knowledge of the anatomy will enable delineation of which lobes are involved in a pathological process.

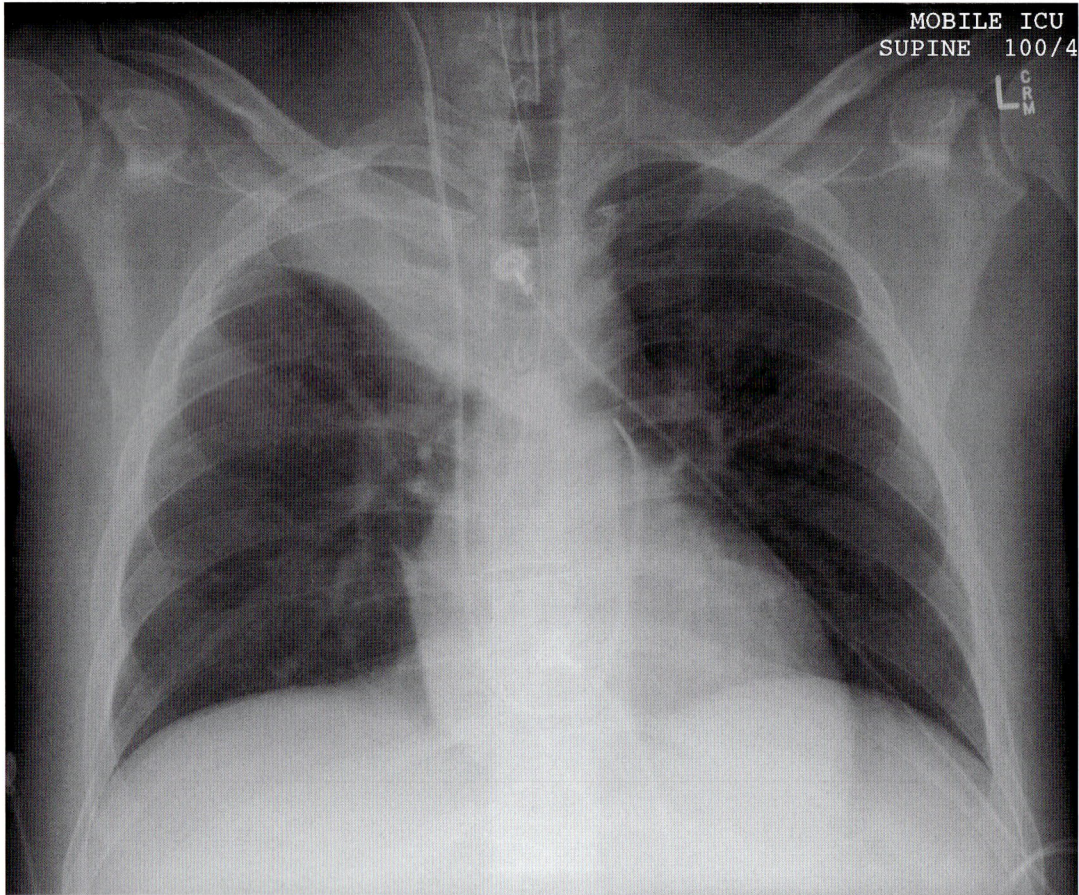

This 32-year-old man presented with septic shock. A pulmonary artery catheter was inserted to guide management. Your junior medical staff are concerned that the findings on this image suggest the pulmonary artery catheter may have caused a pulmonary infarct.

**Q**
What do you think?

# A

The tip of the pulmonary artery catheter appears to be in the proximal pulmonary artery. The appearances in the right upper lobe suggest collapse, as evidenced by:

- homogenous opacification in the right upper zone
- loss of right upper mediastinal border
- creation of a new border at the horizontal fissure
- upward shift of the horizontal fissure

These features are not suggestive of pulmonary infarction.

The endotracheal tube is not too low. Indeed, it is too high, suggesting that it is unlikely to be the immediate cause of the collapse.

## LEARNING POINT

Pulmonary collapse creates traction forces on adjacent structures, often shifting them towards the area of collapse.

With right upper lobe collapse, it is common to find the horizontal fissure shifted upwards. There may also be upwards shift of the right hilum and right upper lobe bronchus and/or shift to the right of the trachea and other upper mediastinal structures. Hyperinflation of the rest of the right lung may occur as it expands to fill up the space left by the collapsed right upper lobe.

## PROBLEM 1.05

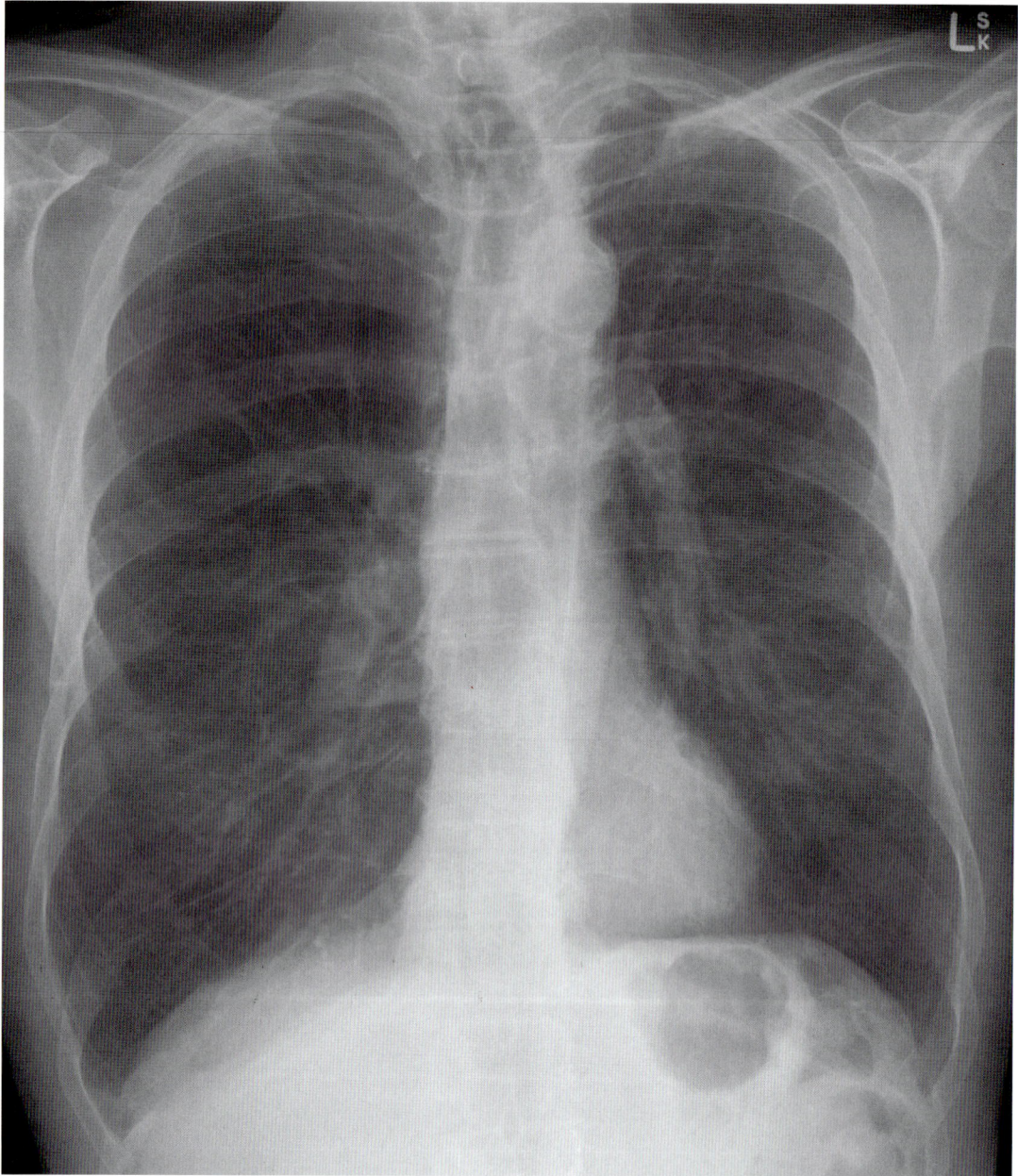

This is the preoperative chest X-ray of a 65-year-old man with a 50-year history of heavy smoking. He is scheduled to have major ENT surgery for a squamous cell carcinoma of the tongue.

**Q**

What two pathological processes are evident?

## A

Two evident pathological processes are:
- hyperinflated lungs suggestive of emphysema: normally, there are six ribs visible anteriorly above the diaphragm and ten posteriorly. In this film, there are seven ribs visible anteriorly above the diaphragm and ten posteriorly; the mediastinum is narrow and elongated and the diaphragm flattened. Lung markings are reduced bilaterally with emphysematous bullae at both apices.

- left upper lobe fibrosis: the left lung hilum is abnormally elevated, suggesting a loss of lung volume in the left lung apex. There are increased reticular markings in the left apex. The differential diagnosis of unilateral upper lobe fibrosis includes lung carcinoma, tuberculosis, trauma, radiation therapy or previous pneumonia (Dahnert, 2007).

## LEARNING POINT

The left hilum is normally only slightly higher than the right. Changes in position of structures may give a clue to otherwise subtle pathology.

## PROBLEM 1.06

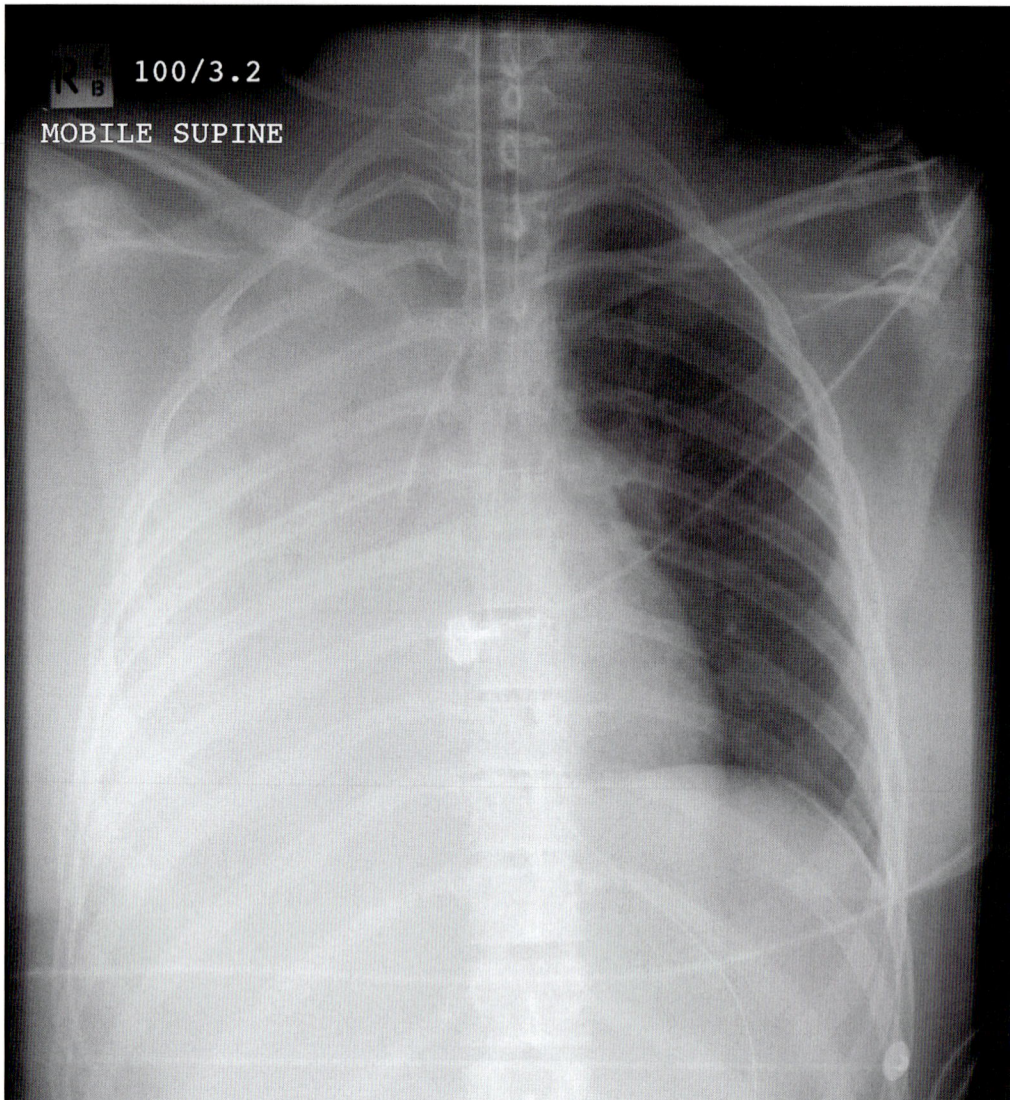

```
100/3.2
MOBILE SUPINE
```

This 18-year-old woman had fevers for one week then became short of breath yesterday. She now presents to hospital with hypoxaemic respiratory failure.

Q
1. What is your differential diagnosis?
2. What is the most likely cause?
3. Why do you favour this diagnosis?
4. What further investigation would help resolve the diagnosis?

# A

1. The differential diagnosis of a unilateral opaque hemithorax includes:
   - consolidation
   - pleural fluid
   - tumour
   - pneumonectomy
   - collapse

2. Consolidation, with or without pleural effusion.

3. In a case like this, it is not certain what process is present. Isolated collapse is unlikely as there is no mediastinal shift. There is no evidence of surgical clips or rib resection to suggest pneumonectomy. If the process involved tumour or pleural fluid causing this extent of opacity, there would usually be contralateral mediastinal shift but, occasionally, secondary lung collapse means this does not occur. Consolidation will often produce air bronchograms, but these are not always seen. There are small lucencies in the right hemithorax, which may represent air bronchograms or early abscess formation.

   This patient had a staphylococcal pneumonia with no effusion.

4. CT scan will be the most helpful. Ultrasound will demonstrate if an effusion is present.

---

## LEARNING POINT

On a plain chest X-ray, it is not always possible to make a definitive diagnosis. Other investigations may be needed.

## PROBLEM 1.07

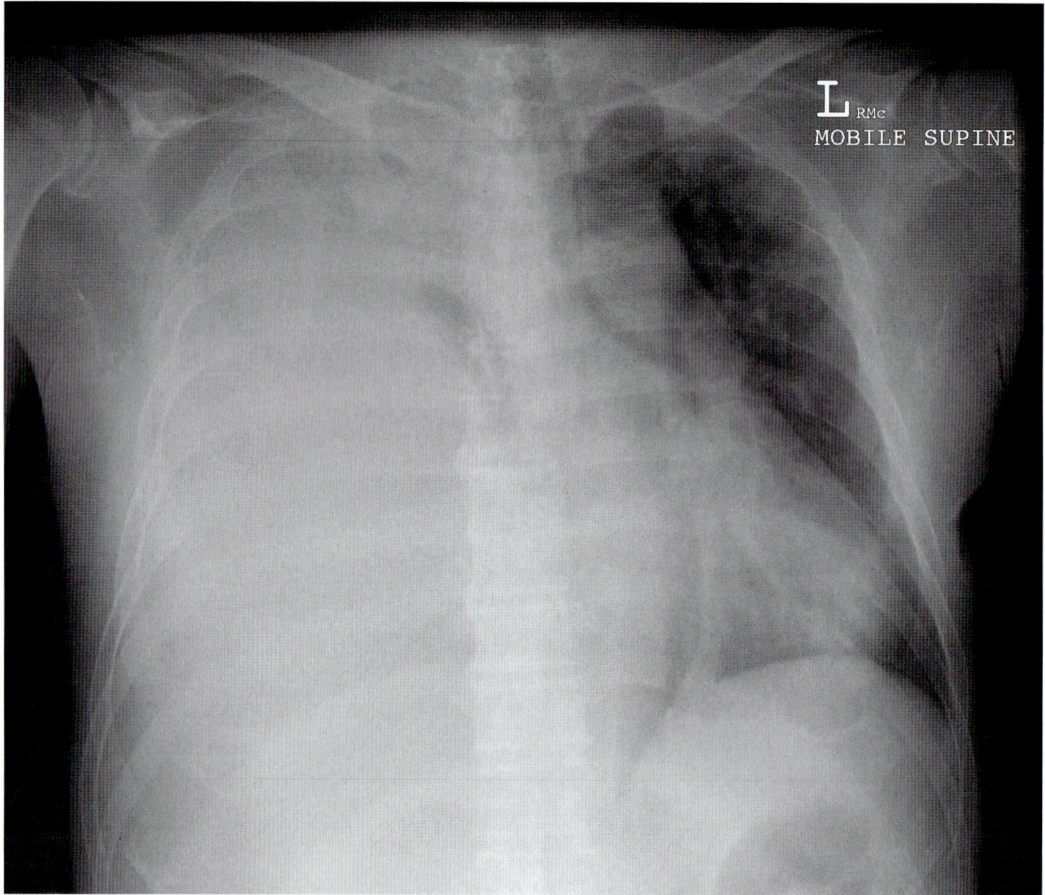

This 70-year-old man presented with hypotension and dyspnoea. He gave a history of progressive fatigue and shortness of breath over the previous two weeks.

## Q

1. What is the most likely cause of the opaque right hemithorax?
2. What findings on the X-ray support your diagnosis?

## A

1. In this chest X-ray, there is pleurally based opacification of the right hemithorax with contralateral mediastinal shift. The most likely cause of this is a collection of pleural fluid under tension. Other possibilities include a pleurally based tumour, such as a mesothelioma or metastases.

2. Findings that support this diagnosis are:
   - homogenous opacification of the right side of the chest
   - mediastinal shift away from the pathology (contralateral shift)
   - no signs of bony trauma to suggest a haemothorax

## LEARNING POINT

The direction of shift of the medistinal structures is a clue to the underlying pathology. With pathological processes that produce loss of lung volume (collapse, fibrosis, pneumonectomy), there is shift of the structures towards the affected area.

In contrast, with processes that produce mass effect (pleural collections, most tumours), the shift is away from the affected area. Consolidation does not usually produce significant shift of structures.

## PROBLEM 1.08

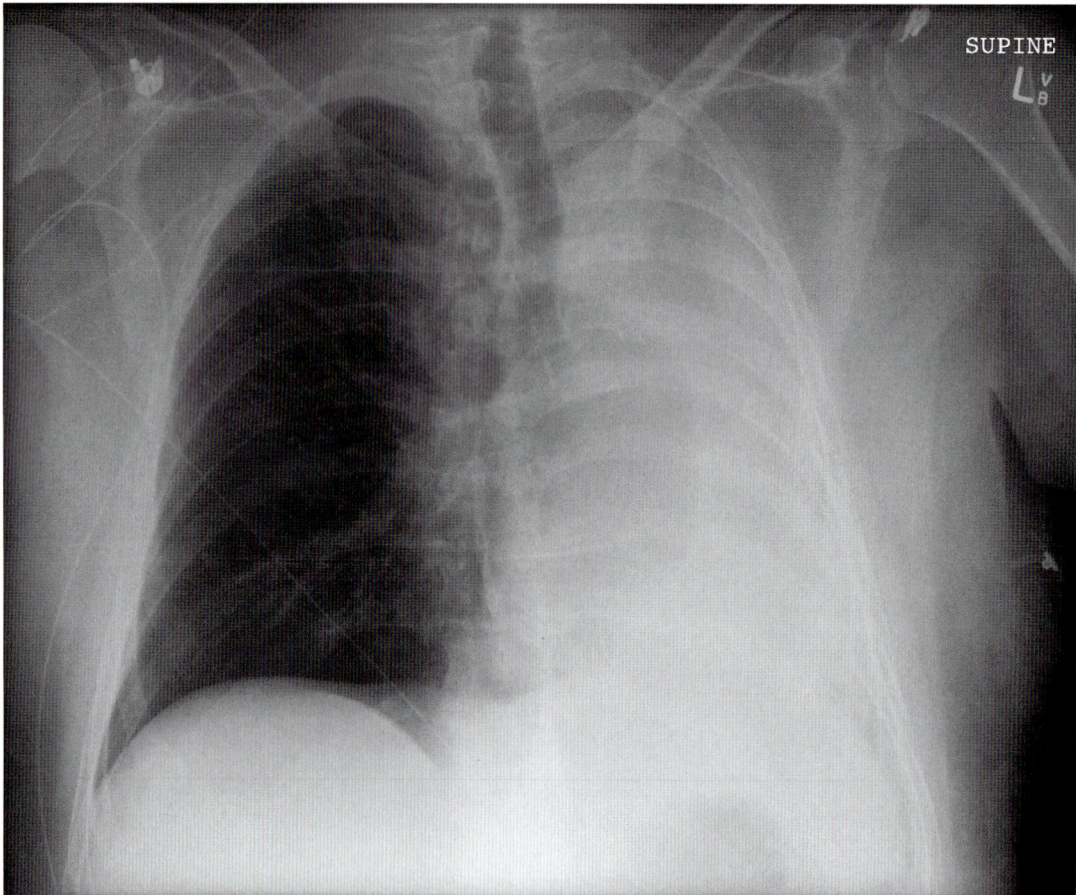

This 54-year-old man was in a car crash today, sustaining lower limb fractures. You are shown this chest X-ray by a resident working on the surgical ward. He wants to know what size chest drain to insert.

**Q**

1. What is the most likely cause of the opaque left hemithorax?
2. What findings on the X-ray support your diagnosis?

## A

1. Prior pneumonectomy.

2. Findings on the X-ray that support this diagnosis include:
   - narrowing of intercostal space between the sixth and seventh left ribs posteriorly
   - homogeneous opacity in left hemithorax with loss of diaphragmatic and cardiac borders
   - surgical clips in region of left hilum
   - hyperinflation of right lung, which herniates across the midline to the left side
   - shift of mediastinal structures towards the pathology (ipsilateral shift)
   - abrupt cut-off of left main bronchus

### LEARNING POINT

The clinical history, including past surgical procedures, is important when generating the differential diagnosis of appearances on imaging.

## PROBLEM 1.09

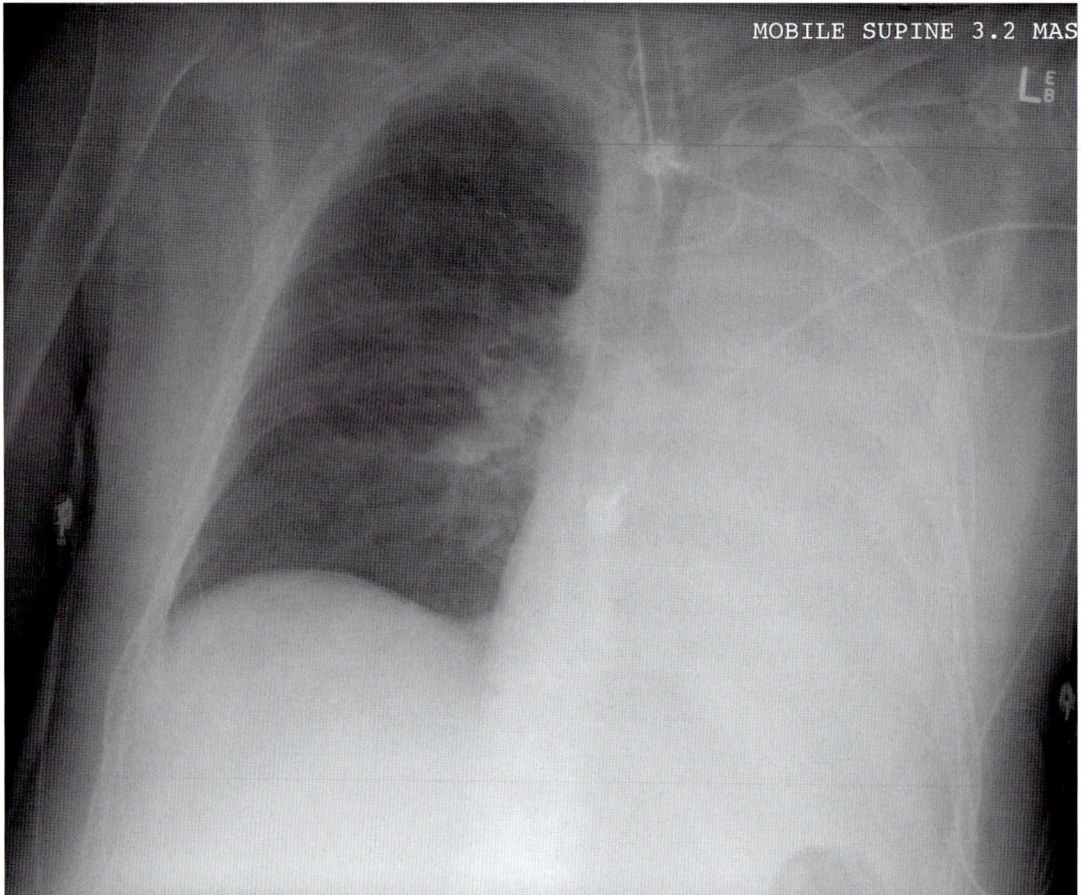

This 43-year-old man sustained a C5 vertebral injury during a car crash. He has been in the ICU for seven days and is quadriparetic.

**Q**
1. Why is there an opaque left hemithorax?
2. What findings on the X-ray support your diagnosis?

# A

1. Collapse of the left lung.

2. Findings that support this diagnosis include:
   • homogeneous opacity in left hemithorax with loss of diaphragmatic and cardiac borders
   • narrowing of rib spaces in left hemithorax
   • mediastinal shift towards the pathology
   • abrupt cut-off of left main bronchus

# LEARNING POINT

Lung collapse is associated with shift of the mediastinal structures towards the side of pathology.

## PROBLEM 1.10

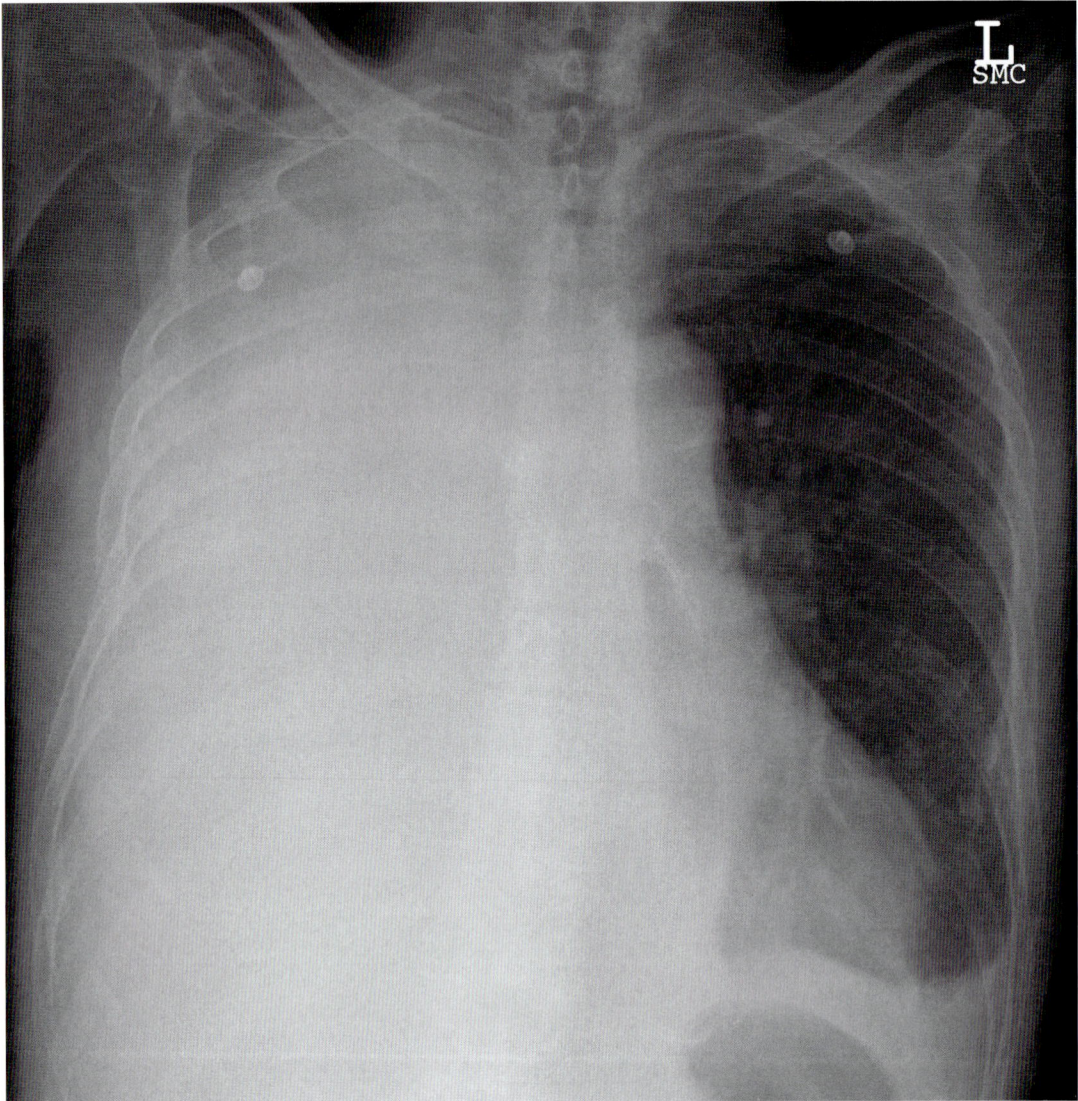

This 63-year-old man has had increasing short-ness of breath for two months, associated with malaise and four kilograms of weight loss.

**Q**

Suggest a differential diagnosis.

## A

The entire right hemithorax is opacified. The opacification is homogeneous with no visible lung markings present. There is some mediastinal shift to the opposite side. The differential diagnosis for these findings include:

- pleural fluid
- neoplasm
- pneumonia with empyema

Other findings present on this image are a smaller left pleural effusion, left pleural calcifications and an oesophageal stent. The most likely diagnosis is mesothelioma. Clues are the presence of pleural calcification (consistent with prior asbestos exposure) and less mediastinal shift than expected with this amount of pleural opacification. The latter is due to the fibrotic nature of the tumour, resulting in volume loss of the involved hemithorax. If this was all pleural fluid, more mediastinal shift would be expected.

## LEARNING POINT

The cause of an opaque hemithorax cannot always be determined with certainty by a chest X-ray. Other imaging, such as CT or ultrasound, may be required.

## PROBLEM 1.11

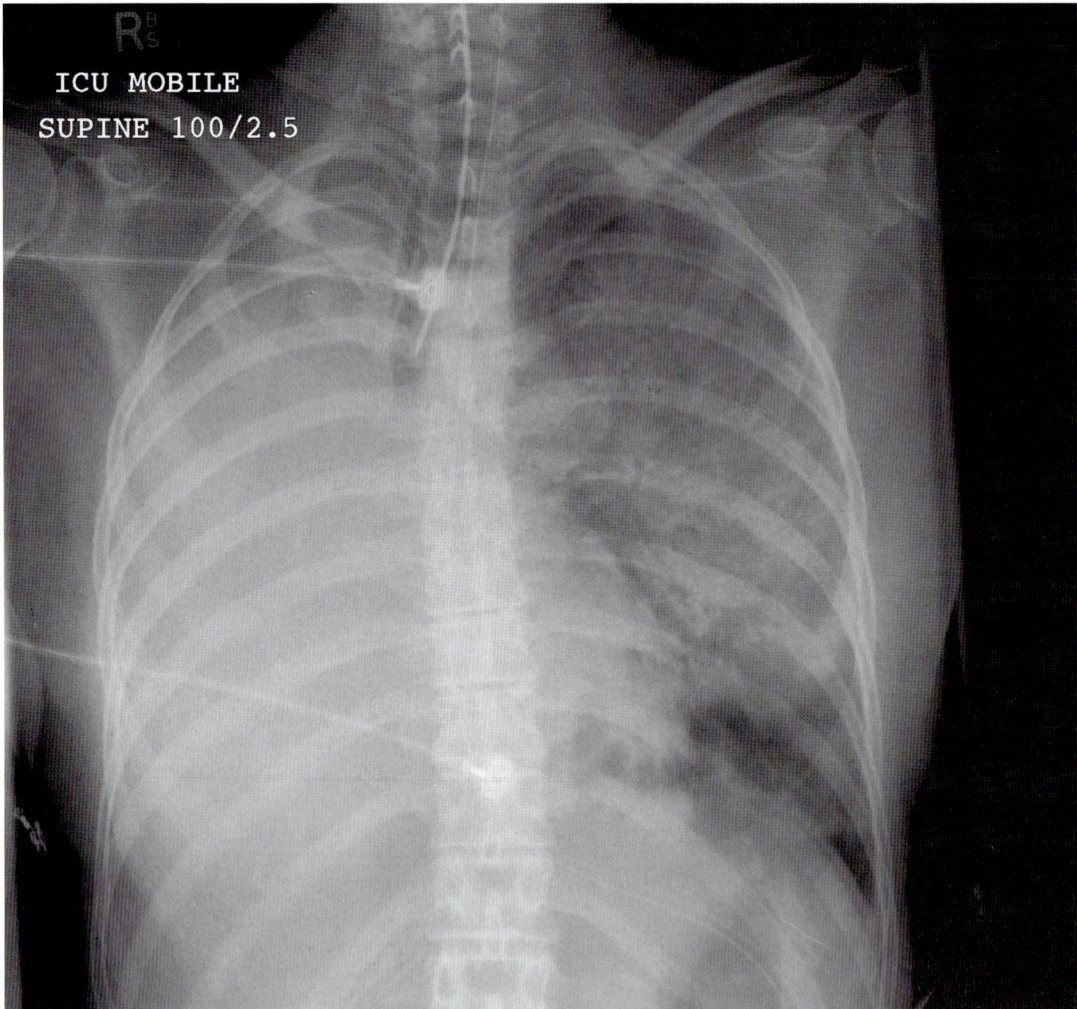

This 60-year-old woman presented with hypox-aemic respiratory failure and was intubated in the emergency department 12 hours ago. The gas exchange has deteriorated over the last two hours.

**Q**
Why is the gas exchange so poor?

# A

The gas exchange is poor because:

- The entire right hemithorax is homogeneously opacified and no underlying lung markings are seen. There is an abrupt cut-off of the right main bronchus, likely to be due to a mucus plug or blood clot obstructing the bronchus. The mediastinum is shifted to the right. This is in keeping with collapse of the right lung. The endotracheal tube is just above the carina.

- Most of the left hemithorax is opacified, but the opacification is non-homogeneous, with air bronchograms, and appearances suggestive of alveolar shadowing. This would be consistent with pneumonia, but the differential diagnosis is broad.

- There is a paucity of lung vessels in the left costophrenic recess, but no other sign of a pneumothorax.

## LEARNING POINT

Multiple processes may contribute to impaired gas exchange.

## PROBLEM 1.12

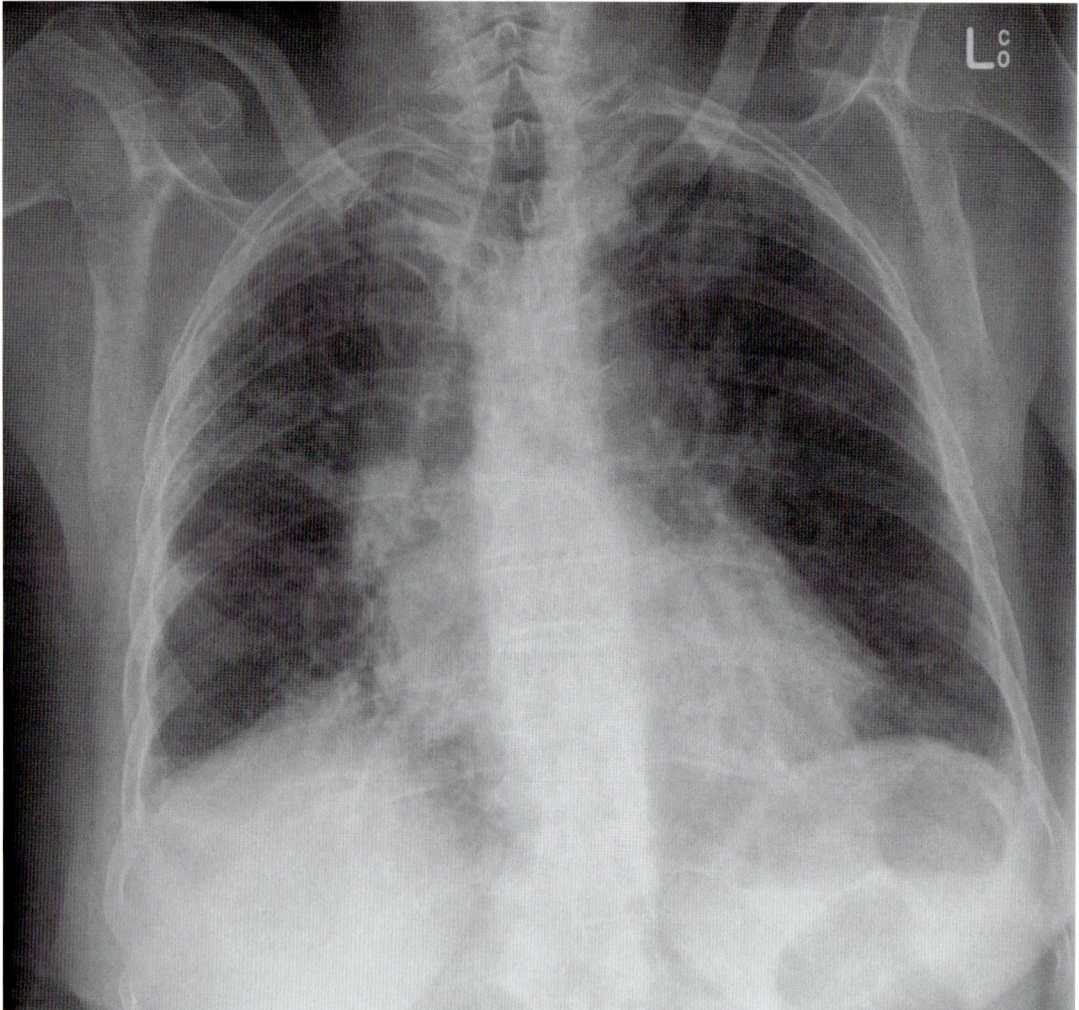

This 68-year-old woman was referred to ICU with respiratory failure and a five-month history of increasing shortness of breath with a dry cough.

**Q**
1. Describe the findings on this film.
2. What is your differential diagnosis?

# A

1. Findings on this film include:
   - increased peripheral interstitial markings in a coarse reticular pattern throughout both lung fields
   - apical pleural thickening
   - tenting of the right hemidiaphragm
   - irregular pleuropericardial interface
   - reduced lung volumes
   - the apparent shift of the trachea is caused by rotation, not a pathological process
   - increased cardiothoracic ratio

2. The differential diagnosis for interstitial lung infiltrates includes (Dahnert, 2007):
   - cardiogenic and non-cardiogenic pulmonary oedema
   - interstitial pneumonitis
   - infection
   - lymphangitis carcinomatosis
   - drug reactions
   - autoimmune diseases
   - sarcoidosis
   - mineral dust inhalation
   - extrinsic allergic alveolitis (hypersensitivity pneumonitis)

   This patient had sarcoidosis, which was proven on lung biopsy.

## LEARNING POINT

The differential diagnosis for interstitial infiltrates on a chest X-ray is broad. The duration of symptoms may be helpful in narrowing the differential.

Reticular infiltrates in acute pulmonary oedema are usually thin, regular, basal and subpleural (Kerley B lines). Chronic reticular infiltrates are usually coarse, with peribronchovascular or peripheral subpleural distribution.

## PROBLEM 1.13

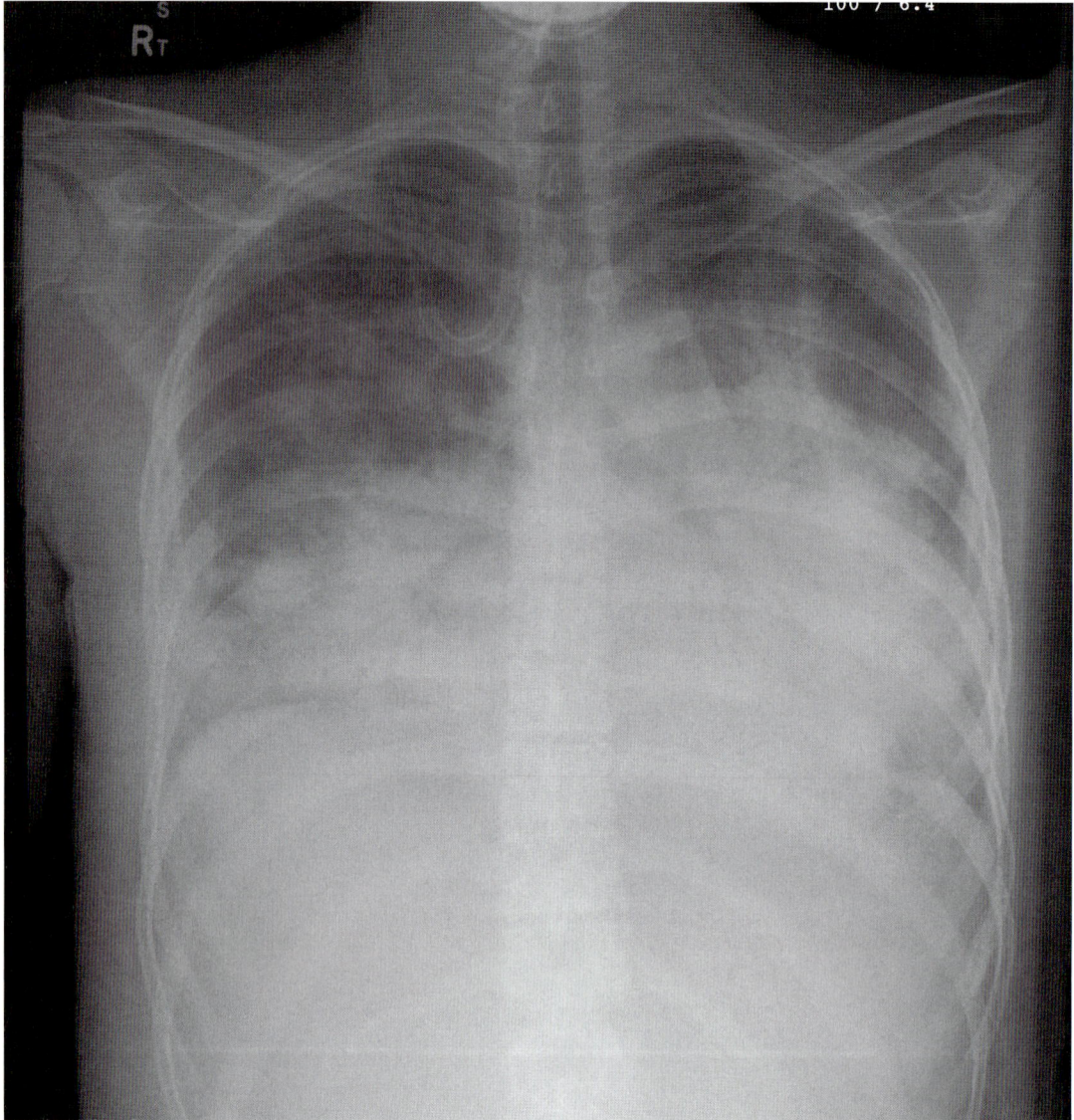

This previously well, 35-year-old female presents to the emergency department with a three-day history of shortness of breath. She is now dyspnoeic at rest and hypoxic despite high-flow oxygen via face mask.

**Q**
1. Describe the findings on this film.
2. What is your differential diagnosis?

# A

1. There is widespread diffuse opacification of both lung fields with relative sparing of the apices and lung peripheries. The opacification has a "fluffy" or "cotton wool" appearance typical of alveolar opacification. Air bronchograms are seen bilaterally, there is loss of the cardiac borders and medial parts of both hemidiaphragms.

   This is a good example of how borders are only seen between tissues of different densities. The diaphragmatic and mediastinal borders are lost because the air spaces in the lung have filled with fluid and are now the same density as the adjacent tissues (silhouette sign). New borders have been created where fluid-filled lung is abutting air-filled bronchi, giving the appearance of air bronchograms.

2. The differential diagnosis should include:
   - cardiogenic pulmonary oedema
   - non-cardiogenic pulmonary oedema (e.g. ARDS, aspiration pneumonitis)
   - pneumonia
   - pulmonary haemorrhage (including pulmonary contusion)
   - primary alveolar proteinosis

   Alveolar cell carcinoma and lymphoma may produce alveolar opacification, but this is typically more localised.

## LEARNING POINT

The differential diagnosis for alveolar infiltrates on a chest X-ray is broad. Diagnoses other than heart failure must be considered.

## PROBLEM 1.14

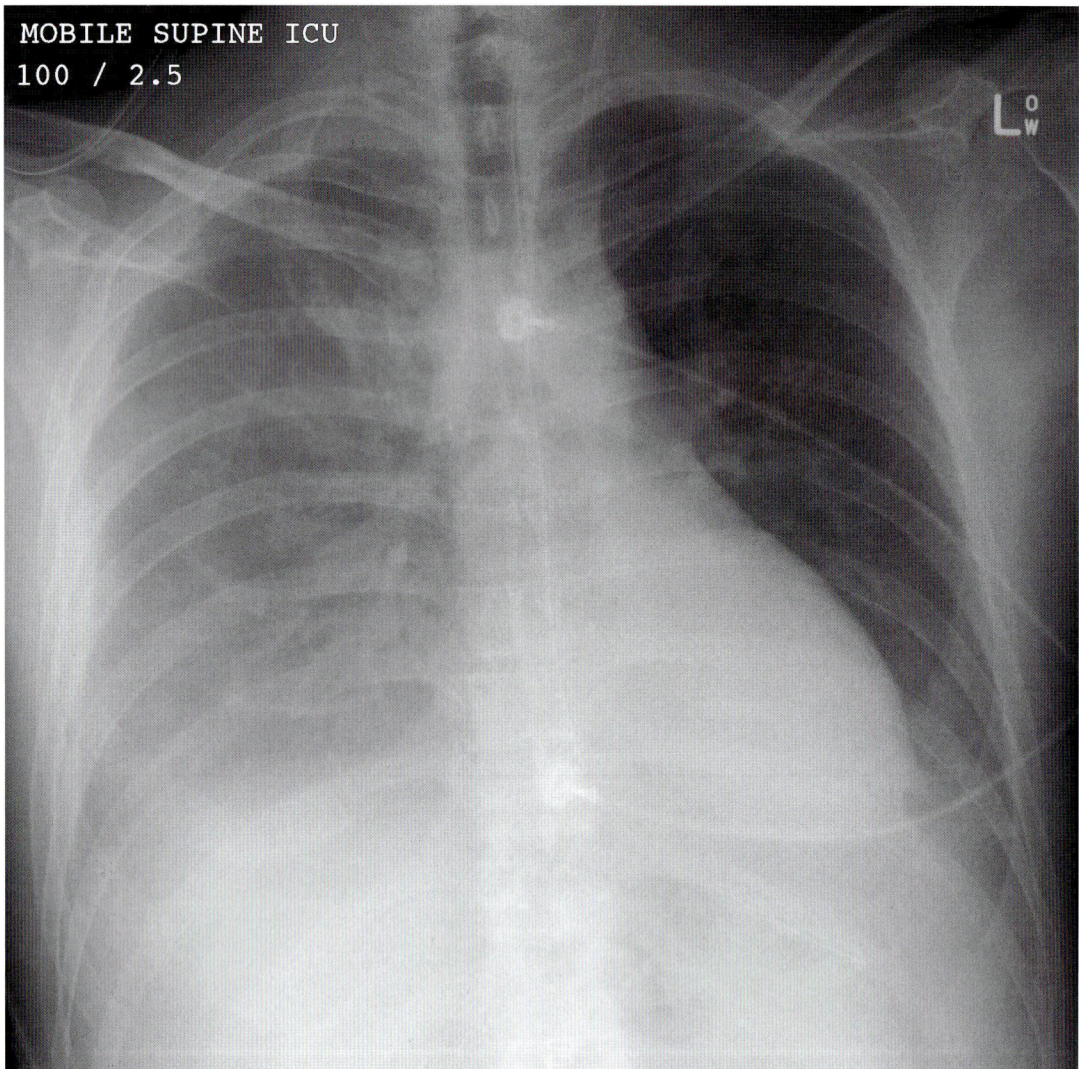

MOBILE SUPINE ICU
100 / 2.5

This 42-year-old man complained of mild shortness of breath, but otherwise felt well.

**Q** What processes are evident on the X-ray that may explain the shortness of breath?

## A

On the right side, there is:
- homogenous opacification throughout the entire hemithorax
- underlying lung markings that appear normal
- a rim of opacity around the periphery of the lung
- loss of mediastinal and diaphragmatic borders
- mediastinal shift to the left

These findings are consistent with a moderate to large pleural effusion. Lung floats on pleural fluid so, in the supine position, pleural fluid lies posterior and to the sides of the lung giving this characteristic appearance.

On the left side, there is:
- loss of the diaphragmatic border
- retrocardiac opacification
- haziness at the base, outside of the cardiac shadow

These findings suggest left lower lobe collapse, probably with a small left pleural effusion.

## LEARNING POINT

The appearance of a pleural effusion on a supine X-ray is different from that on an erect X-ray.

## PROBLEM 1.15

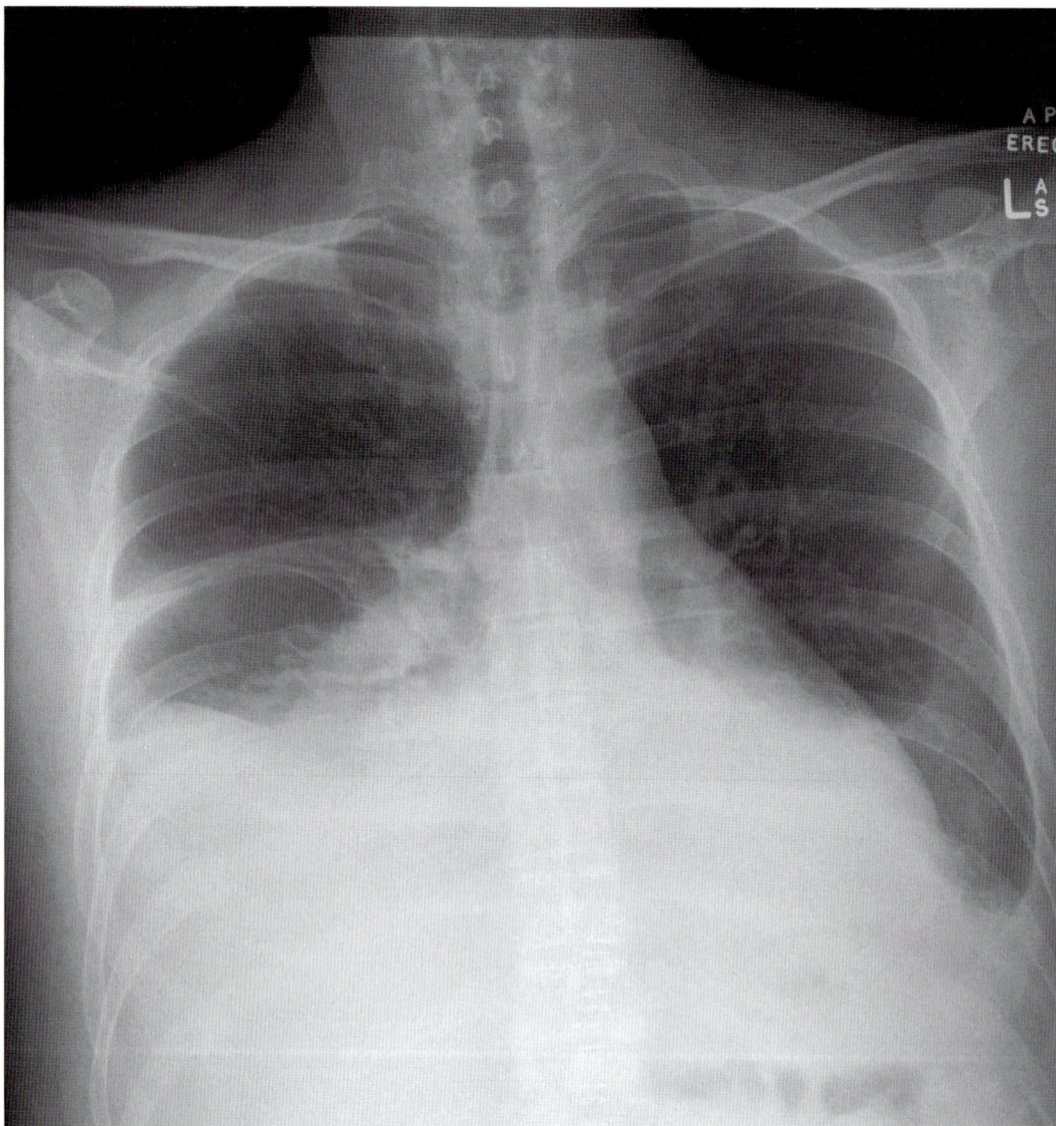

This 42-year-old man is mildly short of breath.

**Q** What processes are evident on the X-ray that may explain the shortness of breath?

# A

On the right side, there is:
- dense opacification at the base with haziness extending up to the midzone
- fluid extending into the horizontal fissure
- an abnormal contour of the "diaphragmatic border", which is flattened and the apex shifted laterally

These findings are consistent with a moderate right, predominantly subpulmonic pleural effusion.

On the left side, there is:
- loss of the diaphragmatic border
- retrocardiac opacification
- haziness at the base and obliteration of the costophrenic angle
- mediastinal shift to the left

These findings suggest left lower lobe collapse with a small left pleural effusion. This is the same patient as in Problem 1.14, but imaged in an erect position.

## Learning point

Pleural fluid moves with gravity as the patient changes position.

## PROBLEM 1.16

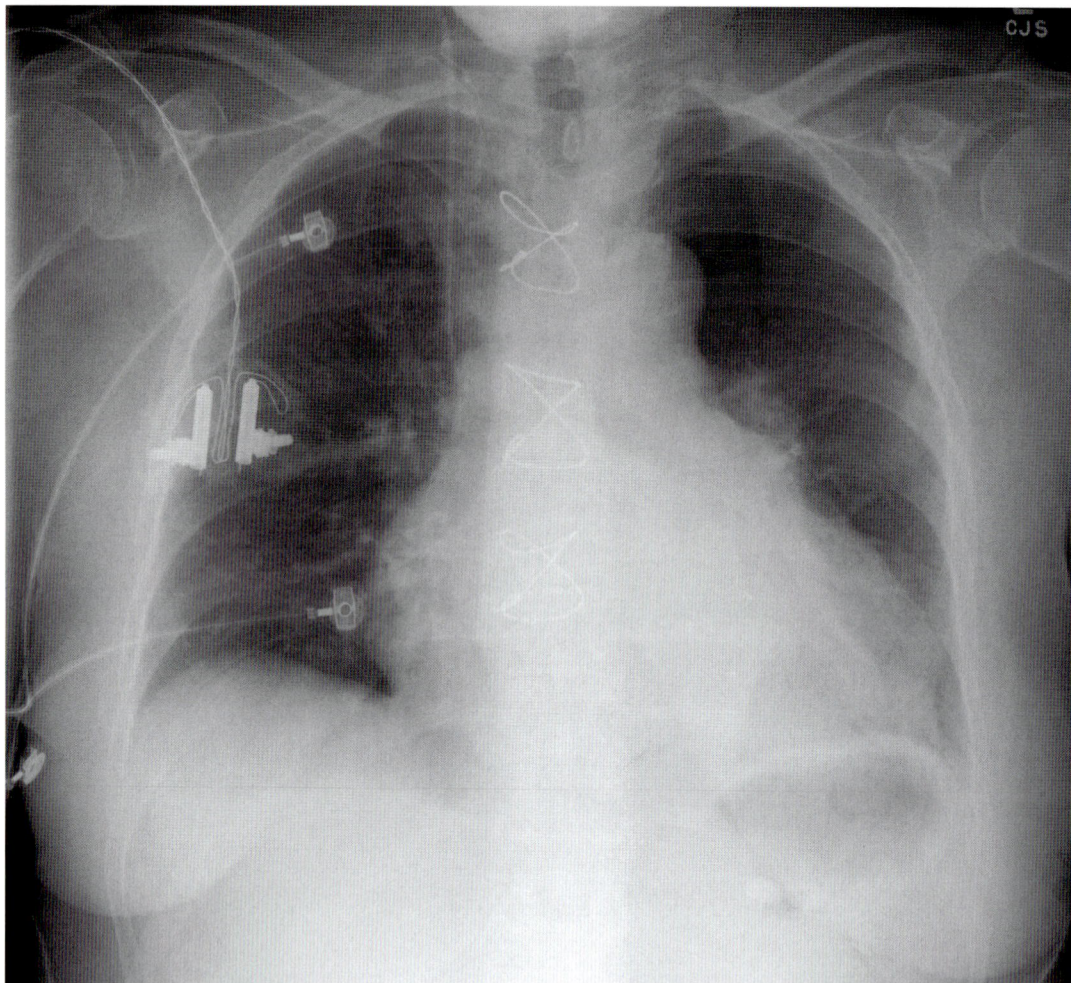

This is a routine erect postoperative film of a 60-year-old woman who had a mitral valve replacement and coronary artery bypass grafting performed yesterday.

**Q** What abnormality is present that may need intervention?

# A

There is a left apical pneumothorax.

Air is lighter than lung so tends to collect in non-dependent areas of the pleural cavity: the apex in the erect patient and anteriorly in the supine patient.

A relatively subtle pneumothorax can easily be missed if the lung edge is not clearly visible. It is important when reviewing chest X-rays to look globally at the film before focusing on the detail, otherwise relatively obvious findings can be missed. On a global inspection of this film, two findings are evident:

- The left upper zone is darker than on the right side. As the right upper zone appears normal, this suggests hyperlucency in the left upper zone.
- Cardiomegaly.

Closer examination of the left upper zone reveals that the upper mediastinal border and aortic knuckle are much sharper than on the right side. This is because, on the right, the interface is between air-filled lung and "tissue density" mediastinum while, on the left, it is between free pleural air and mediastinum. This is strong ancillary evidence of a pneumothorax. In addition, there is an absence of vascular markings in the hyperlucent area. Closer inspection reveals a lung edge, although this could easily be missed without the global inspection.

Other findings on the film include:

- sternal wires
- mitral valve replacement (the three struts are visible)
- linear atelectasis in the left lower lobe

# LEARNING POINT

It is important to stand back and look at the X-ray globally to avoid missing obvious pathology because of a focus on detail.

## PROBLEM 1.17

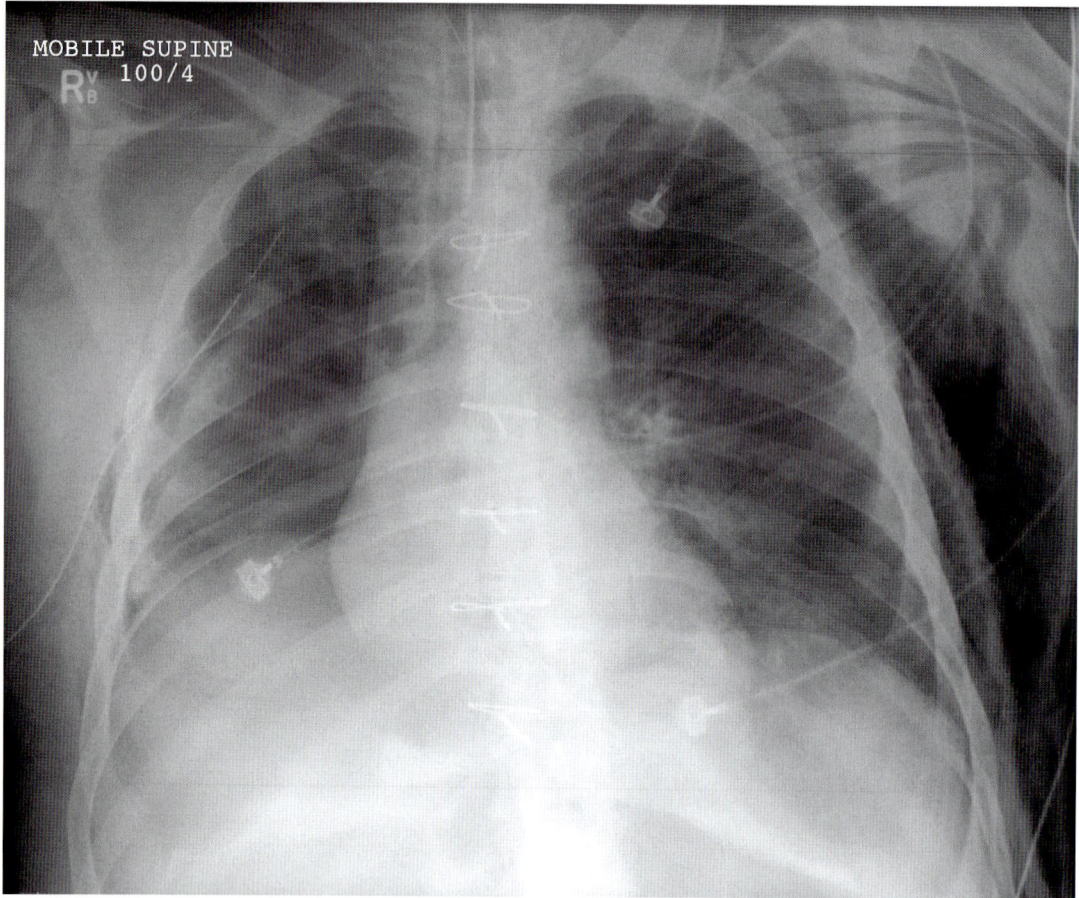

This 40-year-old man was admitted to the ICU following a polypharmacy drug overdose. There was some difficulty with inserting the central venous catheter. The patient now has a high arterial-alveolar oxygen gradient.

**Q** What problems does the X-ray demonstrate?

## A

On the left side, there is:
- extensive surgical emphysema in the subcutaneous tissues of the chest wall and in the pectoral muscles
- a deep sulcus sign at the costophrenic angle
- a lucency over the upper abdomen, not explained by any normal structure
- a lobular mediastinal-based shadow inferomedial to the cardiac apex is due to a new border forming between displaced pericardial fat and the adjoining pneumothorax
- mediastinal shift to the right

These findings strongly suggest a left tension pneumothorax despite the absence of a visible lung edge. In the supine position, air will collect anterior to the lung as this is the non-dependent area of the pleural cavity.

On the right side:
- a lung edge is seen
- the cardiac and diaphragmatic borders are very sharp, suggesting pleural air
- there is lucency over the liver

This demonstrates the presence of significant residual pneumothorax despite what appears to be an appropriately placed chest drain.

Sternal wires are present, suggesting a previous sternotomy.

## Learning Point

In the supine position, a lung edge may not be visible, even with a tension pneumothorax. Other features of a pneumothorax must be sought.

An inferior pneumothorax may produce a sharp outline of the pericardial fat, also known as a "pericardial fat tag" sign (Ziter, 1981).

## PROBLEM 1.18

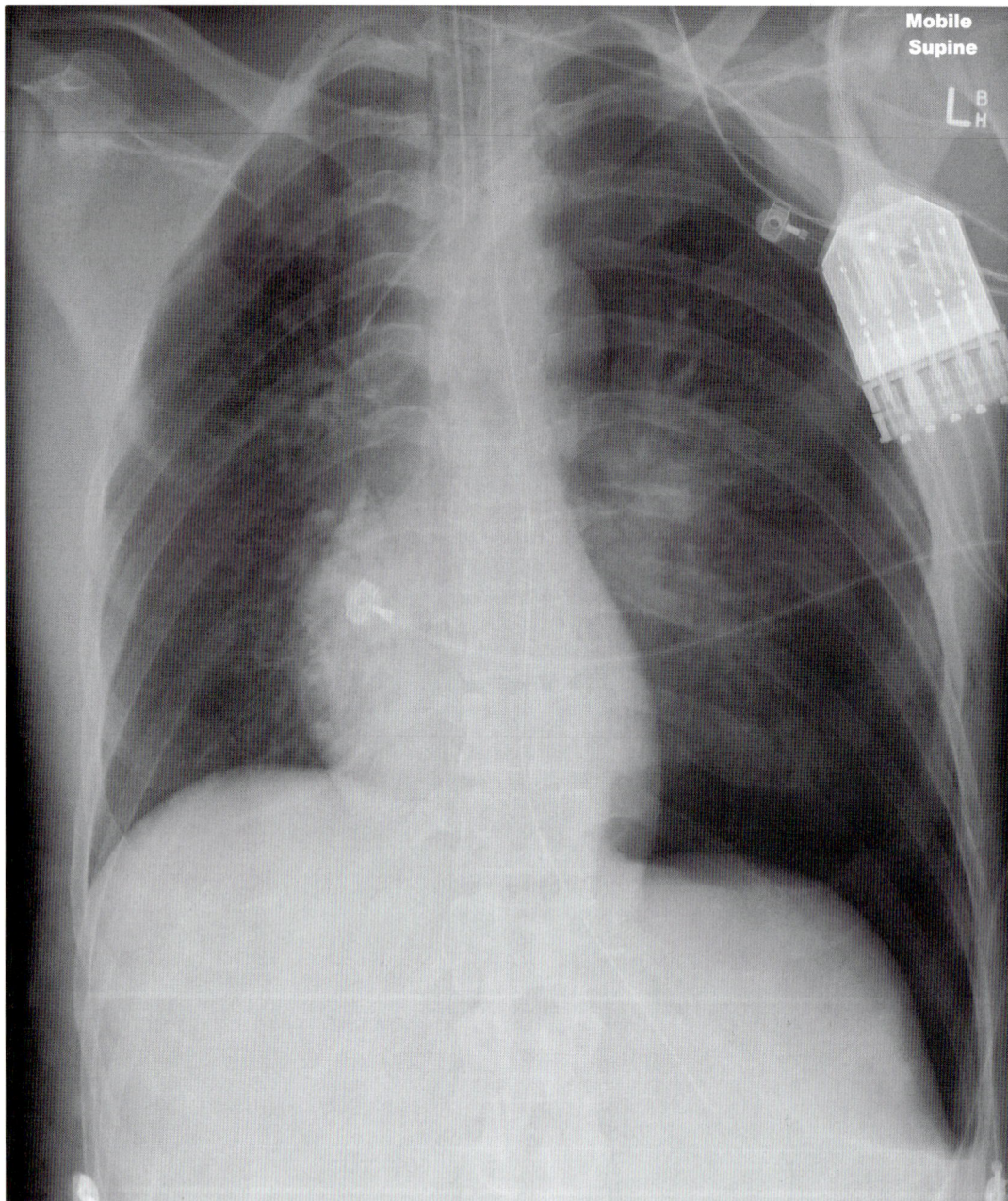

This 40-year-old man with a severe head injury has been in the ICU for four days. He has suddenly become hypotensive and hypoxic.

**Q** Describe the findings on this film.

## A

The findings on this film include:
- left-sided tension pneumothorax (evidence for this includes a visible lung edge with no lung markings beyond the edge; mediastinal shift to the right; depression of the left hemidiaphragm with a deep sulcus sign)
- a small amount of subcutaneous emphysema
- the left lung is partially collapsed
- the left-sided central line, endotracheal and nasogastric tubes are well positioned
- a fine-bore pleural drainage catheter adjacent to the lung edge. This is best appreciated in the DVD images.

## LEARNING POINT

The presence of a pleural drainage catheter does not exclude a significant pneumothorax.

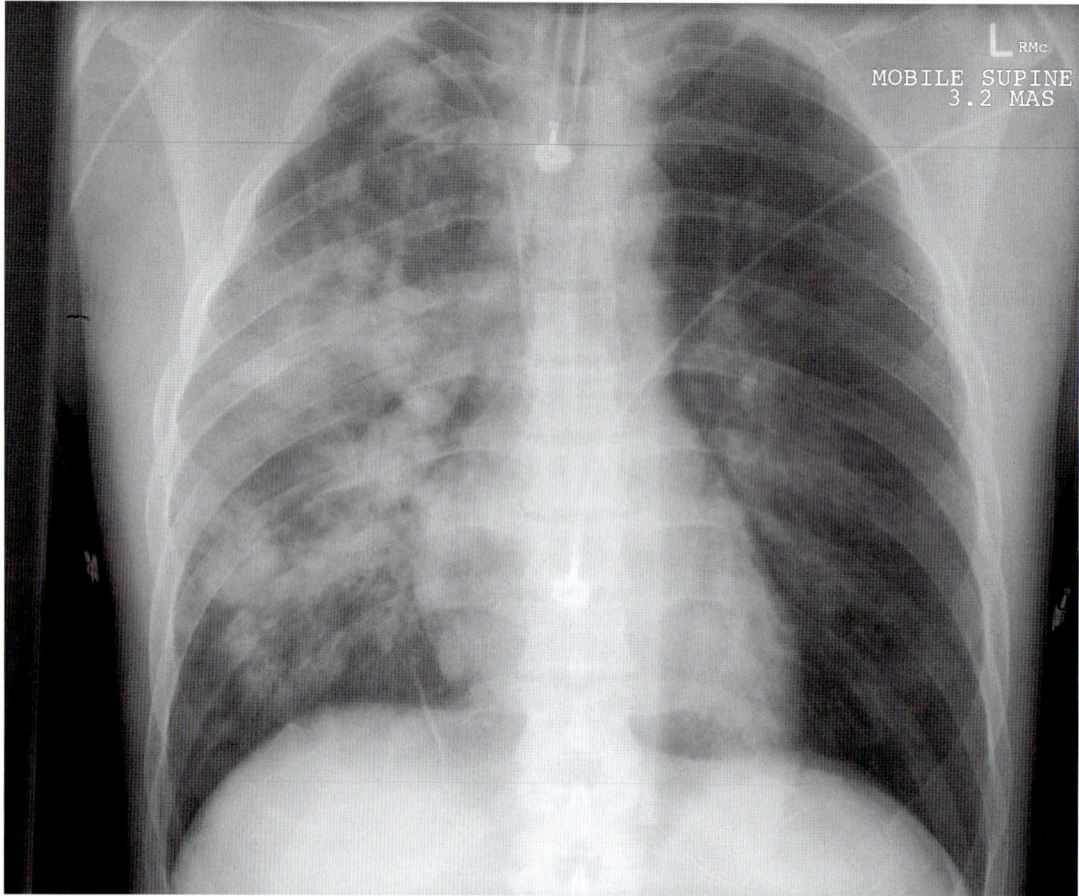

This 35-year-old man had a liver transplant two years ago. He presents with a 36-hour history of fever and rapidly progressive shortness of breath.

**Q** What is the likely diagnosis?

## A

Pneumonia is the most likely diagnosis. There is patchy alveolar opacification throughout most of the right lung field, with alveolar nodules as well as areas of confluent homogeneous consolidation. There is some perihilar opacification on the left.

Fungal infection can cause nodular opacities and this immunosuppressed patient is at increased risk. Metastatic disease could be considered, but is unlikely because of the unilateral appearance and the confluent homogeneous component.

## LEARNING POINT

Although some chest X-ray features may suggest particular causative organisms in a patient with pneumonia, they cannot provide certainty in diagnosis.

Alveolar nodules appear on the chest X-ray as ill-defined opacities greater than 1 cm in size.

## PROBLEM 1.20

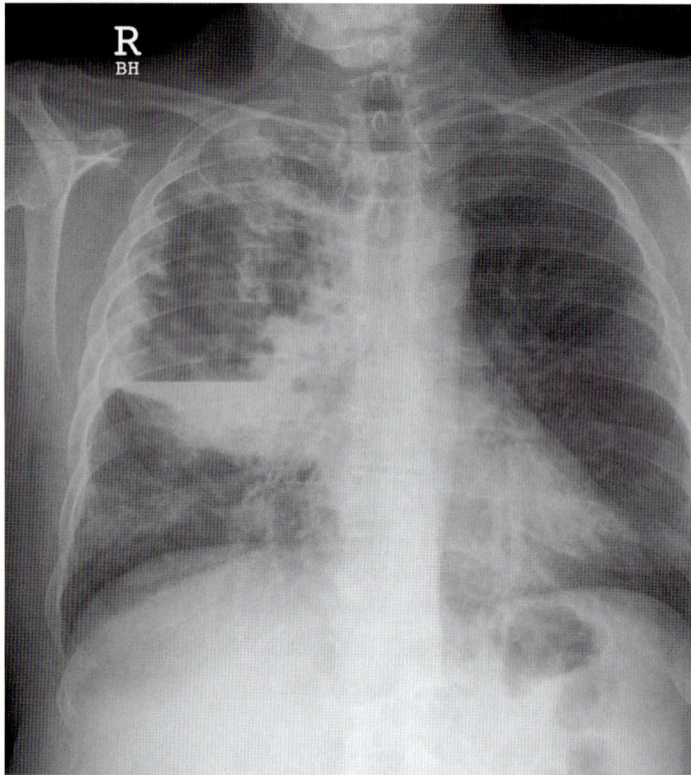

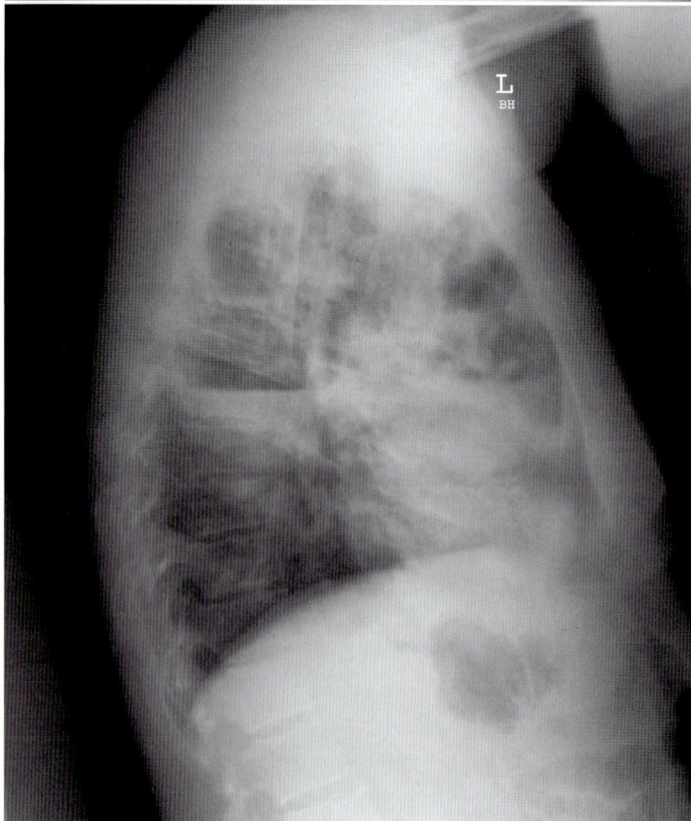

This 66-year-old homeless alcoholic man had a three-week history of fever and cough.

## Q

What is the most likely diagnosis?

## A

There is a cavity in the apical segment of the right lower lobe with a fluid level within it. In this clinical scenario, this is highly suggestive of an abscess. There is extensive patchy opacification throughout the rest of the right lung. This suggests a pneumonic process, which could be either the cause or the result of the abscess.

## LEARNING POINT

The apical segment of the right lower lobe is a very common site for aspiration. It is likely that this lung abscess is the result of aspiration.

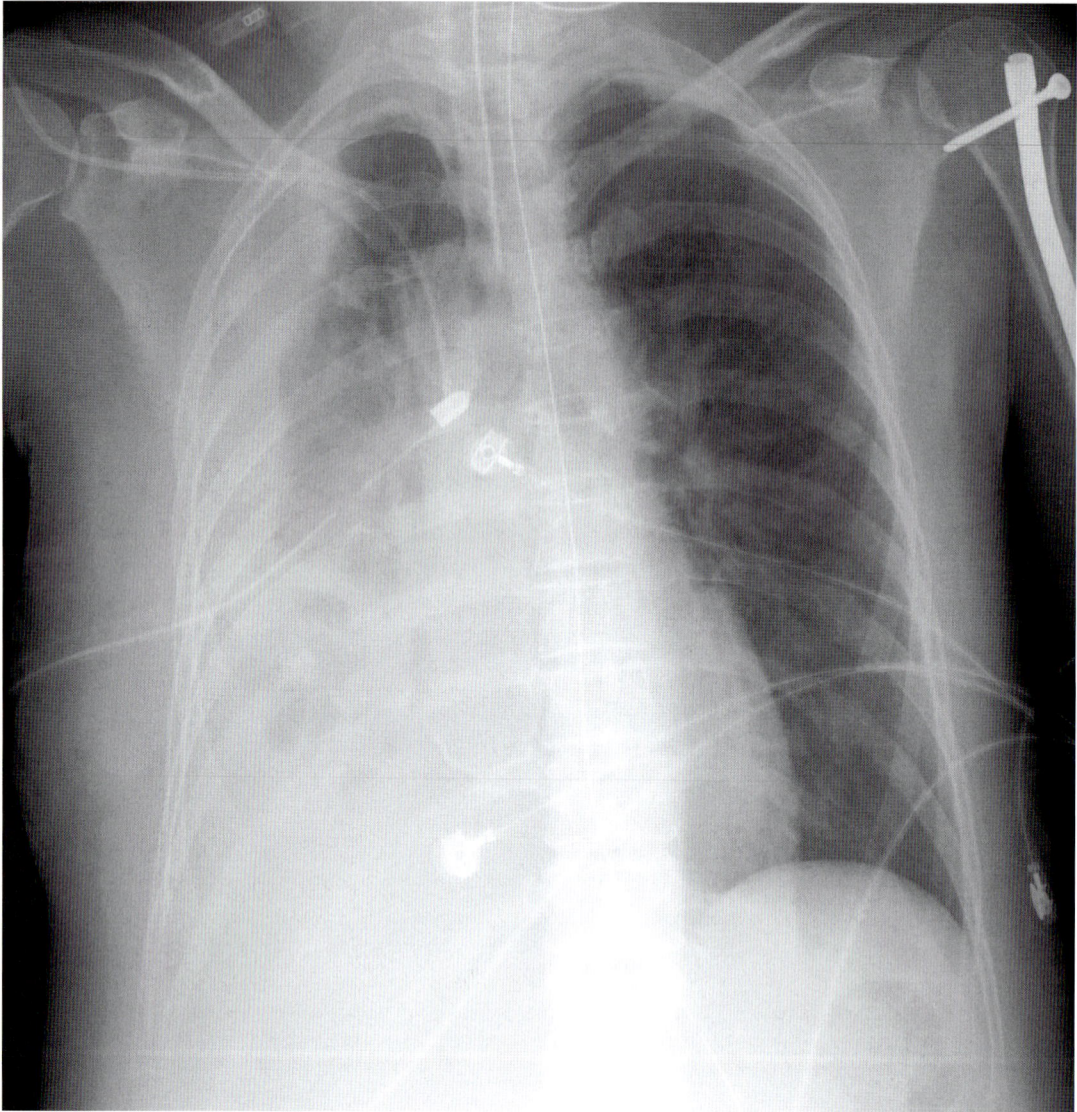

This 49-year-old woman presented with a two-week history of productive cough, fever and worsening shortness of breath.

**Q**
1. What diagnosis is suggested by this image?
2. How will you manage this problem?

# A

1. There is a large pleurally based collection, which has not been adequately drained by an appropriately placed chest drain. In this clinical scenario, the likely diagnosis is empyema. Parapneumonic effusion should also be considered.

2. A CT scan should be performed to confirm the diagnosis of empyema and to check the position of the intercostal catheter. Empyema would be supported by the presence of thickened, contrast-enhancing, parietal pleura. If empyema is confirmed and the intercostal catheter is appropriately positioned, surgical decortication should be considered.

## LEARNING POINT

Empyemas are often loculated and, therefore, may not adequately drain with an intercostal catheter.

## PROBLEM 1.22

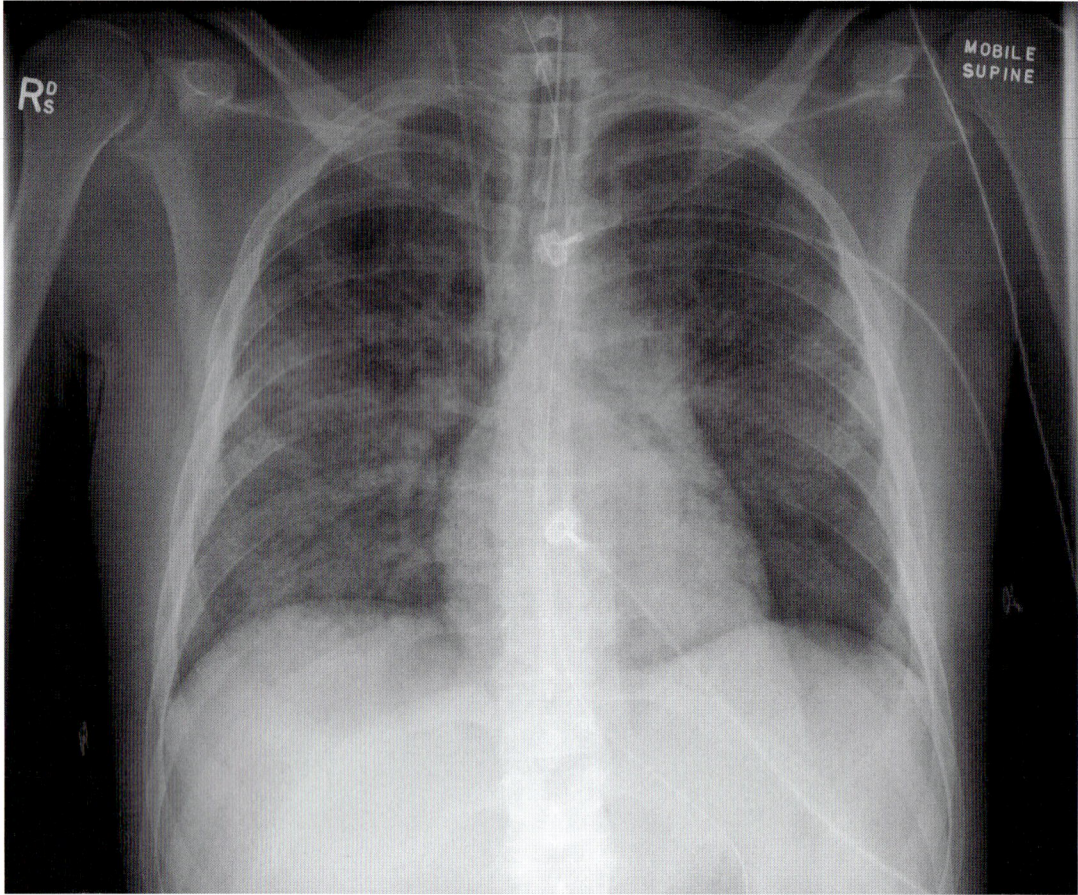

This 30-year-old man lived in India until two months ago. He now presents with fever and shortness of breath.

**Q** What is the most likely diagnosis?

# A
Miliary tuberculosis.

There are small, well-defined nodular opacities, the size of millet seeds, throughout the lung fields; this is the pattern of interstitial nodular opacity. In contrast, alveolar nodular opacities are larger and less defined. There is a thin-walled cavity in the right upper zone.

The differential diagnosis of miliary nodules includes (Dahnert, 2007):
• infection (tuberculosis or histoplasmosis)
• neoplasia (renal cell carcinoma, thyroid or testicular cancers, melanoma deposits)
• pneumoconiosis (silicosis)
• sarcoidosis

# LEARNING POINT
The incidence of tuberculosis and other infectious diseases varies widely from one community to another. When a patient from outside of the local environment is admitted to hospital, exotic diseases need to be considered.

## PROBLEM 1.23

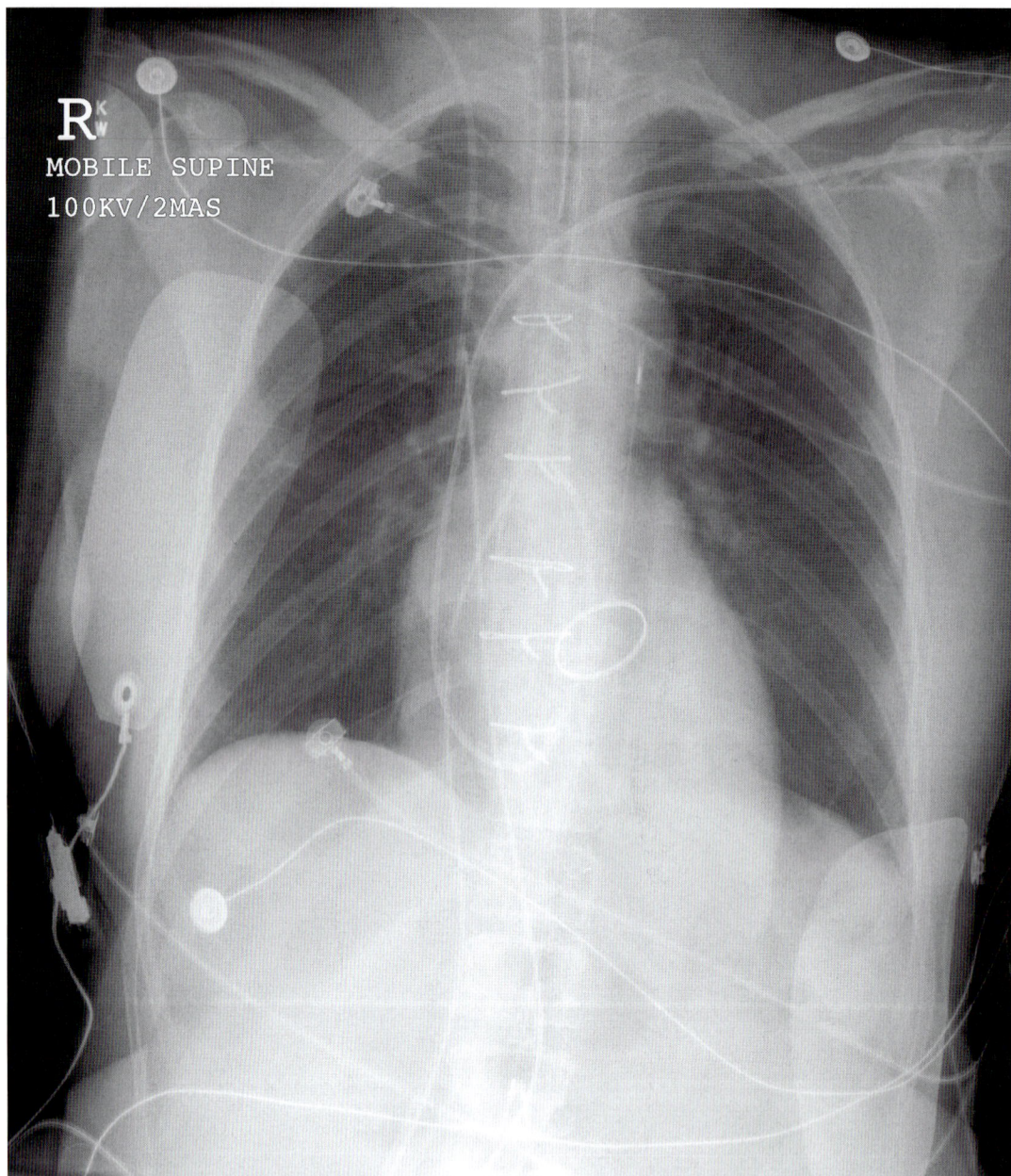

This 68-year-old woman had high-risk elective cardiac surgery 24 hours ago.

**Q**

Comment on the devices present.

# A

The devices present are:
- well-positioned endotracheal tube. The tip is between the medial ends of the clavicles, well clear of the carina, at around the T4 level.
- well-positioned right-sided central venous line. The tip is just above the level of the bronchus in the line of the superior vena cava.
- pulmonary artery catheter. The tip appears to lie in the main pulmonary artery or right ventricular outflow tract. The pressure trace should be reviewed and, if it suggests right ventricular placement, then the catheter should be advanced. The tip of a pulmonary artery catheter should not extend laterally beyond the medial third of either hemithorax.
- intra-aortic balloon pump, which is positioned slightly high. The radio-opaque tip should be located just distal to the left subclavian artery. This corresponds to the tip being just above the left main bronchus, in the second or third left intercostal space anteriorly. The balloon is inflated and is projected as a linear lucency in the left paraspinal region. This should not be mistaken for a pneumomediastinum.
- mitral valve prosthesis
- two surgical drains, which are likely to be mediastinal and pericardial
- sternal wires aligned vertically
- pads for external defibrillation or pacing
- monitoring leads and ECG dots overlying the chest

There is a double right-heart border, consistent with left atrial enlargement from mitral valve disease.

# LEARNING POINT

You need to systematically identify each device and check that the position is correct.

## PROBLEM 1.24

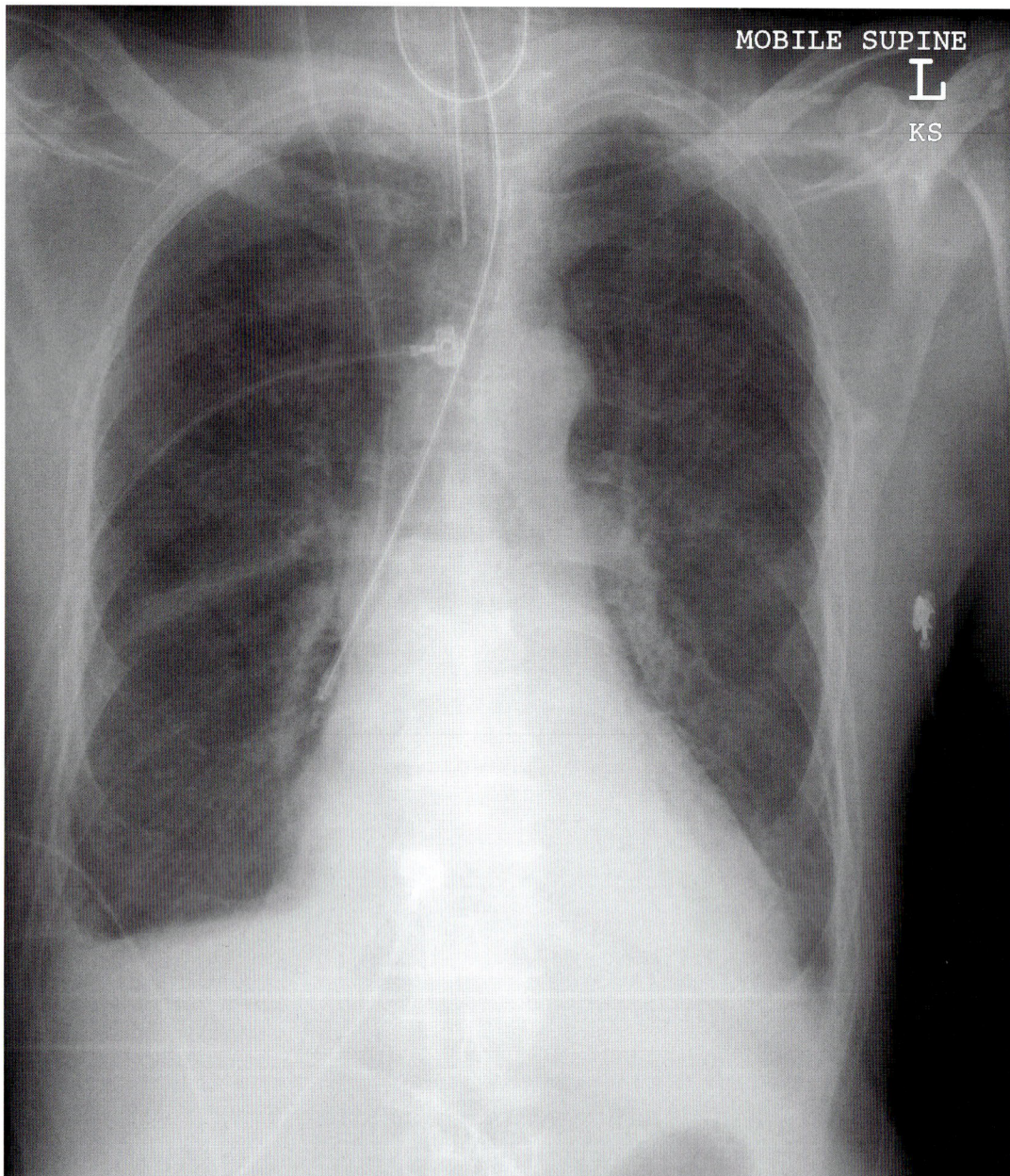

This 64-year-old man has respiratory failure from chronic obstructive airways disease and cardiac failure. He is slow to wean from mechanical ventilation.

**Q** What are the findings on the image?

# A

The feeding tube has been inserted into the right main bronchus. It should be removed immediately. The majority of misplaced feeding tubes go into the right main bronchus.

There are bilateral interstitial infiltrates and pleural effusions with fluid in the horizontal fissure. The right-sided central venous line and the endotracheal tube are in acceptable positions.

## LEARNING POINT

It is important to inspect the position of lines, tubes and other devices on chest X-ray images.

## PROBLEM 1.25

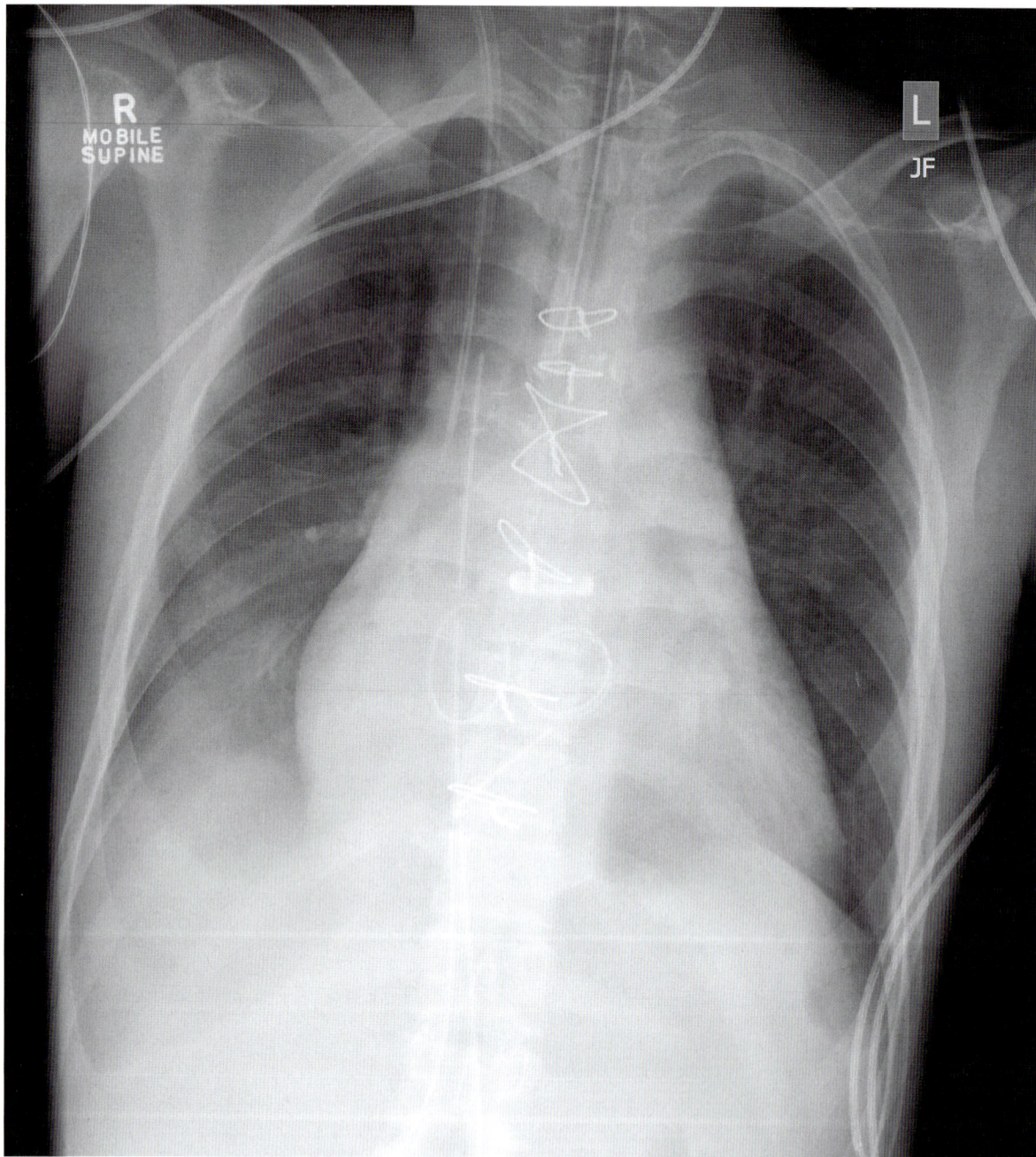

This 19-year-old woman had elective cardiac surgery yesterday.

**Q** Describe the findings on the film.

## A

The findings on the film are:

- At the right lung base, there is hazy opacification with loss of the hemidiaphragm. The horizontal fissure is normally positioned. These findings are suggestive of pleural fluid.
- The medial part of the left hemidiaphragm is unclear and there is increased retrocardiac opacity with some air bronchograms. In this clinical context, this most likely represents atelectasis although consolidation is possible.
- Two surgical drains are present, one of which appears to be kinked.
- The right internal jugular central venous catheter is well positioned.
- The sternal wires are normally aligned.
- There are three ring-like structures seen near the centre of the heart shadow. These represent mitral and aortic valve replacements and a tricuspid valve annuloplasty ring.
- The endotracheal tube is slightly low in position.

## LEARNING POINT

Different prosthetic valves have different appearances on the chest X-ray and some are not radio-opaque. Mitral and tricuspid annuloplasty rings form an incomplete circle and so can be distinguished from valve replacements.

With cardiac disease, the position and orientation of valves may change as the cardiac chambers change their size and position. It is often not possible to be certain which valve has been replaced from the chest X-ray appearance. There are, however, some useful clues based on orientation, valve orifice appearance, perceived direction of blood flow and position (Foot, 2006).

Compared to other valves, aortic valve prostheses tend to have the opening of their ring orientated in a more vertical direction, facing obliquely up and to the right. This gives them an ovoid (in profile) appearance. They are higher than mitral or tricuspid prostheses and tend to be smaller in size. The perceived direction of blood flow across the valve is towards the ascending aorta.

Mitral valve prostheses are lower and more to the left than aortic and oriented in a more horizontal anteroposterior direction. This gives them a more circular (en face) appearance. The perceived direction of blood flow is towards the apex.

Tricuspid valve prostheses are aligned in a more medial-lateral direction and lie to the right of the mitral valve, below the level of the aortic valve.

## PROBLEM 1.26

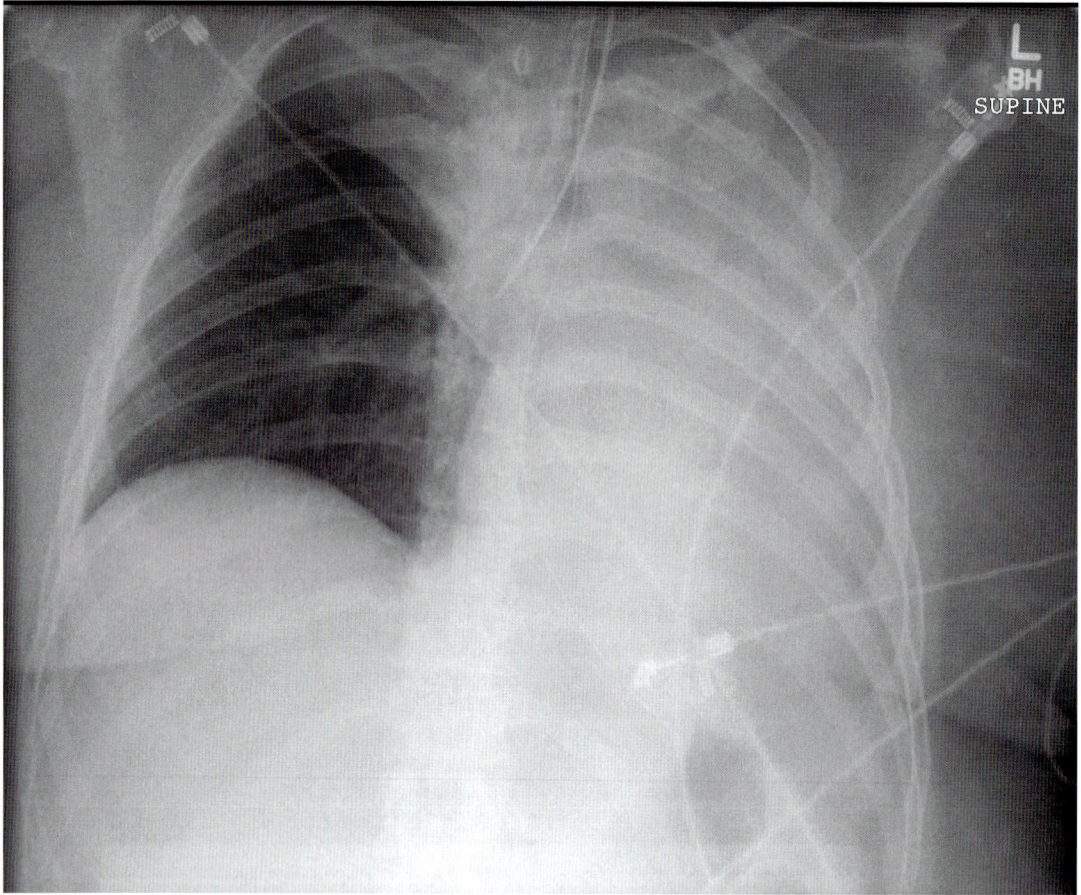

This 42-year-old woman was admitted to ICU following surgery for multiple trauma. This supine chest X-ray was taken 15 minutes later. A haemothorax has been diagnosed and preparations are being made for inserting a chest drain.

**Q**

What is the most likely cause of the opaque left hemithorax?

## A

The endotracheal tube is in the right main bronchus. The left hemithorax is opacified, with shift of the mediastinum to the left, which are features consistent with left lung collapse. In addition, there is at least a partial collapse of the right upper lobe, suggesting the endotracheal tube is occluding the right upper lobe bronchus.

## LEARNING POINT

An opaque hemithorax following trauma is not always due to haemothorax.

## PROBLEM 1.27

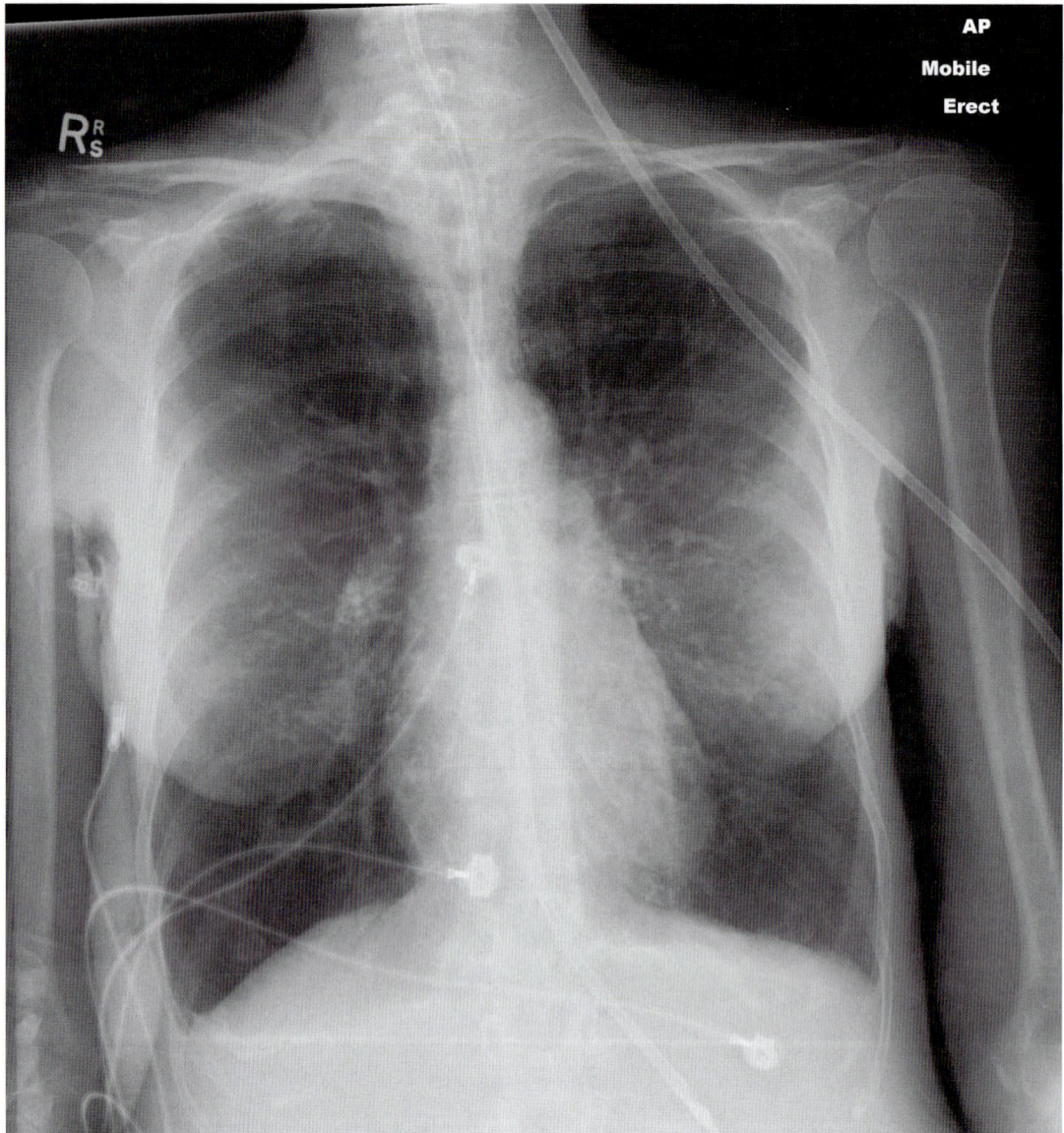

Two weeks ago this 57-year-old woman was admitted to ICU with hypercapnic respiratory failure.

**Q**

Why is this patient difficult to wean from mechanical ventilation?

## A

The lungs are hyperinflated with flattened diaphragms, consistent with chronic obstructive airways disease. The bilateral midzone opacities are due to breast implants.

The patient is most likely difficult to wean because of chronic obstructive airways disease.

## LEARNING POINT

Breast implants may be confused with pulmonary-based opacities.

## PROBLEM 1.28

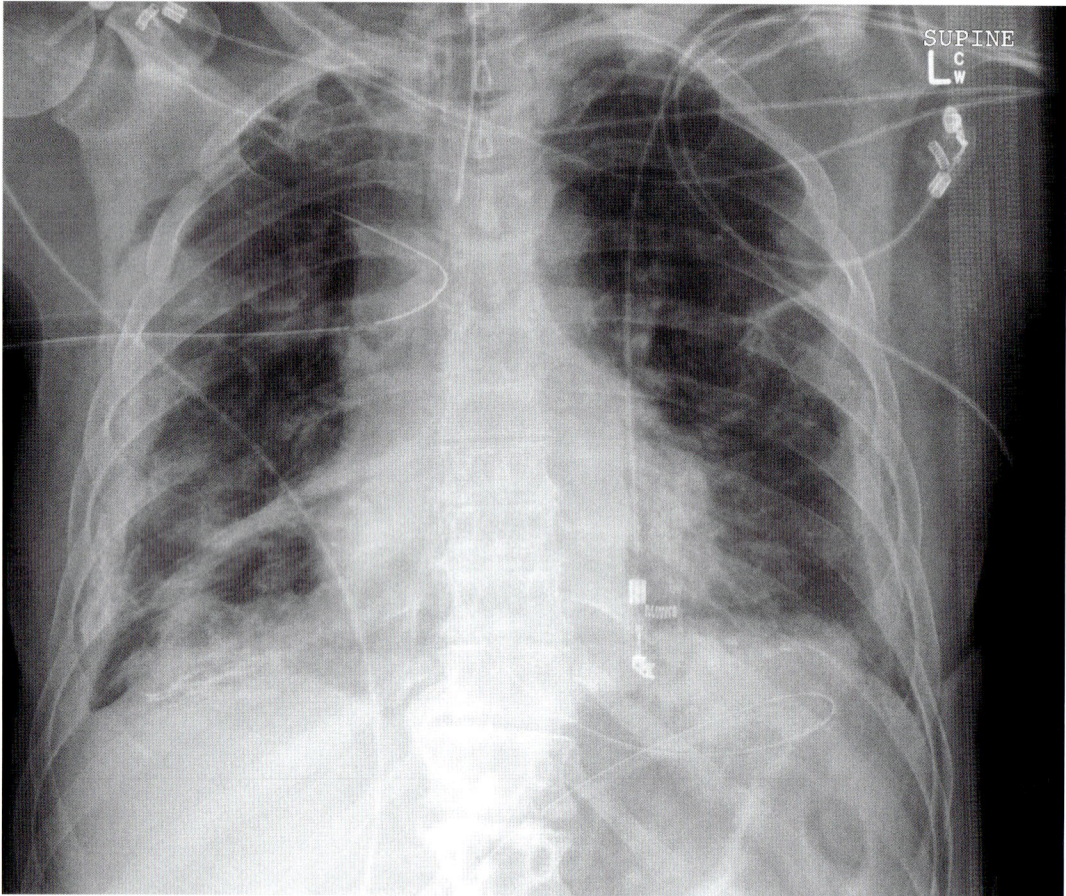

This 62-year-old man fell three metres while working on a building site. He landed on his head and has been unconscious since then. A drain was inserted into the right chest because a haemothorax was thought to be present, but nothing has drained.

**Q**

What pathological process does this image suggest?

## A

There are bilateral calcified pleural plaques with marked pleural thickening on both the diaphragmatic surface and chest wall. These are strongly suggestive of asbestos exposure. There is underlying interstitial opacification consistent with pulmonary fibrosis, which in the presence of pleural plaques is likely to be due to asbestosis. No rib fractures or other evidence of chest trauma is seen. The endotracheal tube is well positioned. The chest drain has been inserted too far.

## LEARNING POINT

Not all pleurally based opacities are a haemothorax or pleural effusion.

## PROBLEM 1.29

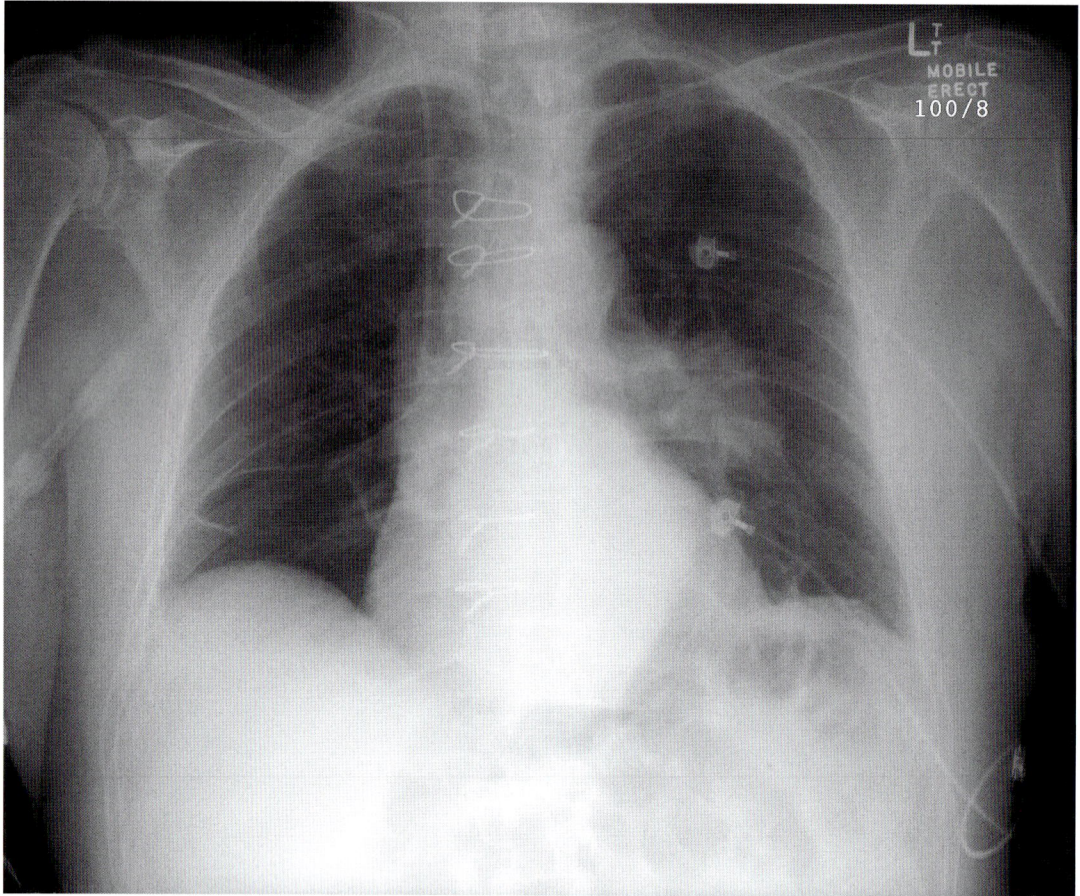

This is the routine postoperative X-ray of a 63-year-old man who had elective coronary artery bypass grafting for stable angina with triple vessel coronary artery disease.

**Q**
1. Describe the major abnormality.
2. List three possible causes for this appearance.

## A

1. There is a large, well-defined mass lesion extending from the left hilar region.

2. Three possible causes for this appearance are:
   - neoplasm: primary or secondary
   - infection: pneumonia, abscess, hydatid cyst
   - pulmonary artery aneurysm
   
   The patient had a bronchial carcinoma.

## LEARNING POINT

Routine X-rays may reveal unexpected but important findings.

## PROBLEM 1.30

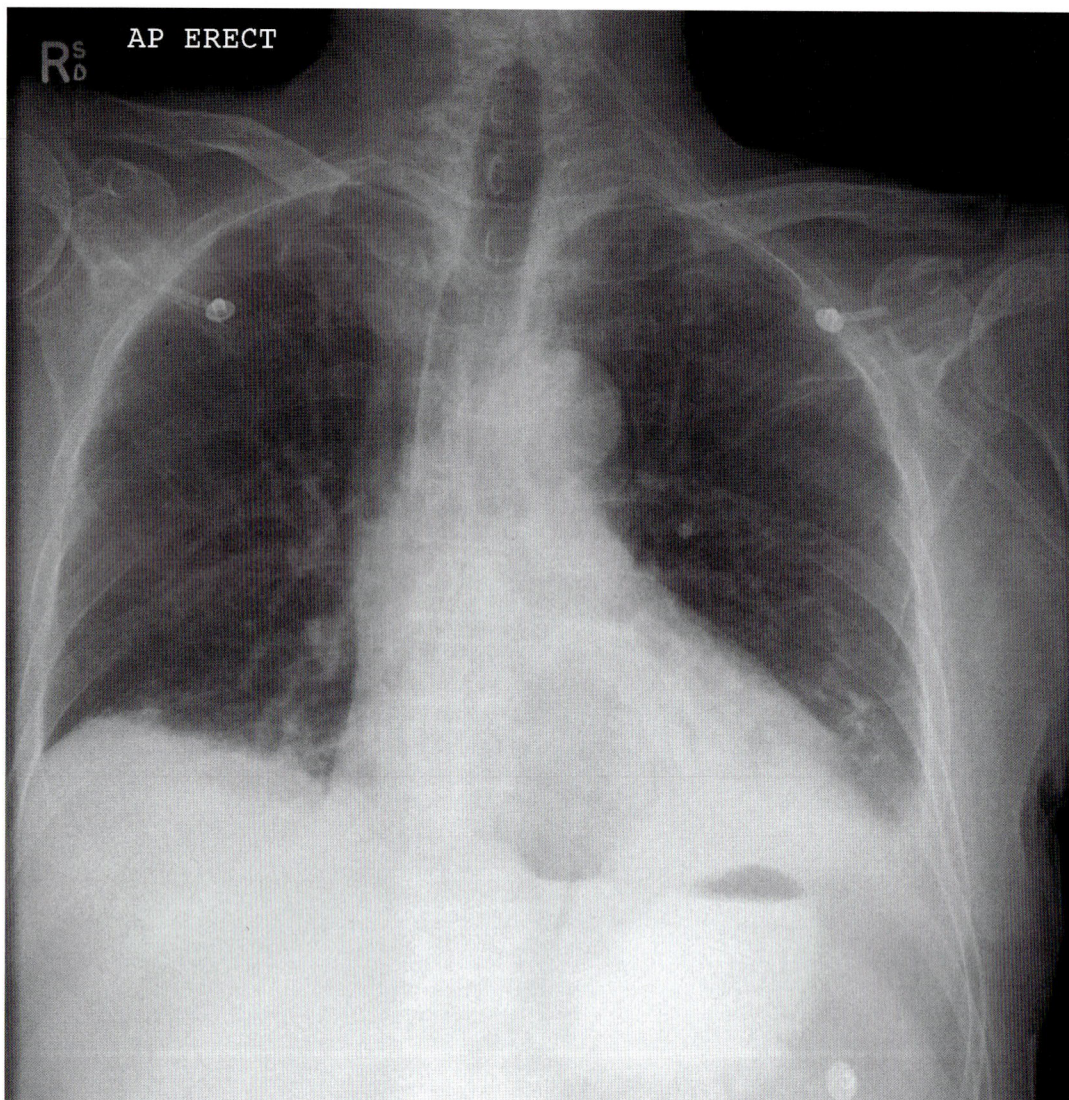

This 79-year-old man suddenly developed severe central chest pain following an alcoholic binge.

Q What is the most likely diagnosis?

## A

The findings on the X-ray are:
- loss of the left costophrenic angle, suggesting a small pleural effusion
- mediastinal air, outlining the left side of the aorta from the top of the arch to below the diaphragm
- atelectasis within the left lower lobe

The combination of pleural effusion and mediastinal air is highly suspicious of a rupture of the oesophagus.

## LEARNING POINT

There is a characteristic appearance of a ruptured oesophagus on a chest X-ray.

## PROBLEM 1.31

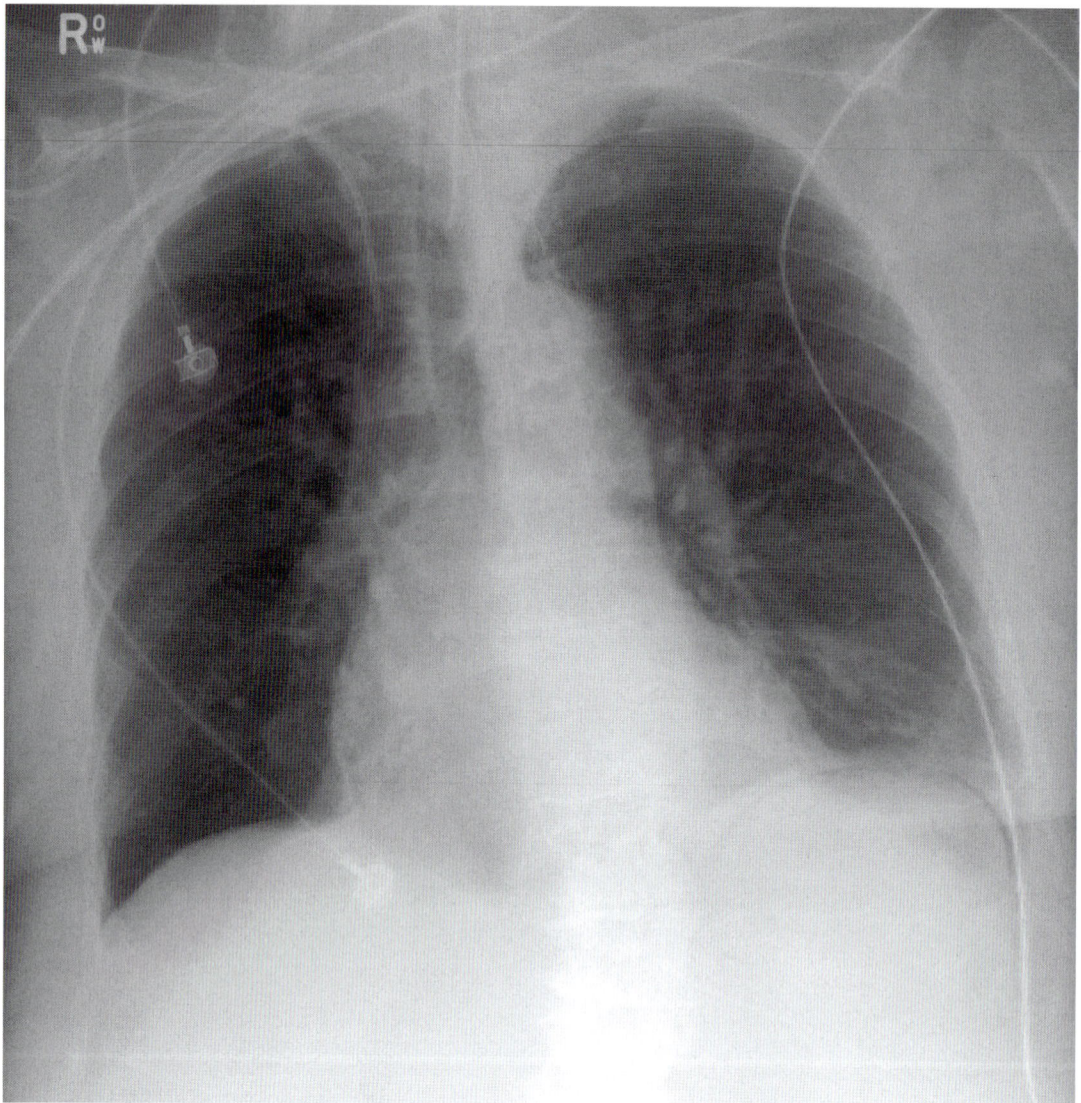

This 75-year-old man was found at home confused and agitated. He was given sedation in the emergency department because of severe agitation, then became obtunded and required intubation.

**Q**

Can you suggest a diagnosis?

## A

There is air under the left hemidiaphragm, as well as a small left pleural effusion. He has septic encephalopathy complicating a perforated viscus.

## LEARNING POINT

Don't forget to look below the diaphragm.

## PROBLEM 1.32

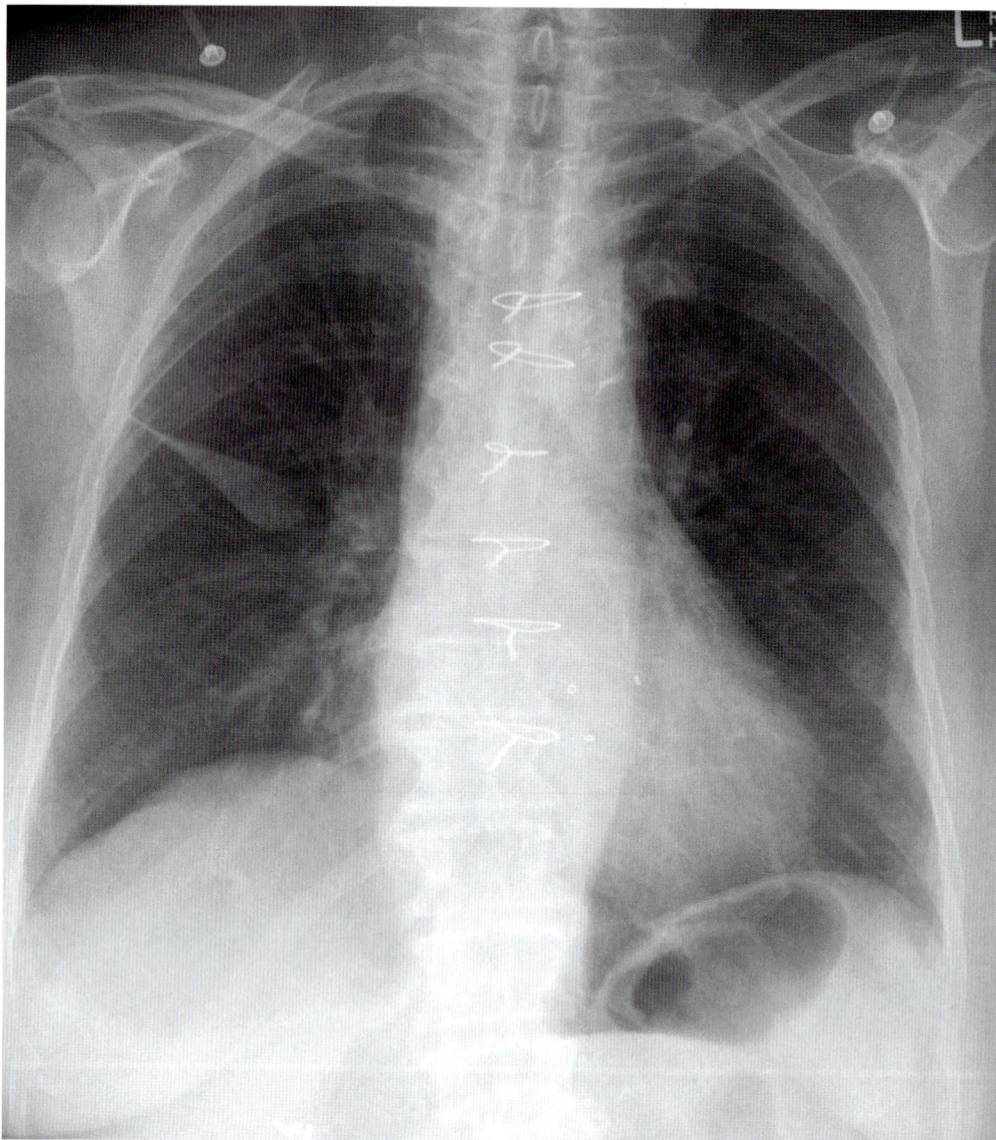

This 68-year-old woman is booked for a needle biopsy of the mass in the right midzone.

**Q** Is this an appropriate course of action?

## A

The appearances on the X-ray are those of a "pseudotumour" caused by encysted fluid in the oblique fissure. There is no indication for needle biopsy.

Other findings on the X-ray include the presence of a mitral valve replacement (seen as three dots to the left of the lower sternal wire) and calcification in the aortic arch.

## LEARNING POINT

Encysted fluid collections in a fissure are often called "pseudotumours" and are easily confused with neoplasms if you are not aware of their characteristic appearance. Pseudotumours may occur in either the horizontal or oblique fissure. A lateral chest X-ray will confirm the oblong configuration, with the long axis of the opacity aligned along the course of the fissure.

## PROBLEM 1.33

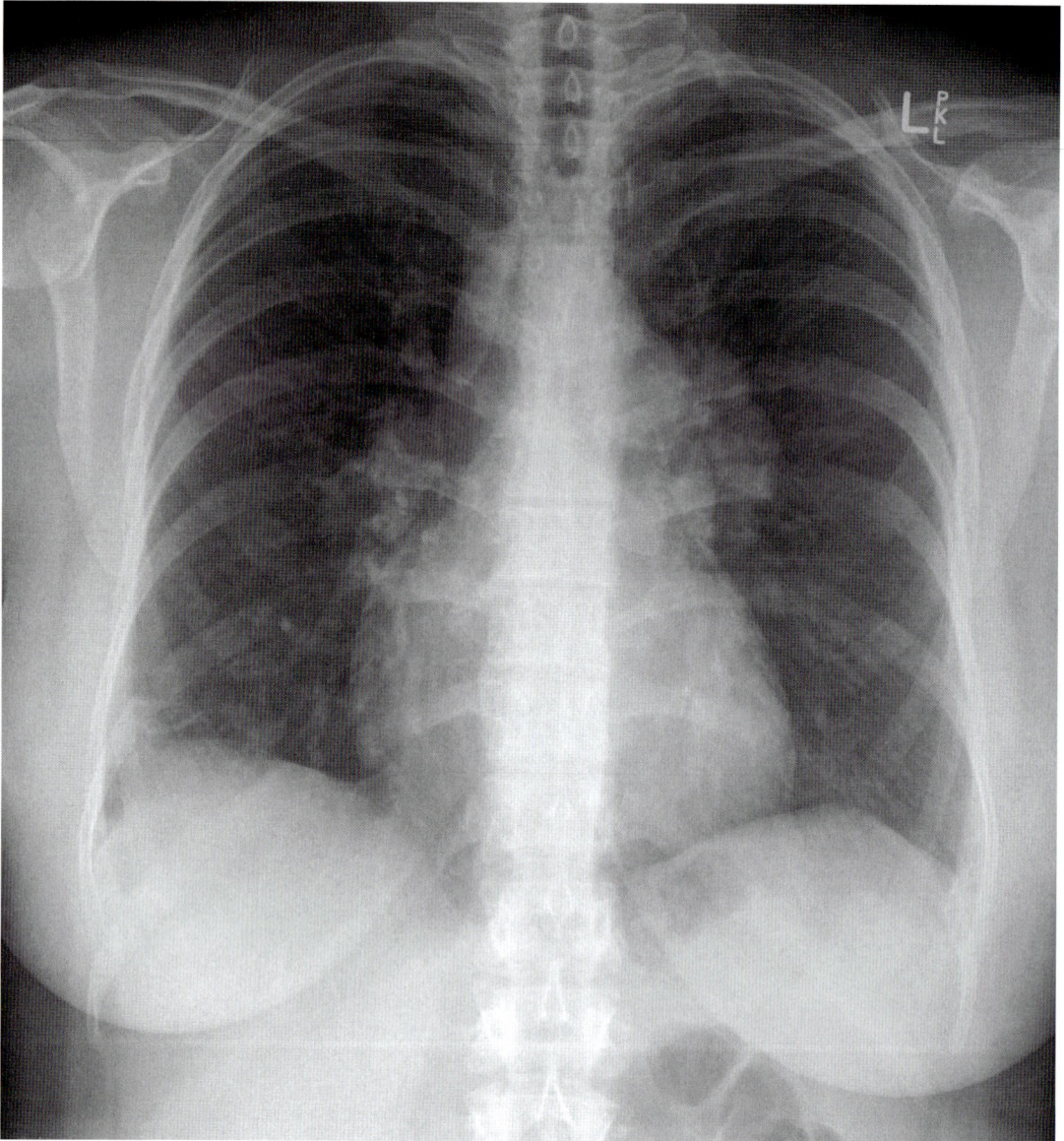

This 38-year-old woman presented with a four-week history of malaise, cough and shortness of breath.

**Q**
Suggest a differential diagnosis.

**A**

There are rounded opacities at both hila. The right paratracheal stripe is thickened. These findings suggest hilar and mediastinal lymphadenopathy, respectively. The differential diagnosis for mediastinal lymphadenopathy includes sarcoidosis, tuberculosis, lymphoma, lung carcinomas and other cancers. There is also minimal patchy opacification at the right base.

**LEARNING POINT**

Not all mediastinal lymphadenopathy is caused by malignancy.

## PROBLEM 1.34

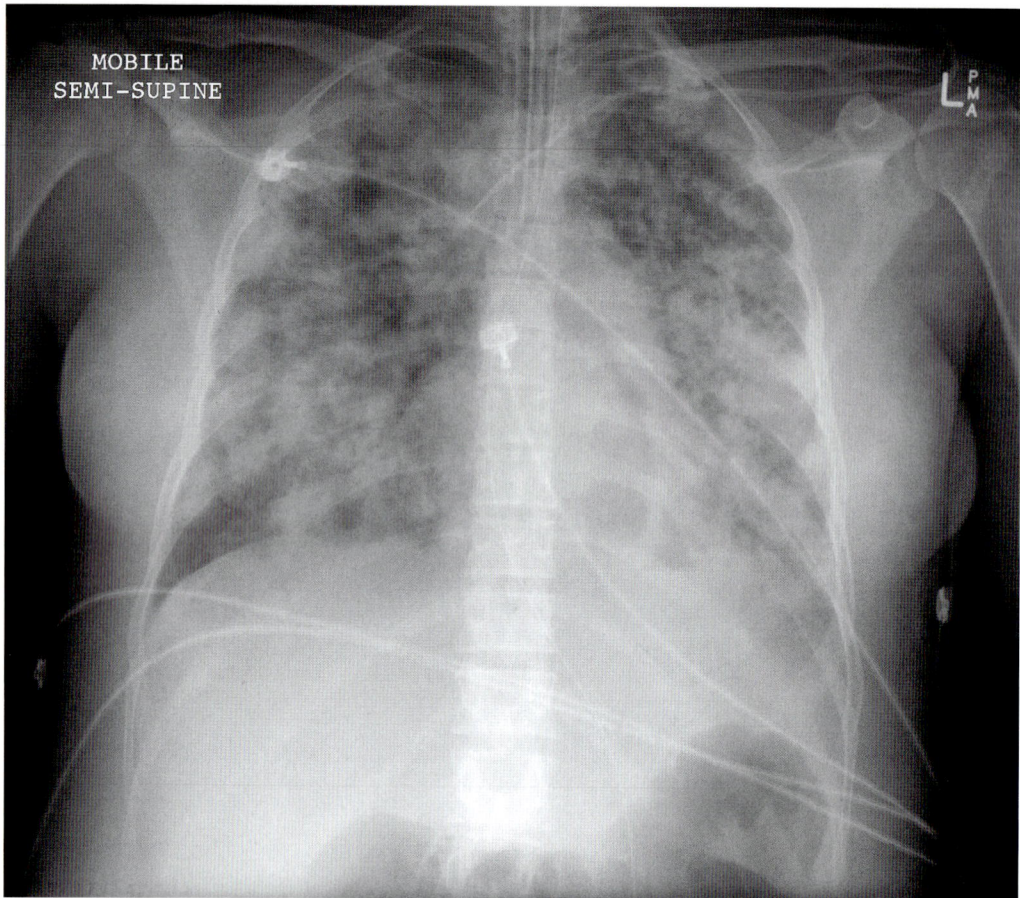

This previously well, 28-year-old woman developed respiratory failure 48 hours after having open reduction and internal fixation of a femoral fracture.

**Q** What is the likely cause of her respiratory failure?

## A

There are widespread patchy alveolar infiltrates throughout both lungs. The cardiac size is normal. Acute respiratory distress syndrome (ARDS) caused by fat embolism syndrome or aspiration is the most likely cause of her respiratory failure.

Without the clinical history, the differential diagnosis would be broad and include cardiogenic and non-cardiogenic pulmonary oedema, pneumonia, pulmonary haemorrhage and primary alveolar proteinosis.

## LEARNING POINT

The chest X-ray must be interpreted in conjunction with the clinical context.

## PROBLEM 1.35

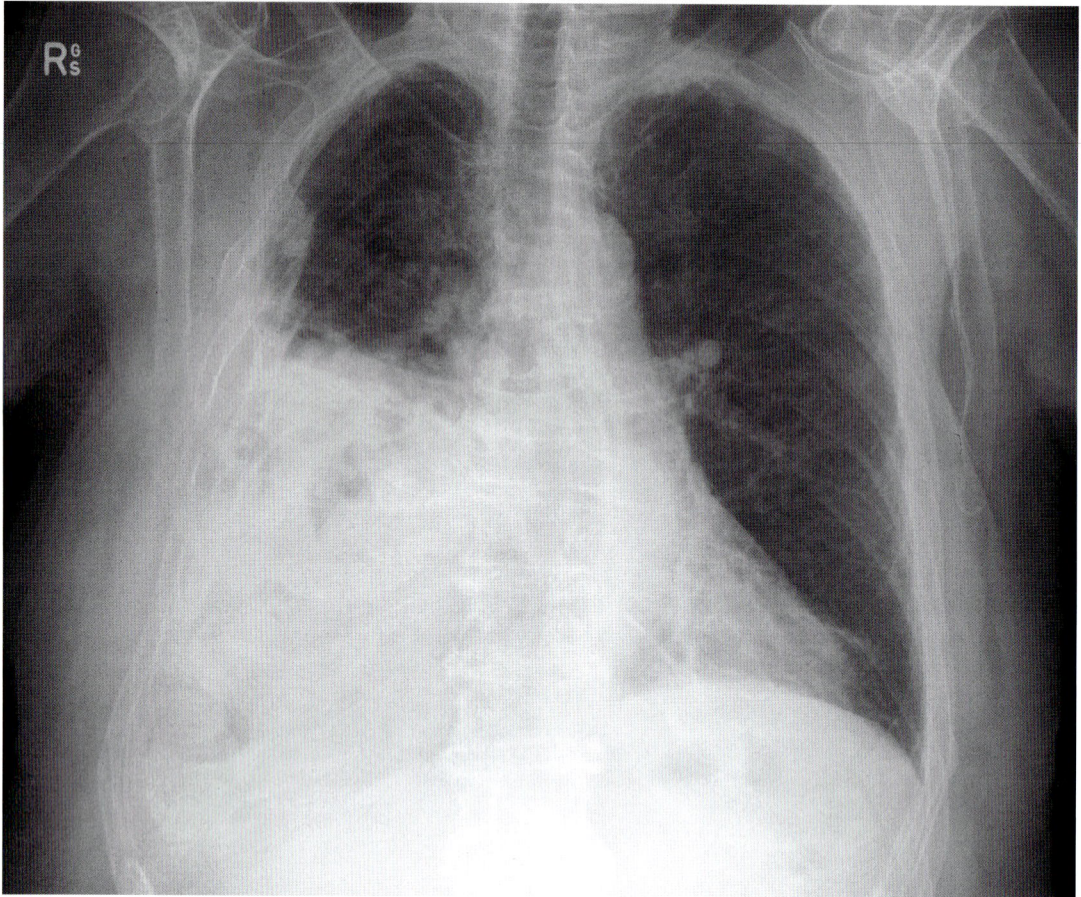

This 75-year-old man complained of increasing dyspnoea over the last six months. Ten years ago, he had a motor vehicle accident requiring ICU admission for two weeks.

**Q** What is the likely cause of the dyspnoea?

## A

The lower and mid zones of the right chest are opacified, with gas density structures seen within this area. There are multiple old rib fractures from previous trauma. There is pleural calcification on the right, which in this clinical context is likely to be due to previous haemothorax.

These findings suggest a traumatic diaphragmatic hernia with bowel herniation into the right chest.

## LEARNING POINT

Following chest trauma, it can take several years for a significant diaphragmatic hernia to develop.

Unilateral pleural calcification may be due to previous empyema or haemothorax. Bilateral pleural calcification usually indicates asbestos exposure.

## PROBLEM 1.36

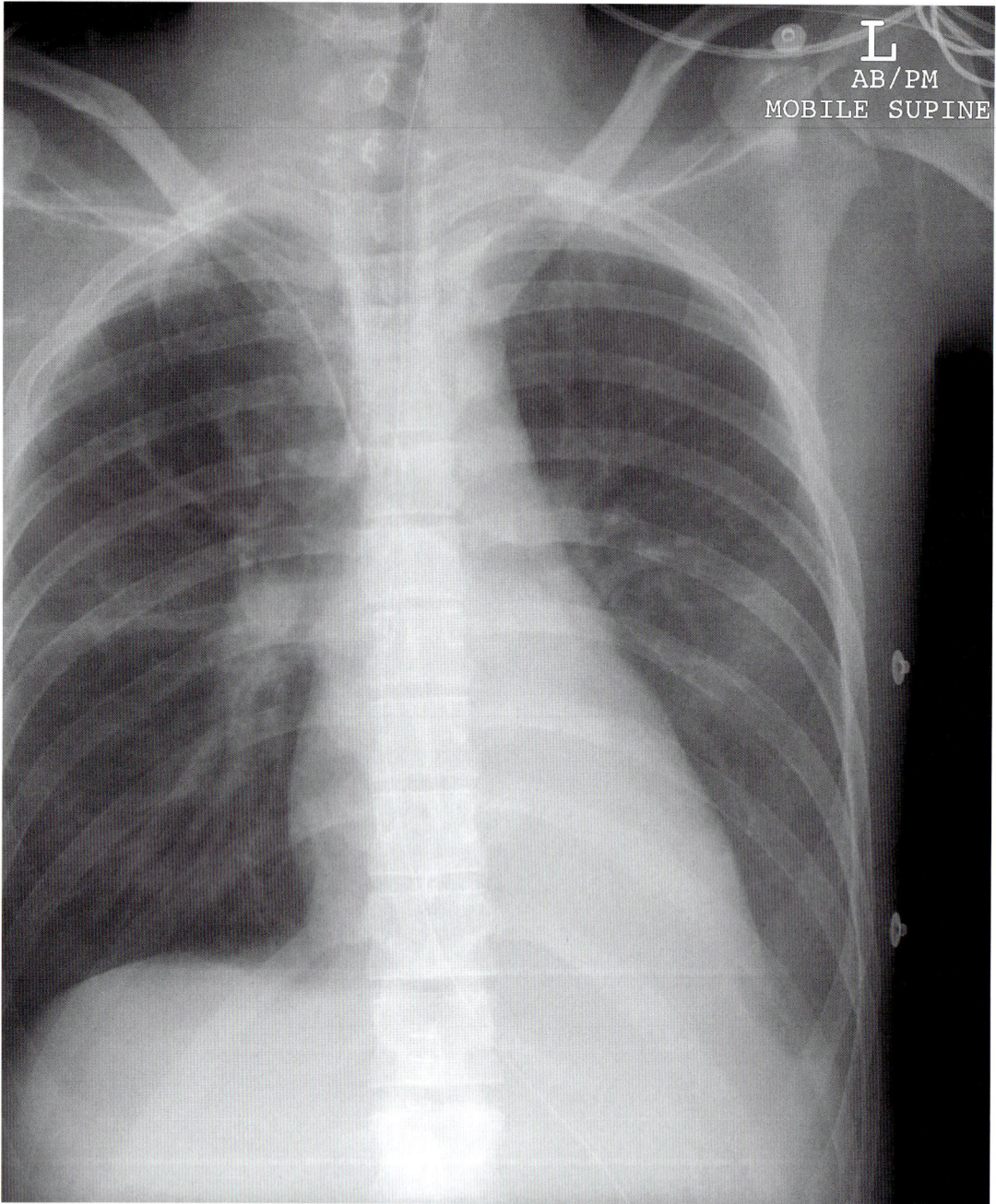

This 26-year-old man presented following a motorbike crash. He is increasingly short of breath and now desaturating on high-flow mask oxygen. He wants to sit up so it is easier to breathe.

**Q**

Are you going to let him sit up?

## A

Although there is left lower lobe collapse, this is not the most important finding on the X-ray. At T4/5 level, there is an alteration in the height of the vertebral bodies and the intervertebral space is not seen. This could be an unstable spinal fracture and he should not be allowed to sit up. Incidentally, there is also an azygous lobe, which is a normal anatomical variant.

## LEARNING POINT

Don't forget to look at the bones on the chest X-ray.

## PROBLEM 1.37

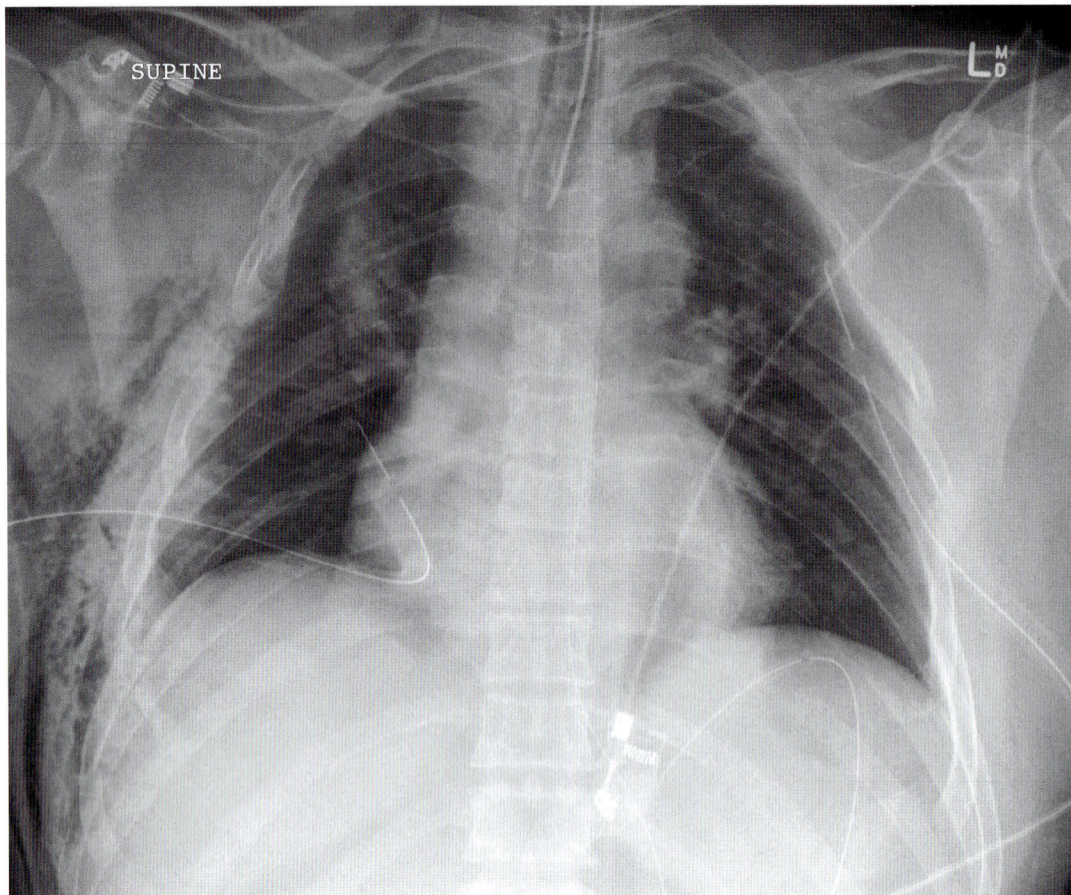

This 42-year-old man was involved in a high-speed car crash and was intubated on the scene for severe respiratory distress.

Q

What features on the image may have contributed to the respiratory distress?

## A

There are multiple fractured ribs bilaterally, so pain may have been a factor. On the left side, there are anterior and posterior fractures, which would be consistent with a flail chest, but this cannot be diagnosed by imaging alone. There is also an opacity in the right midzone, consistent with a pulmonary contusion. Finally, there is surgical emphysema and a chest drain on the right side, suggesting that there may have been a pneumothorax.

## LEARNING POINT

Flail chest is a clinical diagnosis, not a radiological one.

## PROBLEM 1.38

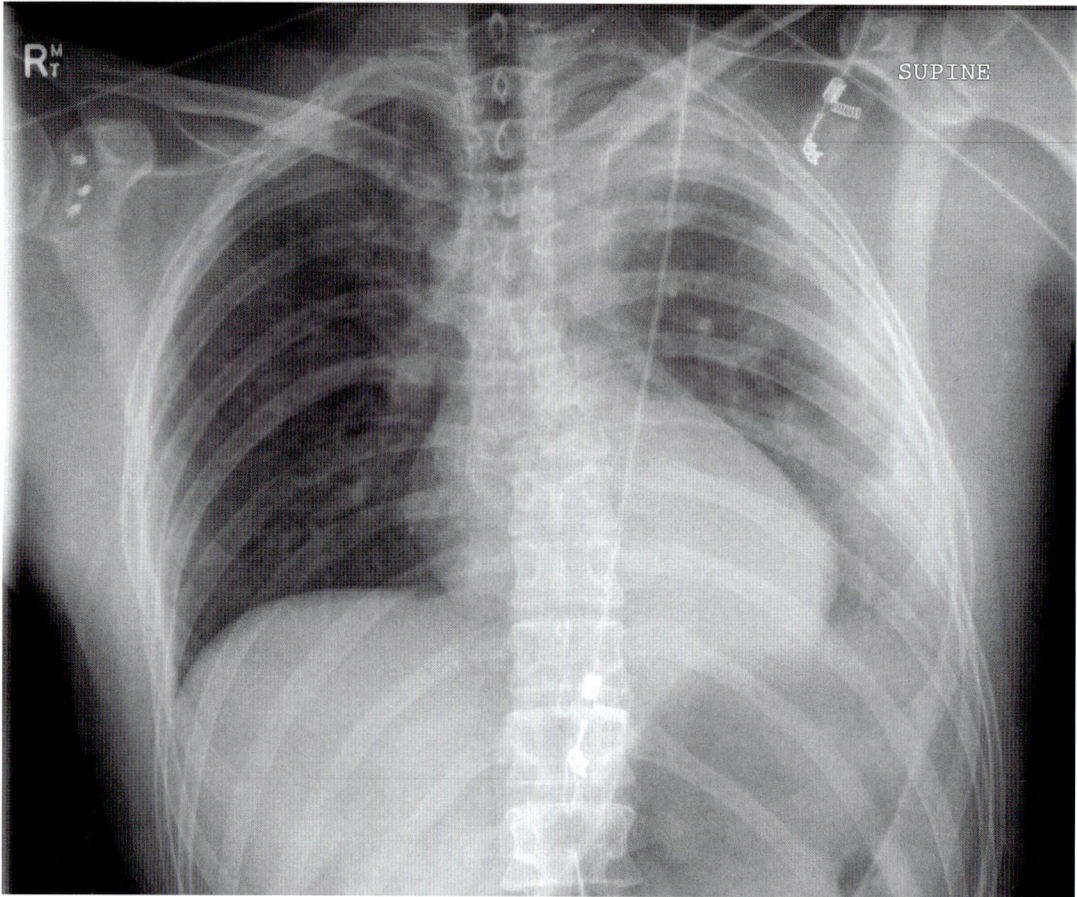

This 28-year-old man had a motorbike crash on the freeway. At the scene, he complained of difficulty breathing.

**Q**

What is the likely source of the haemothorax?

## A

The findings on the image include a pleural fluid collection on the left, gastric distension and a spinal fracture-dislocation at around the T6/7 level. There are no obvious rib fractures. The most likely source of the haemothorax is the spinal fracture. Other possible sites of bleeding are a ruptured aorta, the lung or the chest wall.

## LEARNING POINT

Haemothorax may complicate a thoracic spinal fracture. It is very common to have a haematoma adjacent to the fracture, which may track through the mediastinum giving appearances similar to a ruptured aorta. The haematoma can extend into the extrapleural space, producing the appearance of a pleural cap, or rupture into the pleural cavity, producing a haemothorax.

## PROBLEM 1.39

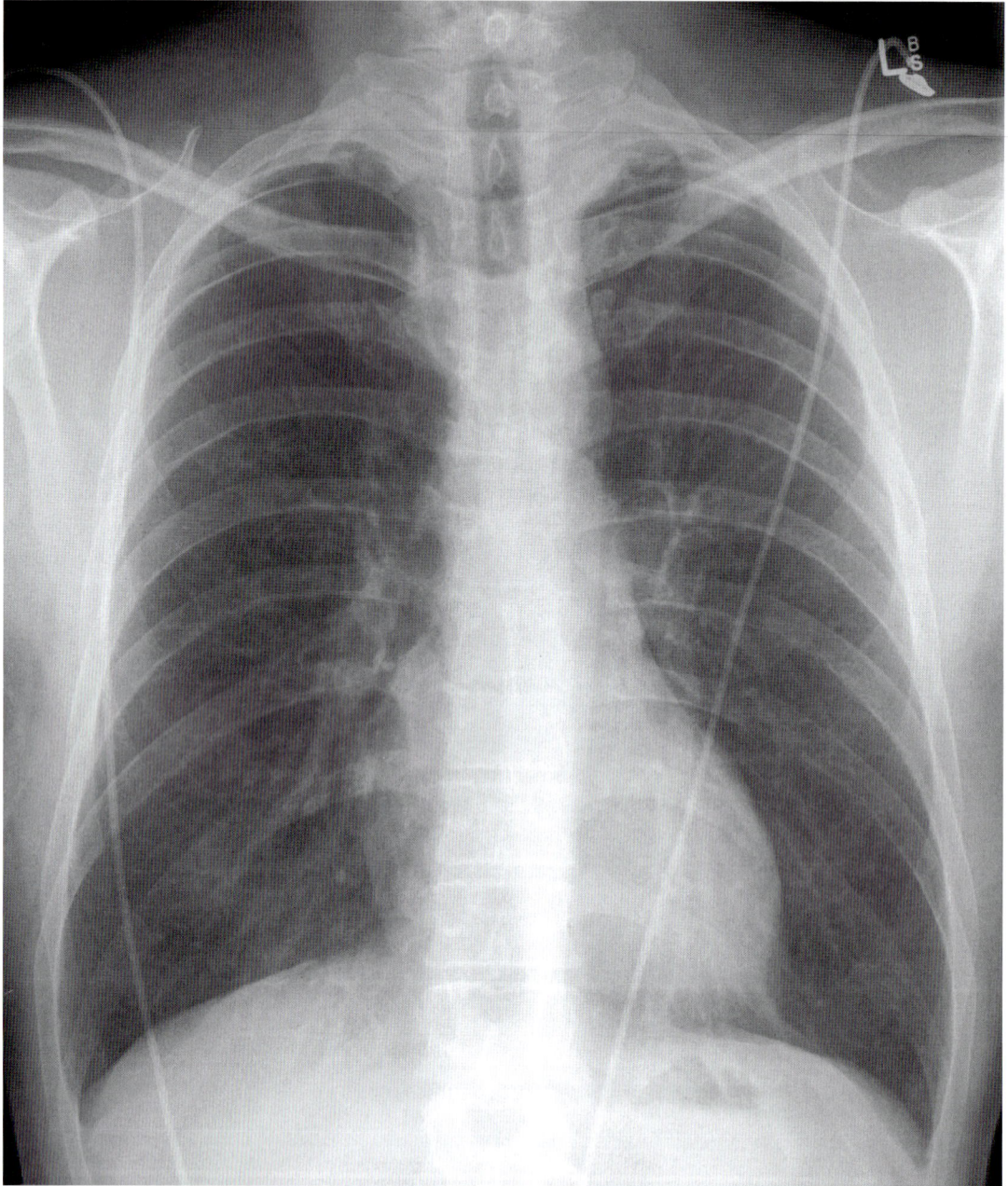

This 25-year-old man has chronic hypertension.

Q
1. What is the diagnosis?
2. What findings on the X-ray support your diagnosis?

# A

1. Aortic coarctation.

2. Findings on the X-ray that support your diagnosis:

- bilateral rib notching from the third to the eighth ribs
- aortic knuckle is small and abnormally shaped

# LEARNING POINT

Subtle signs on the X-ray are easily missed unless the X-ray is systematically examined. A good scheme for systematic examination of a chest X-ray is:
- general overview
- lines and tubes (devices)
- lungs
- mediastinum
- bones
- other soft tissues

## PROBLEM 1.40

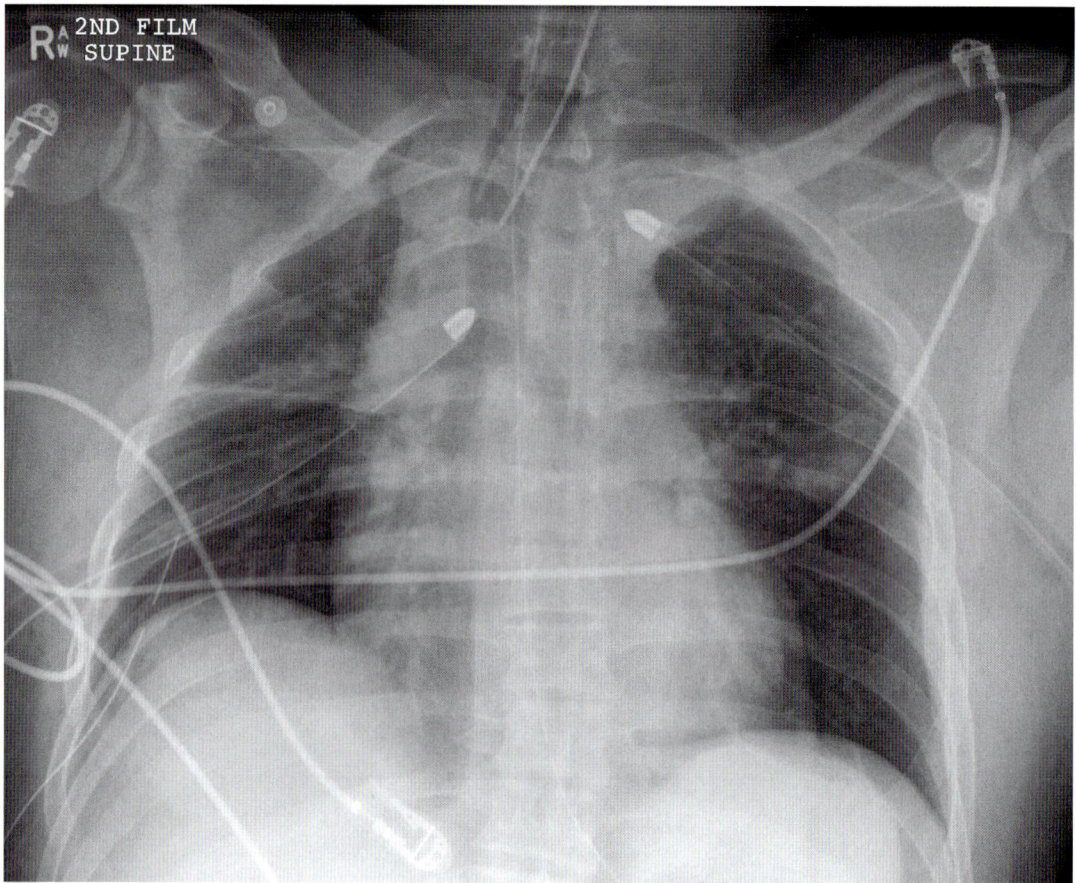

This 29-year-old man was the driver in a high-speed car crash.

**Q**

1. List the abnormalities on this chest X-ray.
2. What further investigation will you do?

# A

1. Abnormalities on this chest X-ray include:
   - endotracheal tube
   - bilateral chest drains (two on right)
   - lower thoracic scoliosis, which raises the question of a spinal fracture

   There are a number of findings on this X-ray suggesting aortic disruption (Clarke, 1997):
   - displacement of trachea and NG tube to right
   - wide upper mediastinum
   - left pleural cap
   - loss of aorto-pulmonary window (the space on the left mediastinal border between the aortic knuckle and the pulmonary artery)
   - indistinct outline of aortic knuckle
   - depression of left main bronchus

   Other features that would suggest the diagnosis of aortic disruption but are not present on this X-ray include:
   - fracture of first or second rib
   - left haemothorax
   - loss of paratracheal stripe

   As is commonly encountered in the ICU, the patient is significantly rotated on this image, which must be considered when interpreting the image.

2. CT angiography, transoesophageal echocardiography or digital subtraction angiography would be acceptable for investigation of a possible traumatic rupture of the aorta. MR angiography may be used, but the requirement for a prolonged investigation in a suboptimally monitored environment limits its usefulness.

## LEARNING POINT

There is a classic constellation of signs on the chest X-ray associated with aortic injury.

## PROBLEM 1.41

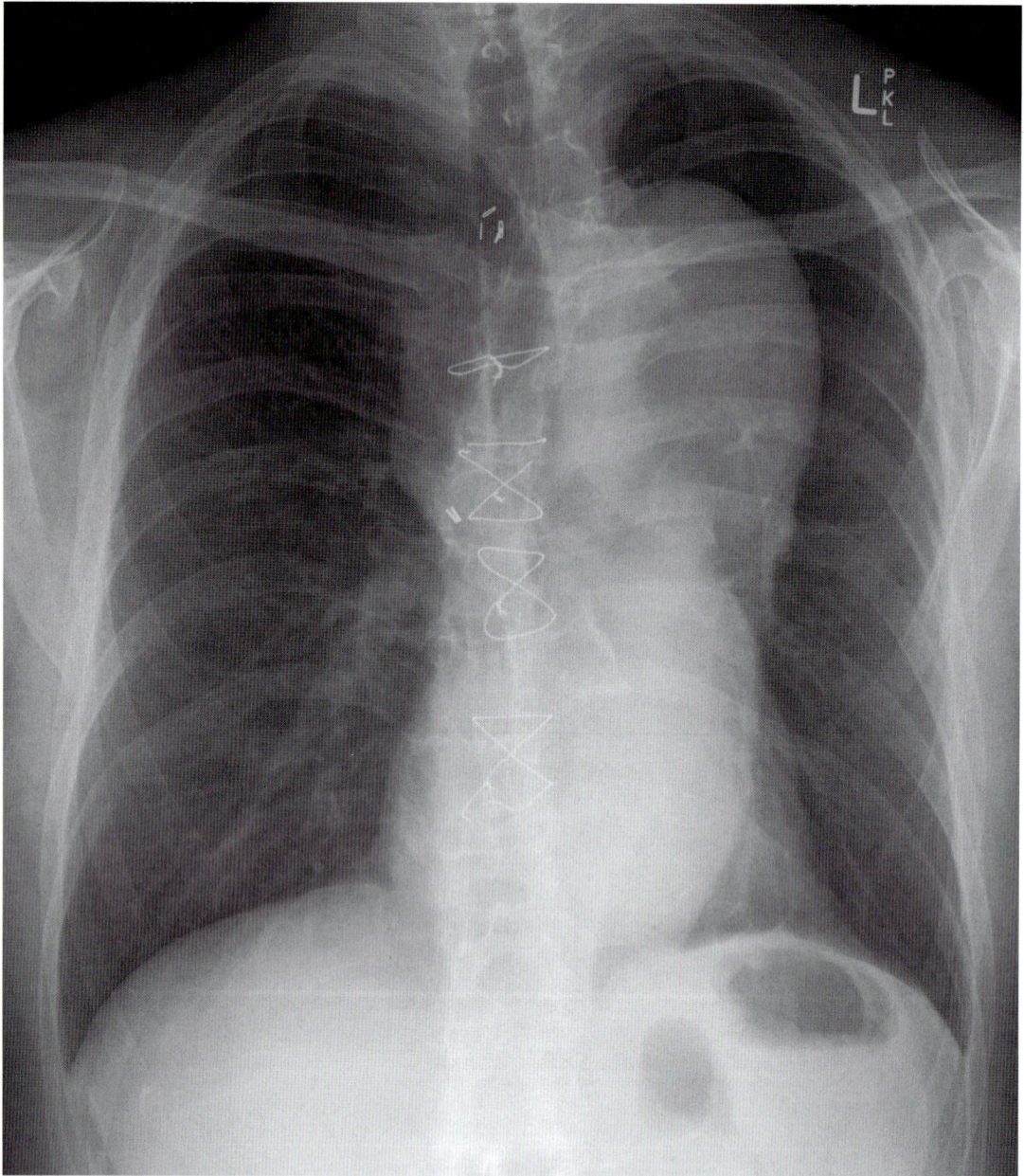

This 33-year-old man presented with sudden onset of chest pain.

**Q**
1. Describe the findings on the film.
2. What diseases are associated with this appearance?

# A

1. There is a superior mediastinal mass. The differential diagnosis for this includes:
   - lymphoma
   - teratoma
   - thymoma
   - thyroid
   - thoracic aortic aneurysm

   In this case, the presence of sternal wires, surgical staples and visible aortic root replacement graft favour a thoracic aortic aneurysm. The border of the "mass" is also contiguous with the aortic wall inferiorly, hence confirming its aortic origin. The thoracic cage is elongated and there is an upper thoracic scoliosis, convex to the left.

2. Conditions associated with thoracic aortic aneurysms include (Dahnert, 2007):
   - Marfan syndrome and other connective tissue disorders
   - hypertension
   - tertiary syphilis
   - previous trauma
   - infection
   - seronegative arthritides

## LEARNING POINT

Thoracic aortic aneurysms in young adults are usually due to Marfan syndrome.

## PROBLEM 1.42

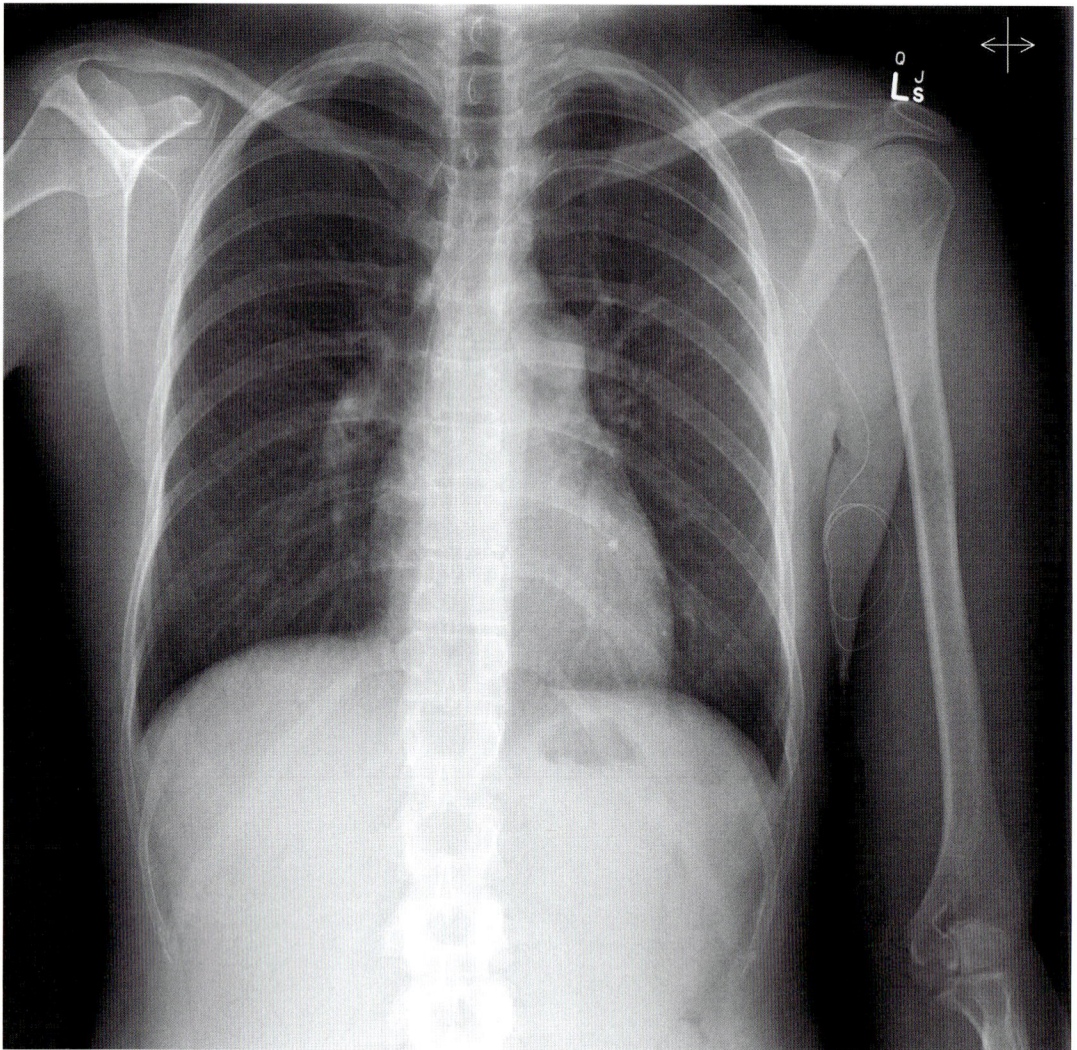

This 25-year-old man presented with shortness of breath and reduced exercise tolerance, which has developed progressively over the last six months.

**Q** What is the likely diagnosis?

## A

The central pulmonary arteries are enlarged and there is peripheral pruning of the pulmonary vasculature. The cardiac shadow and the lung fields appear normal. This suggests primary pulmonary hypertension, but other causes of pulmonary hypertension, such as recurrent pulmonary emboli, need to be excluded. The peripherally inserted central venous catheter is well positioned.

## LEARNING POINT

Peripheral pruning describes an abrupt change in calibre between the lobar pulmonary arteries and their segmental branches. It gives the appearance of a "pruned" tree.

Before making a diagnosis of primary pulmonary hypertension, other causes of pulmonary hypertension need to be excluded.

## PROBLEM 1.43

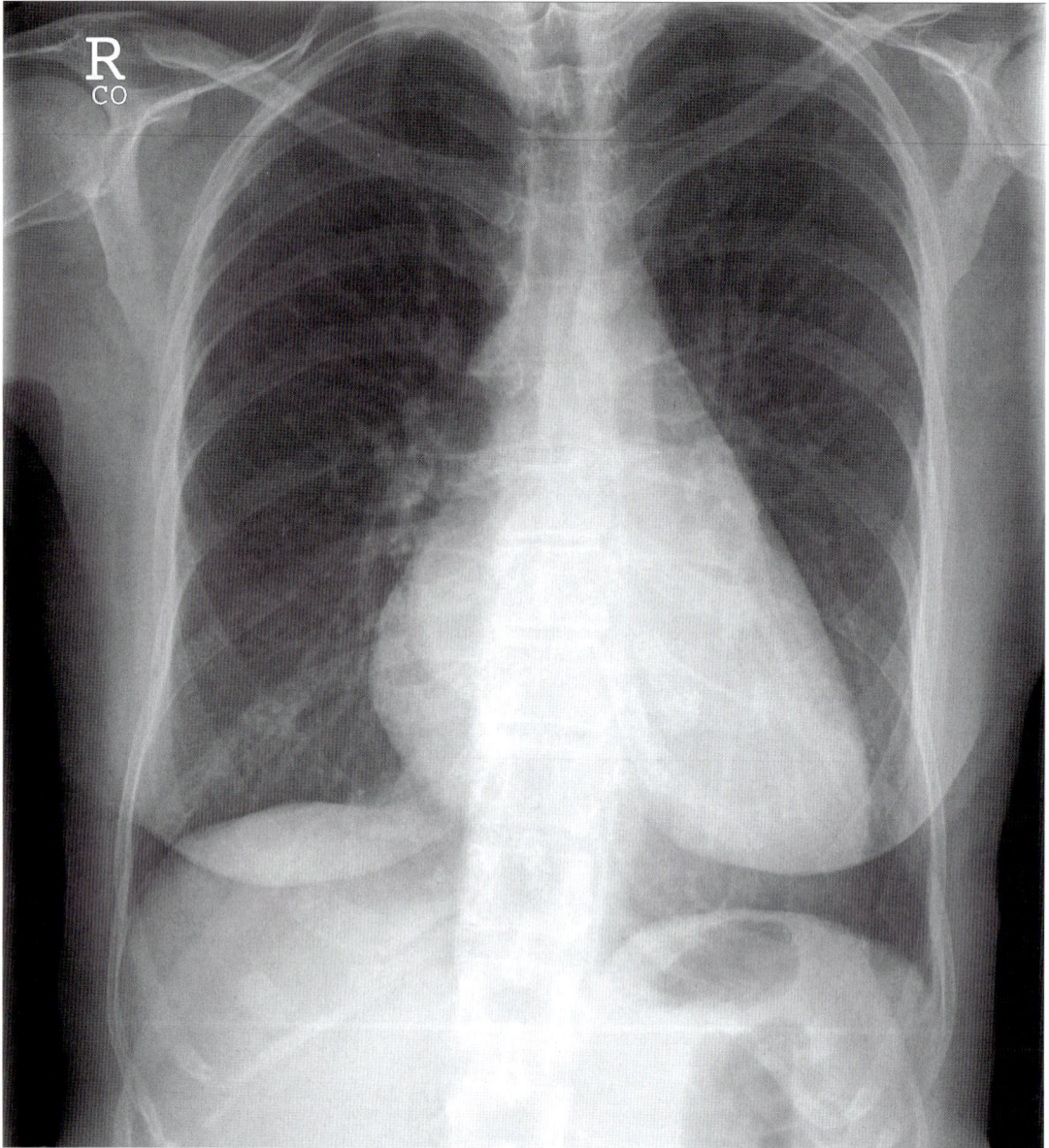

This 62-year-old woman presented with reduced exercise tolerance and episodic shortness of breath, which had been slowly worsening over the last three months.

**Q**

What is the most likely diagnosis?

# A

The key findings are:
- mild cardiomegaly
- an abnormally straight left heart border
- splaying of the carina to over 90 degrees
- a double right-heart border

These findings suggest left atrial enlargement and mitral valve disease. There is no evidence of pulmonary oedema on this film.

## LEARNING POINT

Knowledge of normal anatomy of the heart assists with interpreting the X-ray in cardiac disease.

## PROBLEM 1.44

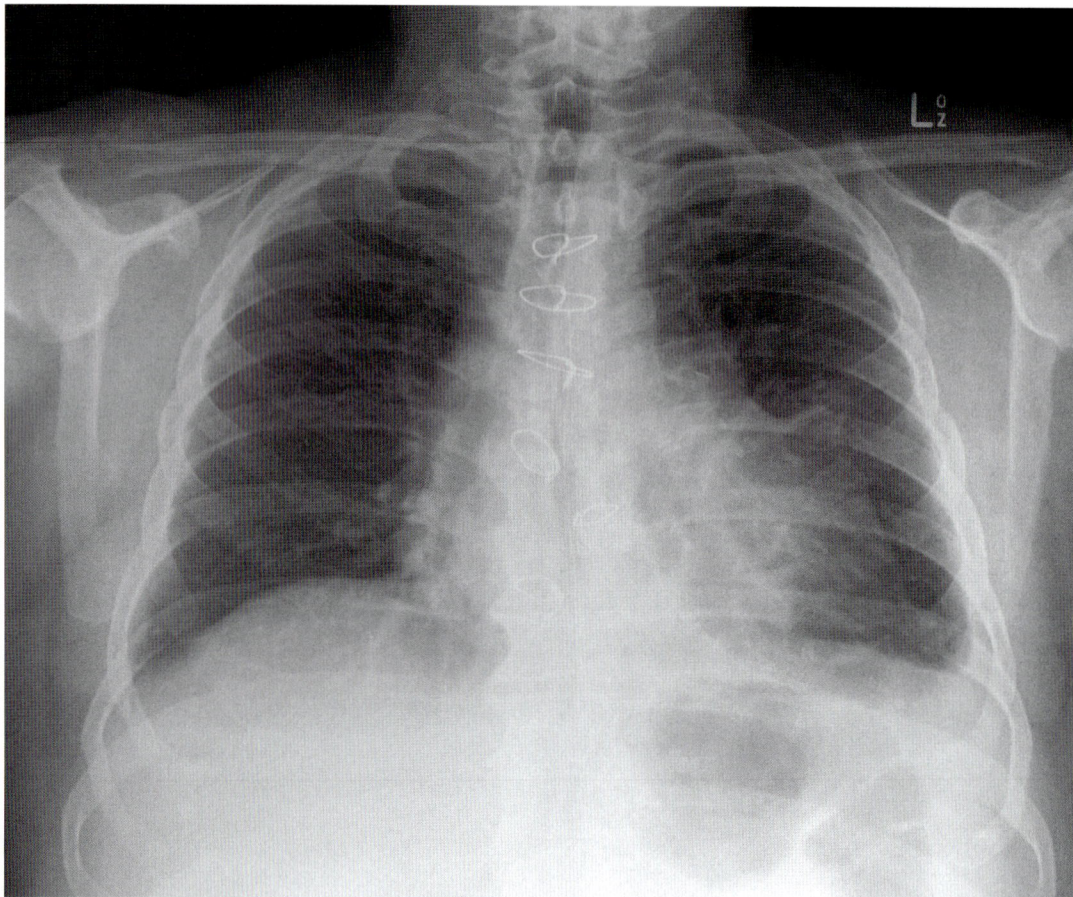

This 62-year-old diabetic man developed fever, shortness of breath and severe chest pain five days after coronary artery bypass surgery.

Q

What is the major abnormality?

## A

The sternal wires are not lined up in the centre of the chest, which suggests sternal dehiscence. Not all sternal dehiscence is caused by infection but, in this clinical context, wound infection and mediastinitis are highly likely. There is also blunting of the left costophrenic angle due to a small pleural effusion.

## LEARNING POINT

Risk factors for sternal dehiscence include bilateral internal mammary artery grafts, diabetes, smoking, obesity and prolonged postoperative ventilation (Losanoff, 2002).

Don't forget to look at medical devices such as sternal wires.

## PROBLEM 1.45

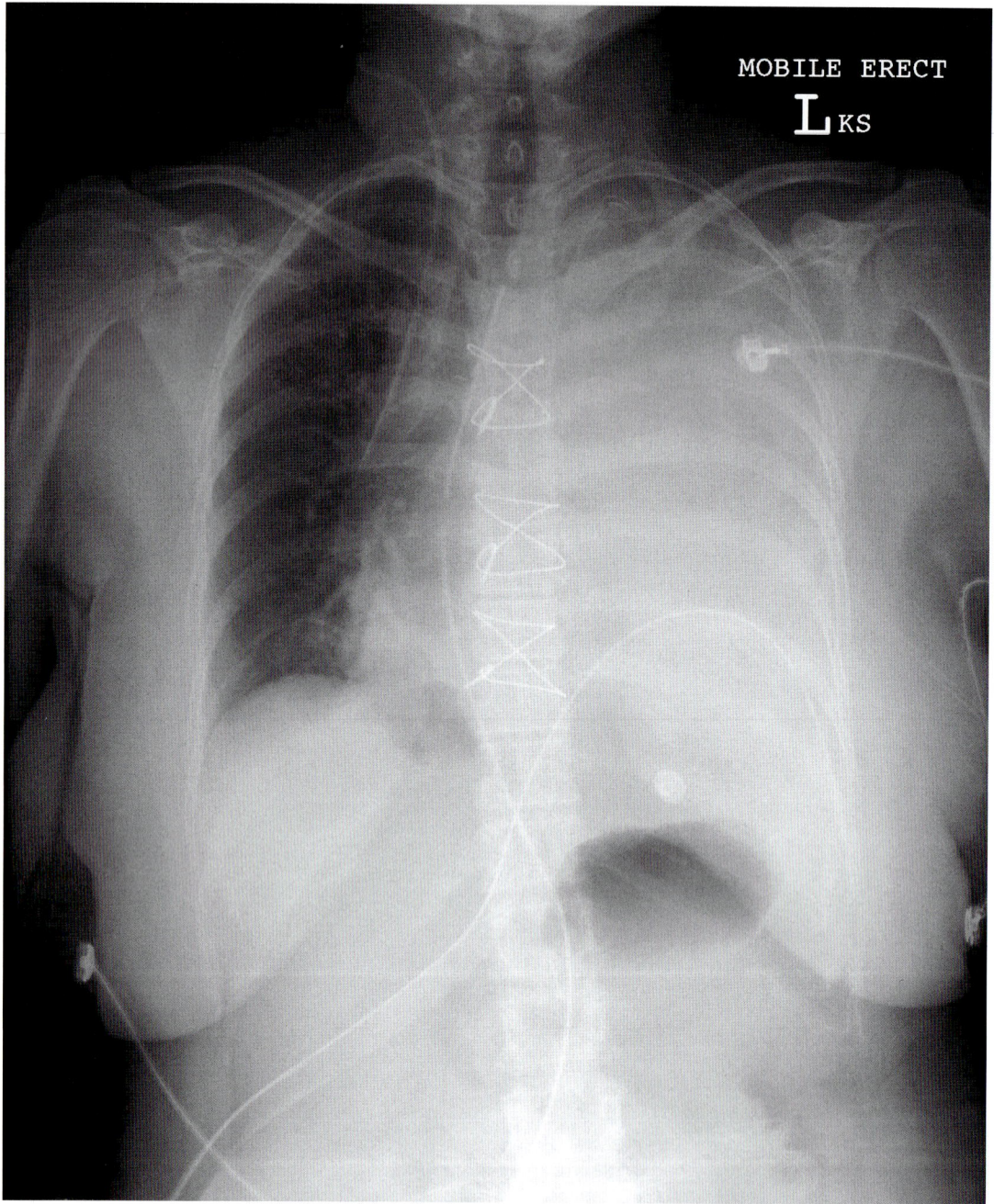

This 59-year-old woman underwent coronary artery bypass grafting yesterday. There was significant bleeding out of the mediastinal drains initially, but this settled after a few hours. Extubation occurred uneventfully this morning.

**Q** What is the likely diagnosis?

## A

There is an opaque left hemithorax with mediastinal shift to the right. The most likely diagnosis is massive haemothorax. The bleeding did not stop, but the drains were blocked and hence a large volume of blood accumulated in the pleural cavity.

If these X-ray abnormalities occurred several days after surgery, then chylothorax from damage to the thoracic duct should be considered.

## LEARNING POINT

Blood does not always come out of the chest drains.

## PROBLEM 1.46

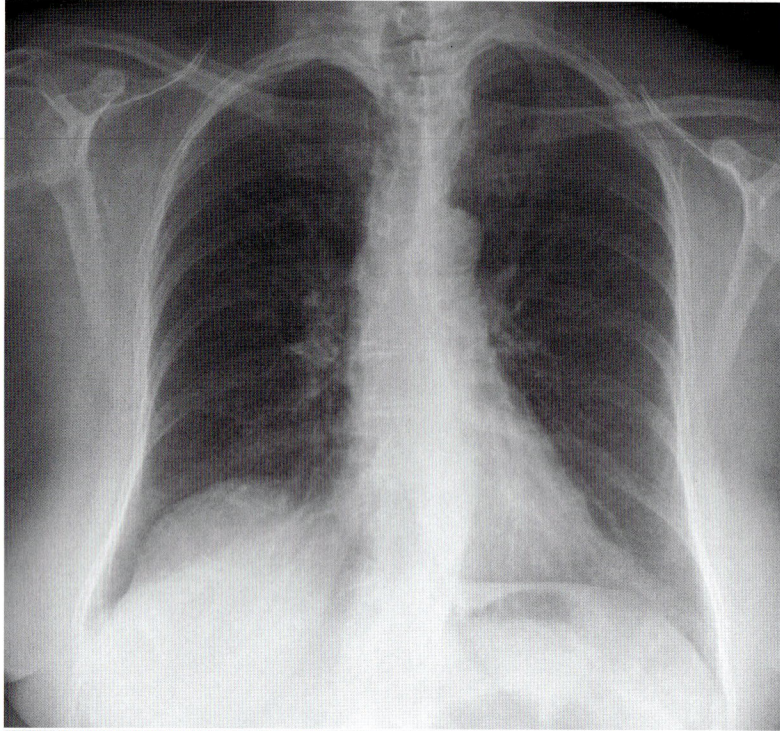

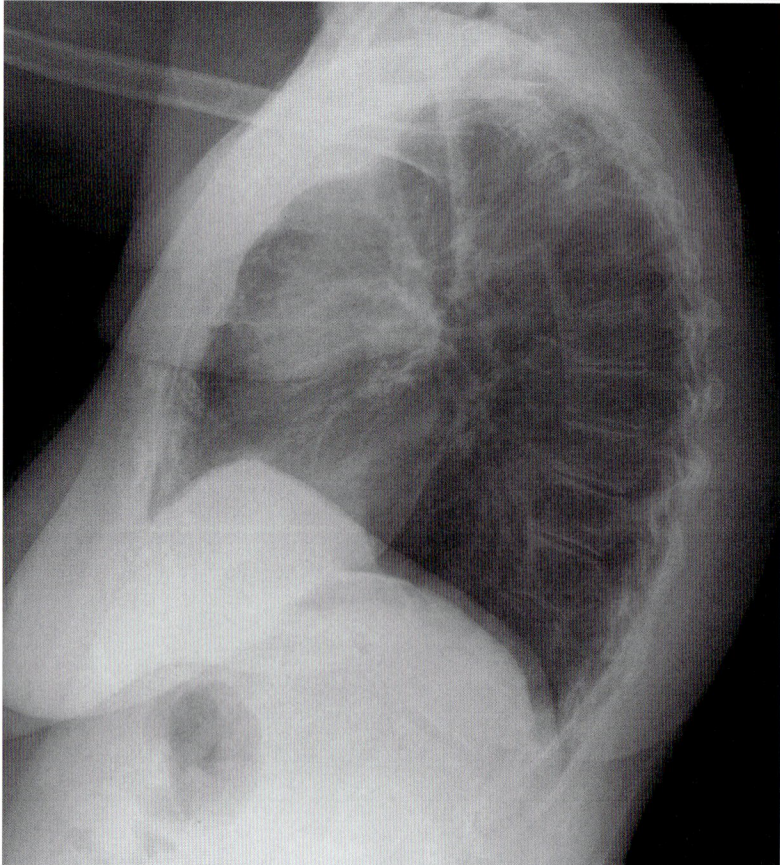

This 68-year-old woman is scheduled for elective hip surgery tomorrow. You have been asked to look at the X-ray because of concerns about the appearances at the right lung base.

## Q
What do you think?

## A
The anteromedial part of the right hemidiaphragm is elevated, consistent with a focal eventration of the diaphragm. There is no need to defer surgery.

## LEARNING POINT
With eventration of the diaphragm, there is an upward displacement of abdominal contents secondary to a thin hypoplastic diaphragm. It is usually asymptomatic but, if large, can cause respiratory compromise. The most common position is anteromedial on the right side (Dahnert, 2007).

## PROBLEM 1.47

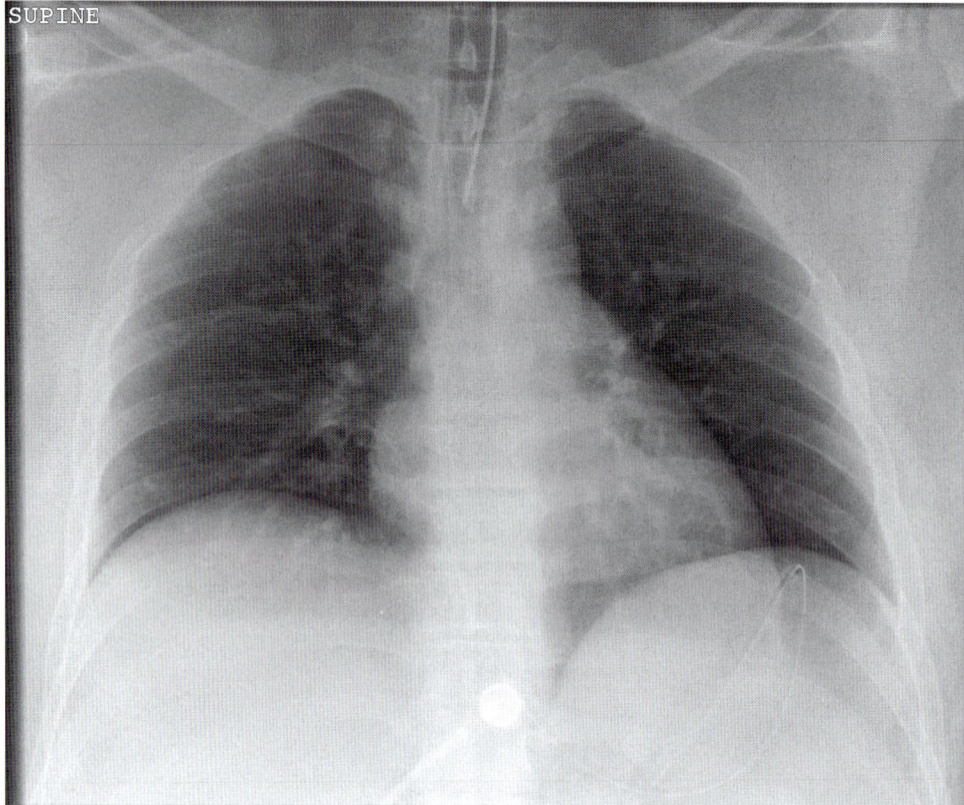

This 29-year-old man was admitted to ICU following open reduction and internal fixation of multiple lower limb fractures. Concerns have been raised that his X-ray has prominent lung markings and that he may have fluid overload or fat embolism syndrome.

### Q
What do you think?

## A

On an appropriately inflated chest X-ray, 10 ribs should be visible above the diaphragm posteriorly and the ends of six ribs anteriorly. In this image, only seven ribs are visible posteriorly above the diaphragm. This chest is significantly underinflated, making the vessels appear more prominent than they would if the film was adequately inflated. No significant pathology is present.

## LEARNING POINT

Technical aspects that need to be considered with interpreting a chest X-ray include:
- correct patient / time / date
- direction of X-ray beam (PA, AP or lateral)
- patient position (erect, supine or decubitus)
- amount of rotation
- positioning of patient on film
- amount of inflation and exposure

# PROBLEM 1.48

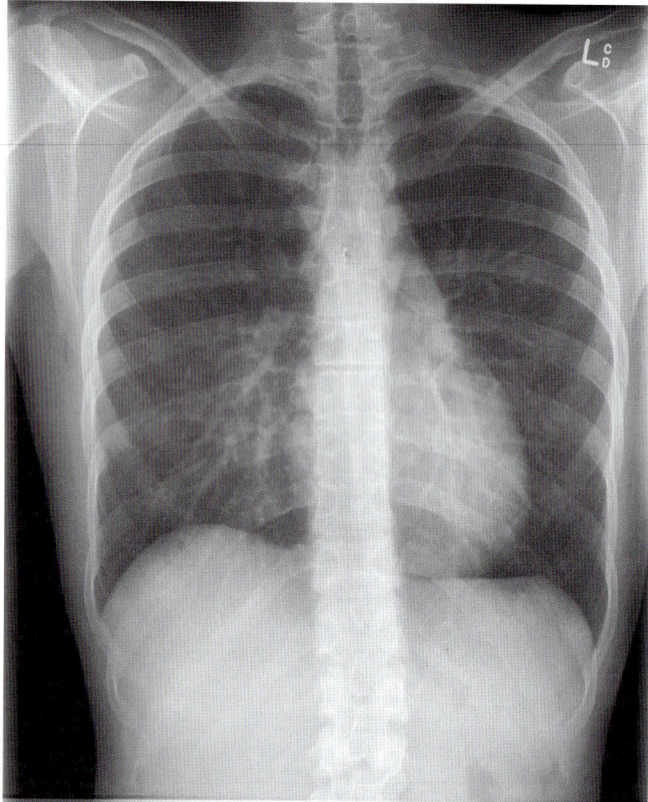

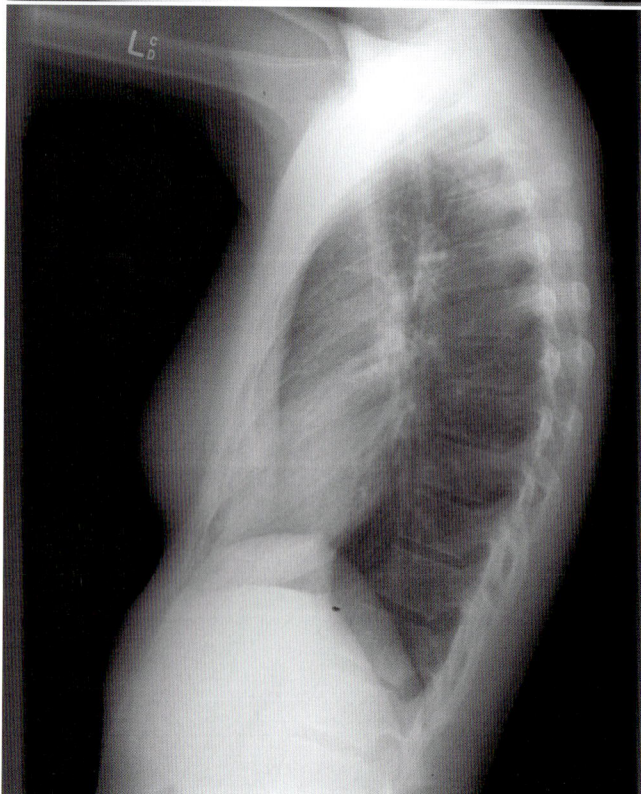

This 25-year-old woman received a blow to the head with a transient loss of consciousness. Review was requested by the neurosurgical team because they think the patient may have aspirated. The patient looks and feels well.

**Q**

What is the likely cause of the appearances on the X-ray?

**A**

Pectus excavatum. The lateral film shows the lower sternum impressing into the chest cavity. There is an accentuated downward course of the anterior portions of the ribs. The PA film shows an indistinct right heart border mimicking a right middle lobe process, a typical appearance with pectus excavatum. The heart may be displaced to the left, mimicking cardiomegaly, but this is not demonstrated in this example (Dahnert, 2007).

**L**EARNING POINT

Pectus excavatum may be confused with pneumonia on the chest X-ray.

## PROBLEM 1.49

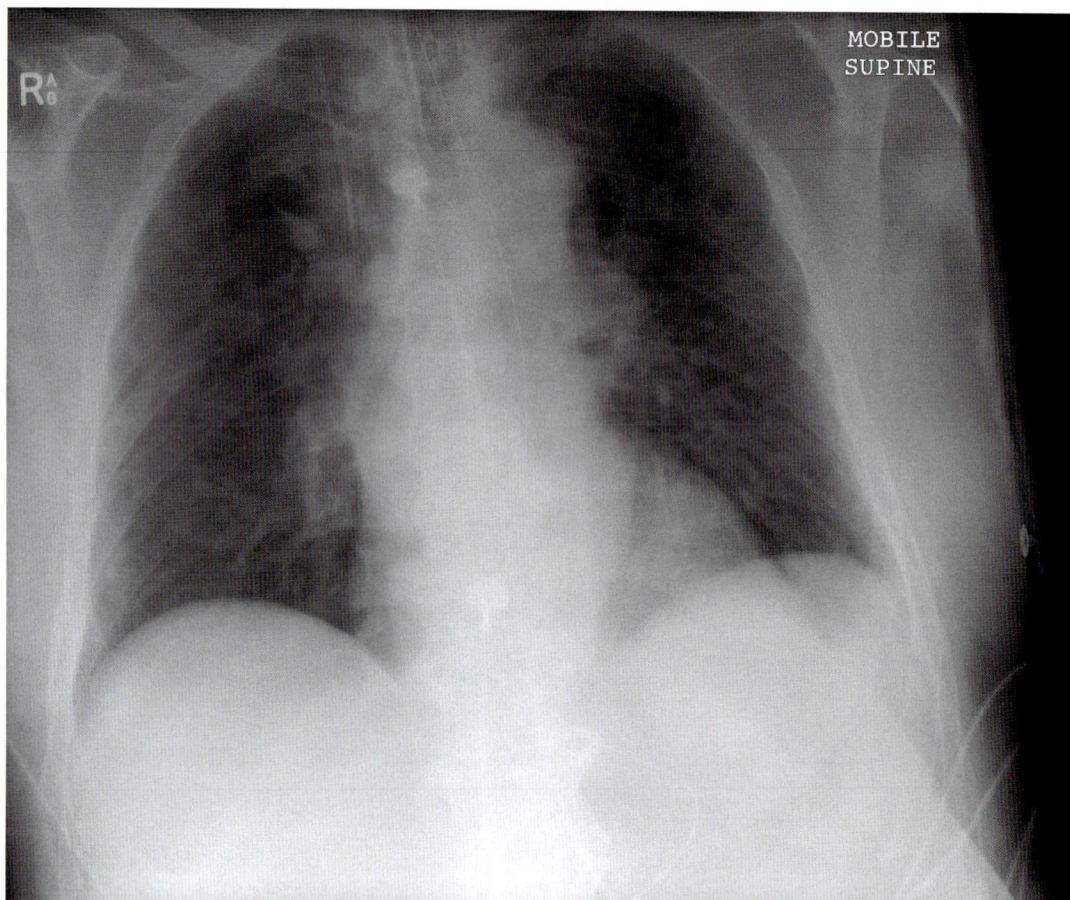

This 79-year-old man was electively admitted to the ICU following major abdominal surgery. Your junior medical staff are concerned about the appearance of the right upper lobe on his post-operative X-ray.

**Q** What do you tell them?

## A

There is an azygous lobe, which is a normal anatomical variant. It is more obvious on this image because there is fluid within the azygous fissure. The azygous fissure also harbours a tear-shaped shadow inferomedially. This is the azygous vein, which is somewhat distended, perhaps because of replete volume status.

## LEARNING POINT

Knowledge of anatomical variants is important in interpreting radiological images.

## PROBLEM 1.50

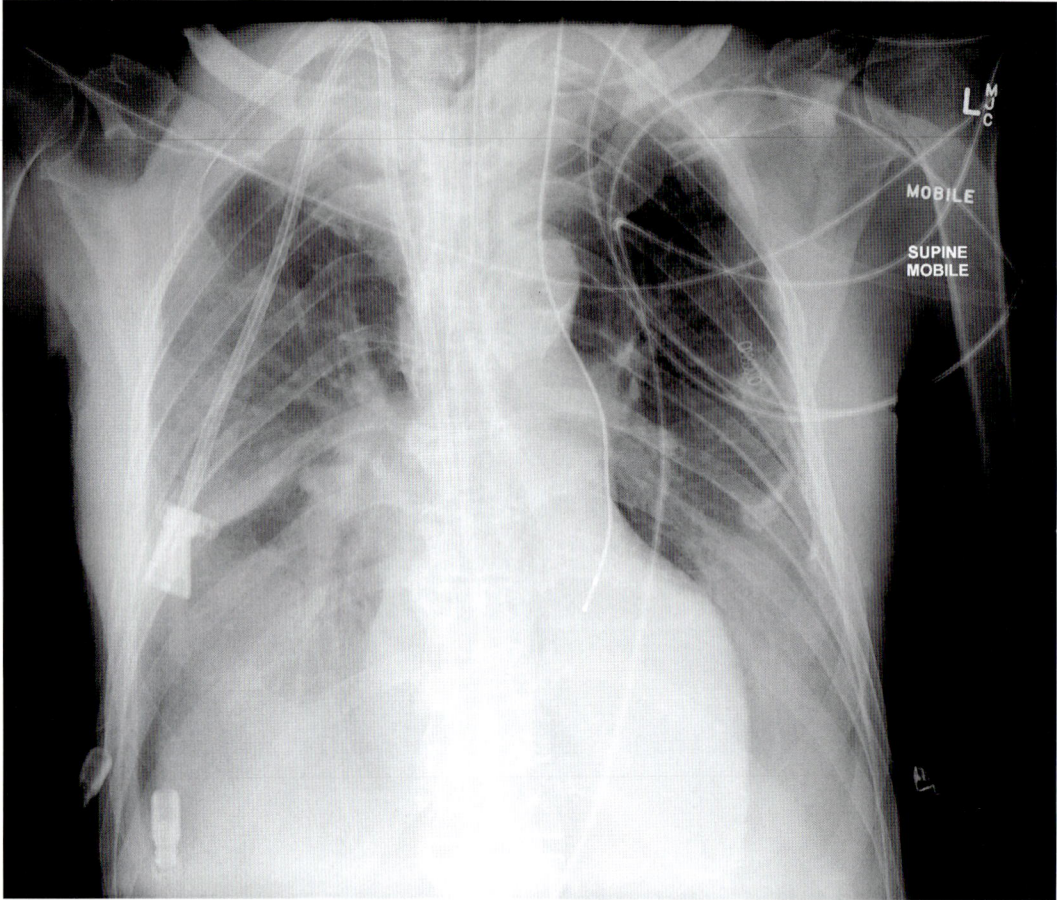

This 60-year-old man has endstage renal failure and went to the operating theatre to have a dialysis catheter inserted. He became severely bradycardic intraoperatively and a temporary transvenous pacing wire was inserted. Capture was achieved with the pacing, though the stimulation threshold was high.

**Q**

Comment on the position of the dialysis catheter and pacing wire.

# A

The dialysis catheter is in an acceptable position with the tip near the junction of the superior vena cava (SVC) and right atrium. It is usually recommended that the optimal position of a central venous catheter is with the tip at the level of the carina, just above the right main bronchus, which places it above the pericardial reflection. Some clinicians prefer that the catheter is inserted further, with the tip at the junction of the right atrium and the SVC.

The position of the pacing wire is somewhat different. It follows the left mediastinal border then turns more medially. The tip appears to be behind the heart. The most likely explanation for this appearance is that the patient has a double SVC system and the pacing wire has been placed in the left SVC with the tip within the coronary sinus. Arterial placement is unlikely, as the wire appears to pass lateral to the descending aorta. Extravascular placement is possible, but the appearance is typical for a device in a left SVC.

## LEARNING POINT

A double SVC system is a normal variant found in 0.3% of the population. It is more common in people with congenital heart disease. The SVC on the left usually drains into the coronary sinus. A single, left-sided SVC is another variant (Minniti, 2002).

## PROBLEM 1.51

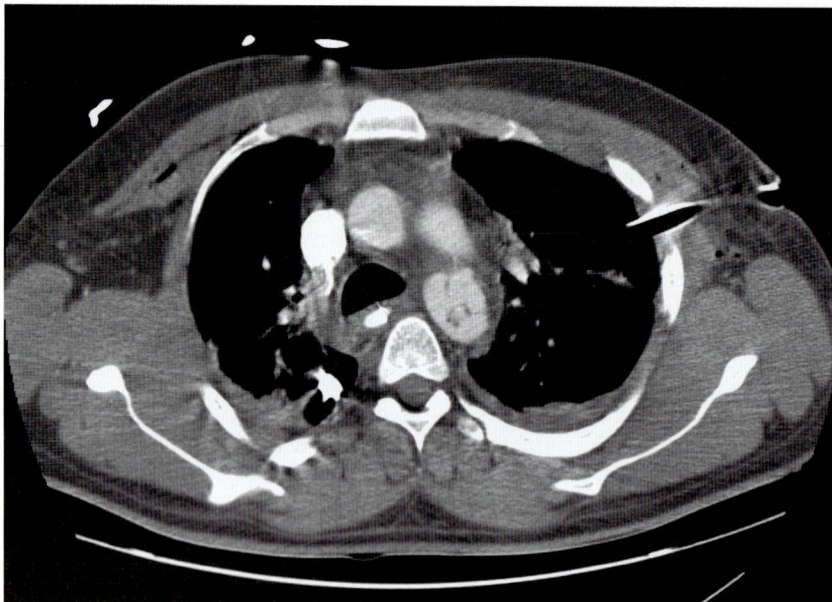

This patient was the front seat passenger in a motor vehicle crash today.

**Q**
1. What diagnosis is suggested by the CT scan?
2. What findings on the CT scan support your diagnosis?

# A

1. Traumatic aortic injury.

2. Findings on the CT scan which support your diagnosis:
   - mediastinal haematoma
   - irregular aortic contour
   - intimal flap

Other signs of aortic injury (Ng, 2006) that are not present on this image are:
- luminal thrombus
- periaortic contrast extravasation (extravasation outside the aortic adventitia, into the mediastinal tissues, suggesting active bleeding)

## LEARNING POINT

CT assessment for possible aortic trauma requires arterial phase images. The commonest site of traumatic aortic injury seen on imaging is at the ligamentum arteriosum.

## PROBLEM 1.52

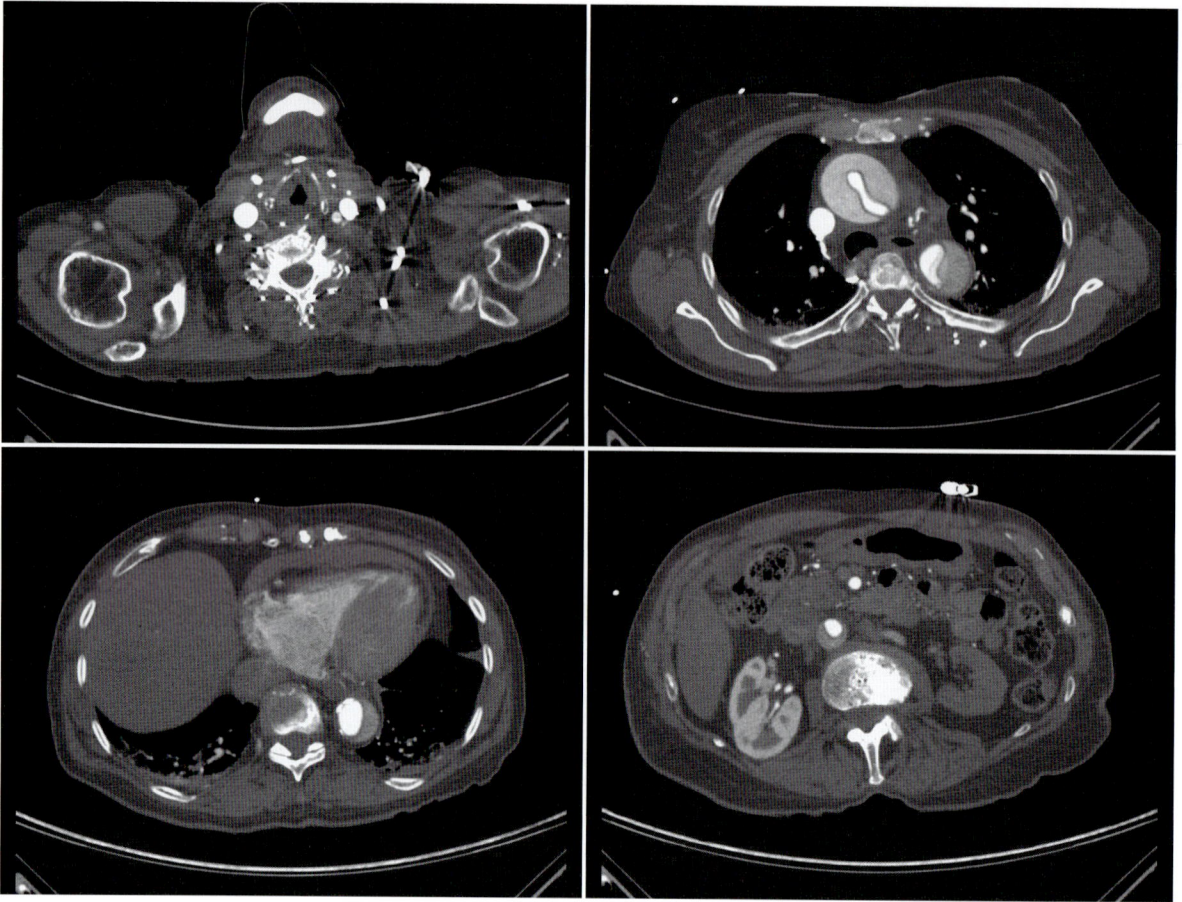

This 77-year-old woman presented with sudden onset of severe chest pain.

**Q**

1. What is the cause of her chest pain?
2. What complications have ensued?

## A

1. There is a Stanford type A aortic dissection.

2. The following complications are visible:
   - The right common carotid artery has not opacified with contrast. This demonstrates that the dissection has compromised flow to this vessel.
   - There is a moderate pericardial effusion, but no clear evidence of chamber compression.
   - The left kidney is not perfused.
   - On the DVD images, the left subclavian artery and the right common femoral artery have not perfused with contrast (the images in the book do not demonstrate these findings).
   - These images are not standard mediastinal windows, but have been modified to more clearly demonstrate the pathological process.

   The DVD images have a chest X-ray with features of an aortic dissection, including a widened upper mediastinum.

## LEARNING POINT

Type A aortic dissections involve the ascending aorta, whereas type B dissections do not (Golledge, 2008). Distinguishing the two types is important, as type A dissections are managed surgically but type B dissections are not operated on unless complications develop.

When a dissection is demonstrated on imaging, the complications of the dissection need to be assessed radiographically and clinically.

## PROBLEM 1.53

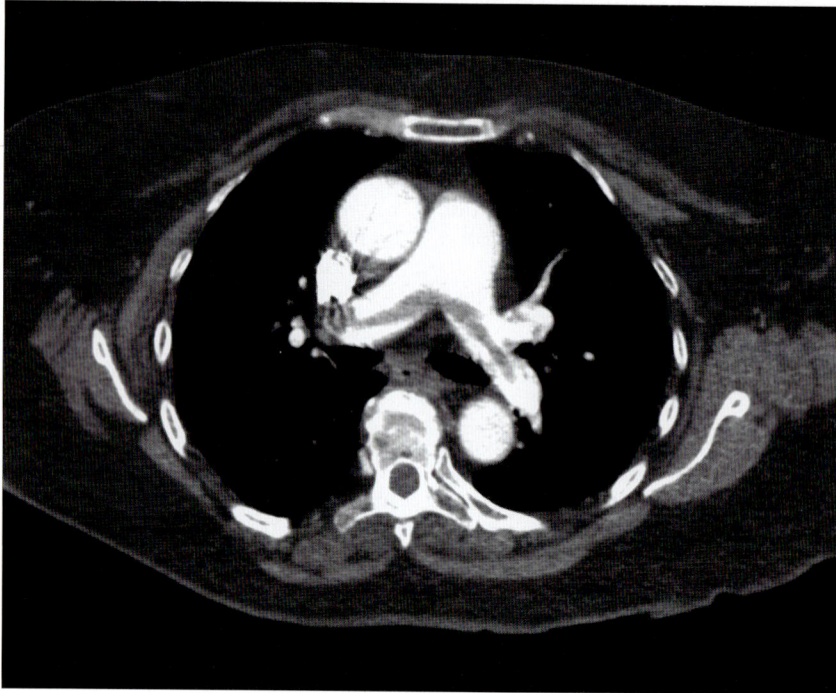

This 72-year-old woman had a hip replacement two weeks ago. She has been admitted to the ICU with chest pain and shock.

**Q**
1. What is the cause of the shock?
2. How will you manage this patient?

# A

1. There is a saddle embolus, seen in the main pulmonary artery, and both right and left main branches. On the DVD extensive involvement of more distal arterial branches is also seen.

2. Heparinisation and supportive care are indicated. As the patient is haemodynamically unstable, consideration should be given to surgical or catheter embolectomy if it is available. Thrombolysis is contraindicated by the recent hip surgery.

## LEARNING POINT

CT pulmonary angiography is a sensitive investigation for large proximal pulmonary emboli, but less so for small peripheral emboli.

## PROBLEM 1.54

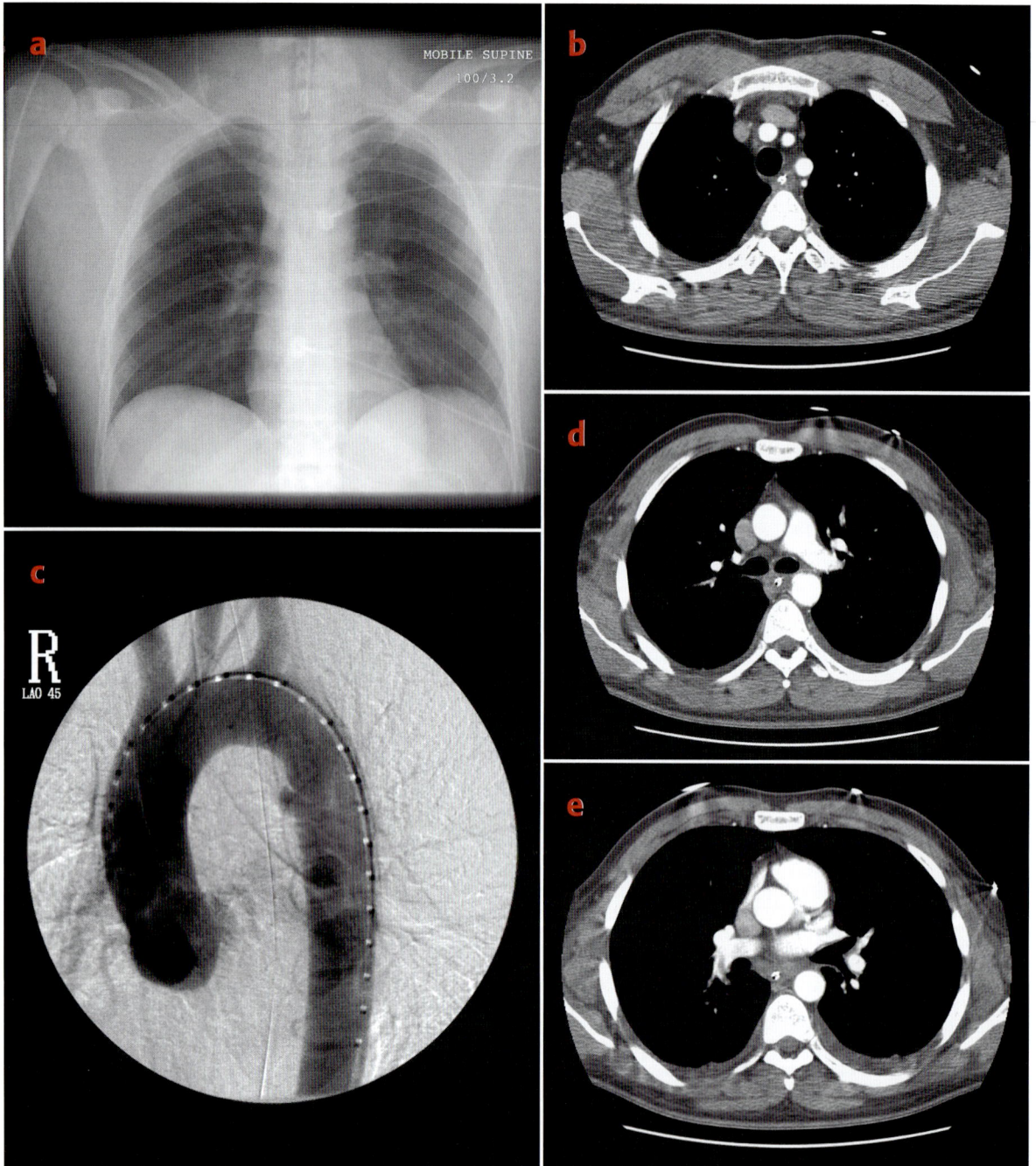

This 28-year-old man was the driver of a car that crashed one week ago.

Q

1. List two pathological processes and one anatomical variant seen on these images.
2. Outline your management plan.

## A

1. Two pathological processes seen on these images are:
   - A small area of contrast extravasation in the region of the ligamentum arteriosum, consistent with aortic disruption. This is seen on the CT angiogram (image d) and the digital subtraction angiogram (image c).
   - A filling defect in the pulmonary artery to the right lower lobe, suggesting a pulmonary embolus (image e).

     The anatomical variant is a left vertebral artery originating directly from the aorta, seen posterior to the left subclavian artery (image b).

2. The dilemma in this case is the desirability of anticoagulation for the pulmonary embolus, but the contraindication of this by the ruptured aorta. Management undertaken was insertion of a stent to the aortic injury, and an IVC filter for prevention of further pulmonary embolic events.

## LEARNING POINT

The chest X-ray in a patient with traumatic aortic rupture may be normal.

Don't stop looking when you find the first abnormality. Multiple problems are common in critically ill patients.

## PROBLEM 1.55

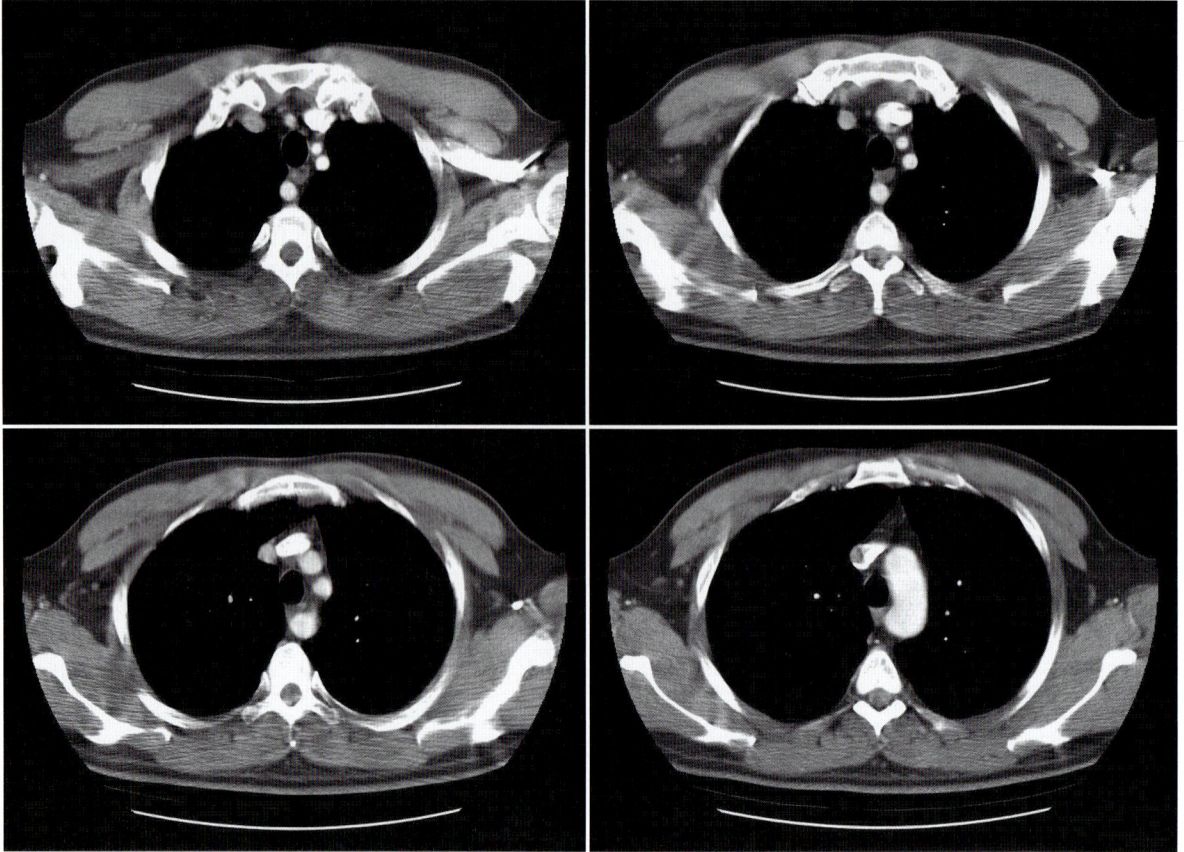

This 28-year-old-man was an unrestrained back seat passenger in a high-speed car crash.

**Q** What anatomical variant is present?

## A

There is an aberrant right subclavian artery, which passes posterior to the trachea and oesophagus.

## LEARNING POINT

Knowledge of common anatomical variants is important when interpreting scans. On a non-enhanced scan, an aberrant subclavian artery may be misinterpreted as a posterior mediastinal mass.

## PROBLEM 1.56

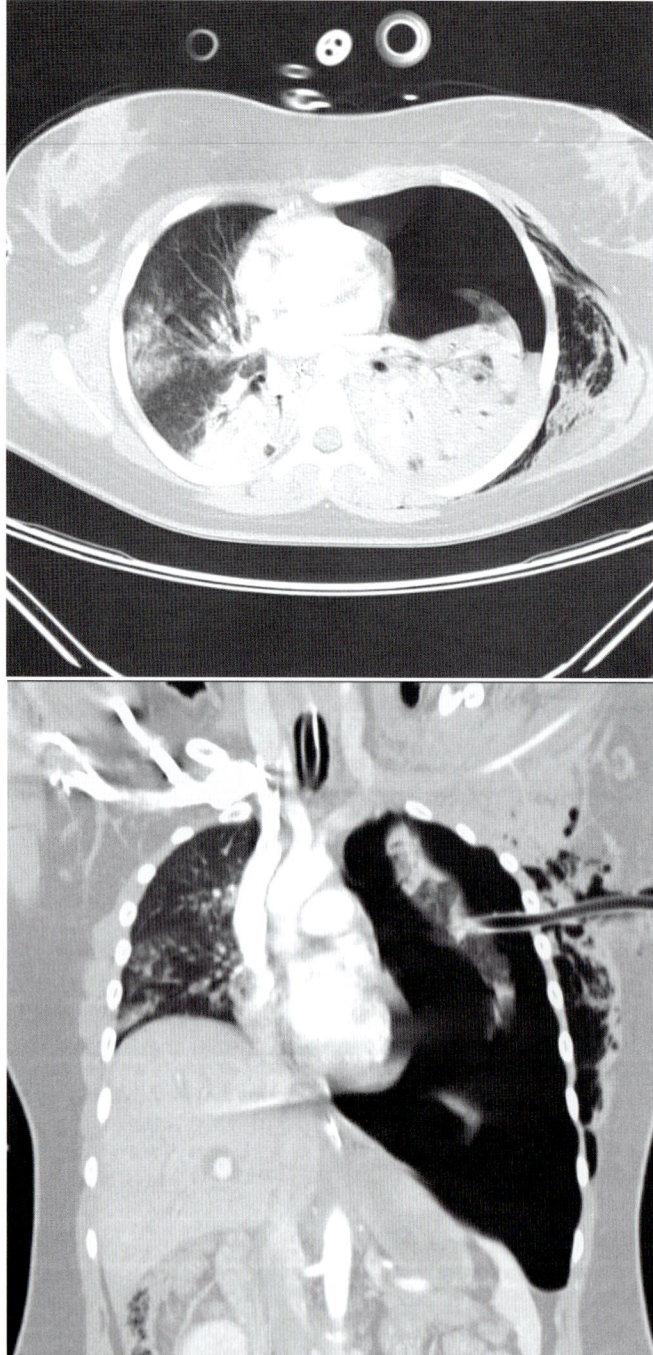

This 19-year-old woman crashed her car on the way to work. She was intubated and ventilated in the emergency department. A chest drain was inserted before she was taken to the CT scanner. She has just arrived in the ICU.

**Q**

What factors are contributing to her poor gas exchange?

## A

There is a left-sided tension pneumothorax with significant depression of the diaphragm but only minor mediastinal shift. The left lung is collapsed and there is a small amount of fluid in the pleural cavity. The right lung has dependent atelectasis and there is patchy peripheral alveolar opacification.

## LEARNING POINT

CT provides significantly more information about the causes of abnormal gas exchange than the chest X-ray. However, the benefits of a more precise anatomic diagnosis must be balanced against the risks of transport to the CT scanner.

## PROBLEM 1.57

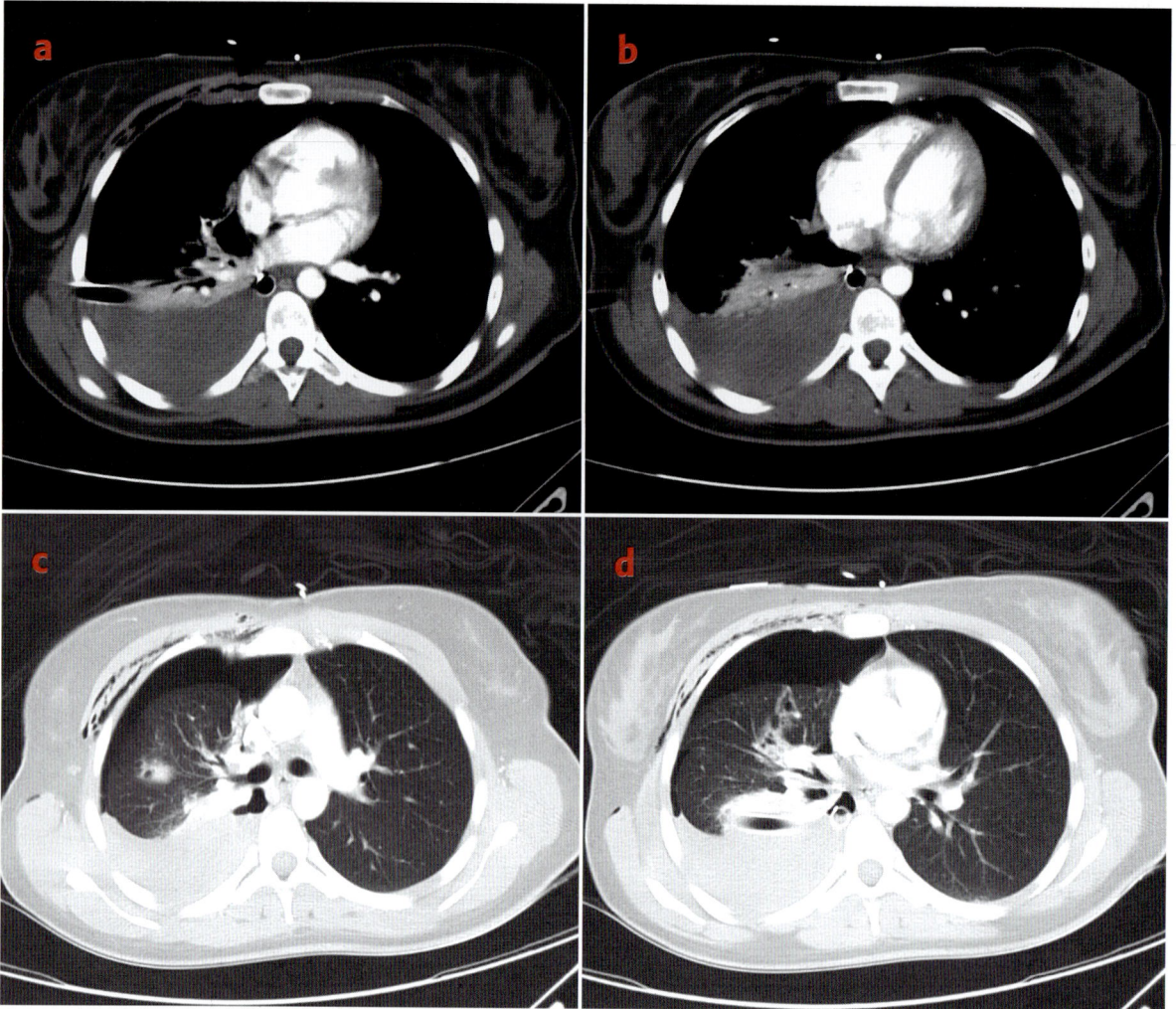

This 25-year-old woman received multiple stab wounds to the chest during a domestic dispute. She presented to the emergency department in respiratory distress with a sucking chest wound. An occlusive dressing has been placed over the wound and an intercostal catheter inserted.

Q
Describe the findings on these images.

# A

A stab wound is seen to enter the right chest wall just lateral to the sternum (image a). It transects the right internal mammary artery (image b) and the laceration extends into the right middle lobe where there is associated pulmonary contusion (images c and d). Other wounds can be seen on the DVD images, but these do not appear to enter the thoracic cavity. There is surgical emphysema in the right chest wall. A large right haemopneumothorax has not been adequately drained by the intercostal catheter and there is partial collapse of the right lung. The chest drain has been inserted too far and is resting adjacent to the posterior mediastinum. On the DVD images, it can be seen that the chest drain is kinked.

## LEARNING POINT

If there is one stab wound, there are often more. These should be actively searched for both clinically and on imaging.

Stab wounds usually have a linear track, which is often evident on CT imaging. Structures adjacent to this track may have been injured, even if damage to them is not obvious on CT images.

Organs may move with respiration or be displaced by the injury, so lacerations to deeper structures do not always lie immediately below the surface wound on the CT images.

# PROBLEM 1.58

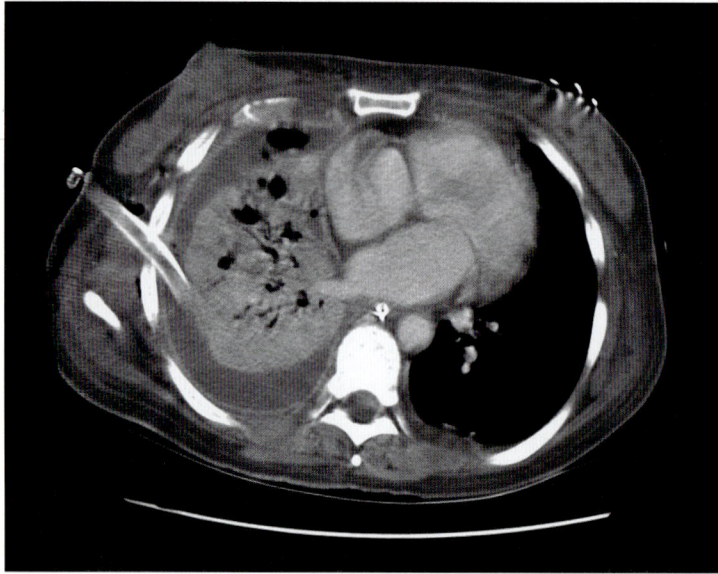

This patient had persisting fevers and malaise following pneumococcal pneumonia.

**Q** What is the likely cause of the fevers?

# A

There is a fluid collection in the right pleural space with a contrast-enhancing rim around it and gas within it. It has not been adequately drained by the intercostal catheter. In this clinical context, this is strongly suggestive of empyema.

No loculations are seen to explain why the fluid is not draining. The gas could be due to gas-forming organisms or was introduced during intercostal catheter insertion. The underlying lung is densely consolidated.

## LEARNING POINT

Empyemas are often loculated and may not respond to simple chest drainage. CT often does not demonstrate septation. Ultrasound is more sensitive for detecting loculations.

## PROBLEM 1.59

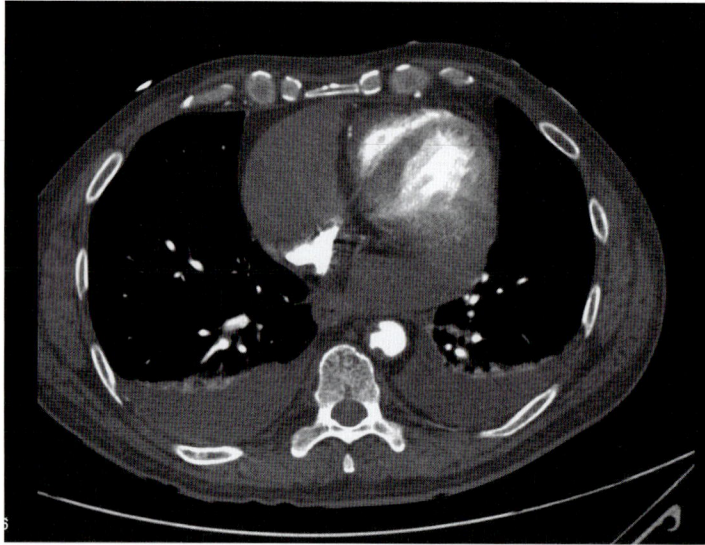

This 62-year-old man gave a history of malaise and lack of energy for one month. He was referred to the outpatient department by his family doctor because of deteriorating renal function. When reviewed in outpatients he was found to be hypotensive. No cause for the hypotension was immediately apparent.

**Q**

Why is this patient hypotensive?

# A

There is a large pericardial effusion posterior and medial to the heart. Chamber compression is difficult to assess on CT but, with such a large effusion, tamponade must be considered.

In this image, there are also moderate bilateral pleural effusions with a small amount of adjacent atelectatic lung. The irregularity in the descending aorta is atheroma, not dissection.

## LEARNING POINT

CT is a good modality for detecting pericardial effusions. It can distinguish between a pericardial fat pad and pericardial fluid, which may be difficult with echocardiography. On the other hand, echocardiography can assess the haemodynamic effects of an effusion, which CT cannot.

## PROBLEM 1.60

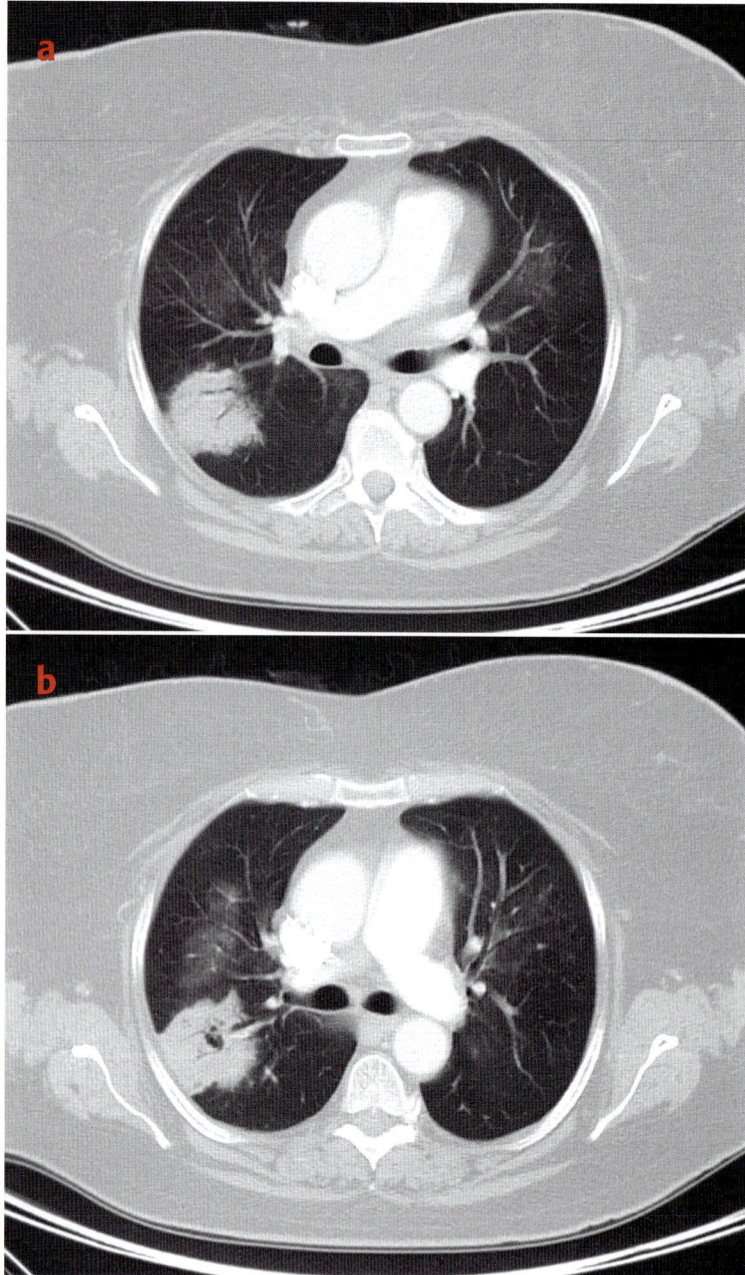

This 58-year-old woman had cough and increasing shortness of breath over 48 hours. There was a past history of chronic liver disease and steroid therapy.

**Q** Describe the changes seen on the CT scan.

# A

There are bilateral perihilar ground-glass infiltrates. In this immunocompromised patient, this could represent *Pneumocystis jiroveci* or viral infection, although the differential diagnosis is broad.

There is a right posterolateral area of consolidation. There is a cavity within the area of consolidation (image b). In an immunocompromised patient, this could represent bacterial infection (*Staphylococcus aureus*, *Klebsiella pneumonia* and *Nocardia* commonly form cavities), or fungal infection (*Aspergillus* or *Cryptococcus*). This is unlikely to be neoplastic due to the visible air bronchograms traversing the lesion. In neoplasia, the traversing bronchi are usually compressed and occluded.

# LEARNING POINT

A ground-glass infiltrate is a hazy increased attenuation that does not obscure visibility of the underlying vascular structures. It is a non-specific finding that can be due to volume averaging of abnormalities too fine to be resolved with high resolution CT, an alveolar process, an interstitial process or a combined alveolar and interstitial process (Gotway, 2005).

In contrast, consolidation is increased attenuation that obscures the underlying vasculature, usually producing air bronchograms (Gotway, 2005). The terms "consolidation" and "alveolar infiltrates" are synonymous. It is a finding that indicates the air within alveoli has been replaced by a substance such as oedema fluid, blood, pus or cells.

## PROBLEM 1.61

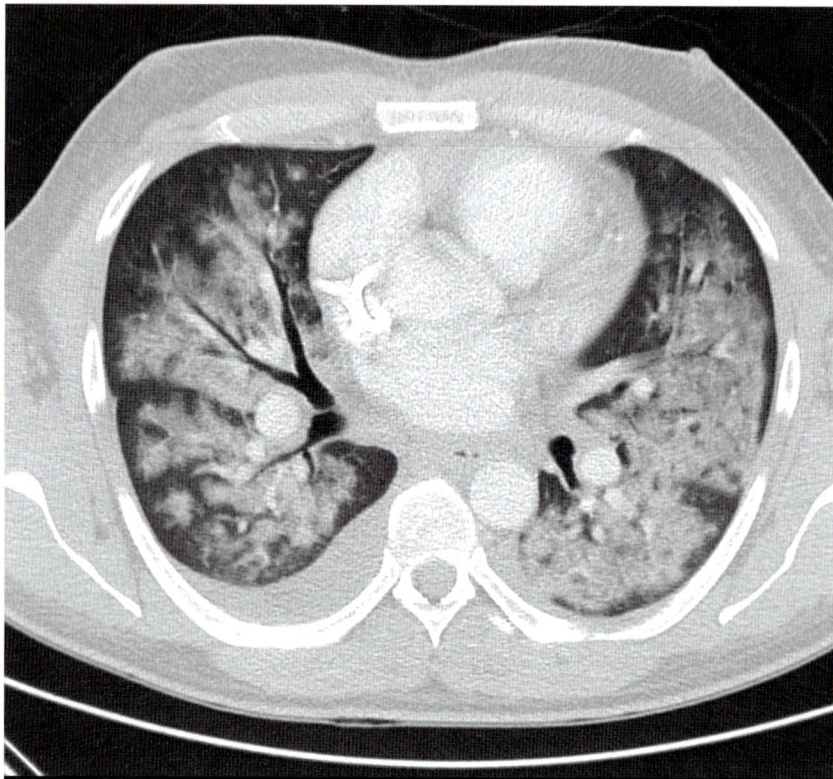

This 32-year-old man with acute myeloid leukae-mia (M3 type) had chemotherapy recently and developed rapidly worsening hypoxaemic respi-ratory failure.

**Q** What is your differential diagnosis?

## A

There is widespread bilateral consolidation with some peripheral sparing. In this clinical context, the differential diagnosis includes ATRA syndrome, cardiac failure, infection (bacterial, fungal, PCP, viral), pulmonary haemorrhage and fluid overload.

Bilateral pleural effusions are also present. Promyelocytic leukaemia (M3 type acute myeloid leukaemia) is commonly treated with ATRA (All-*trans*-Retinoic Acid).

## LEARNING POINT

The differential diagnosis for consolidation is broad and depends on both the clinical scenario and the distribution of the consolidation seen on the CT scan.

## PROBLEM 1.62

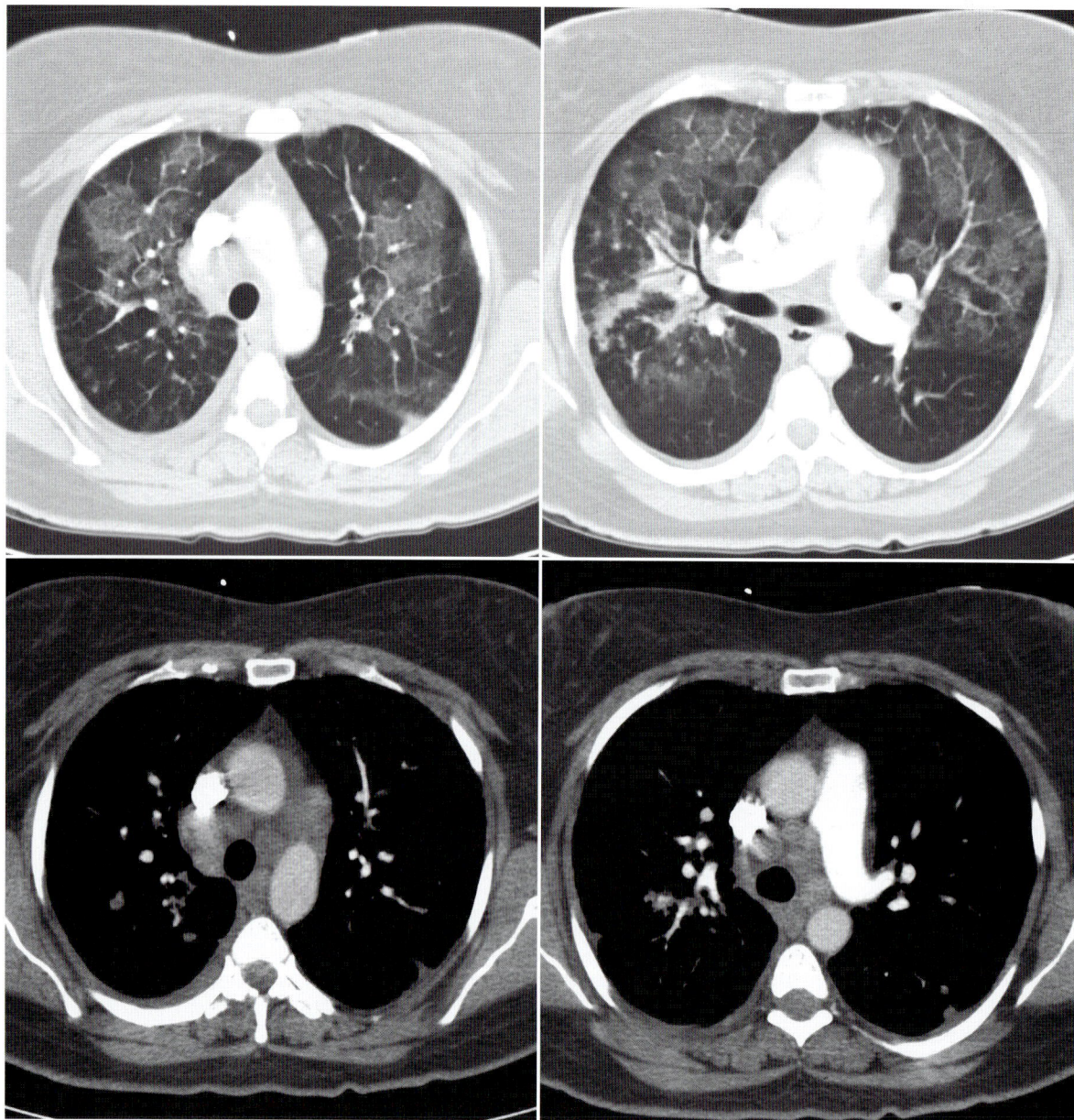

This 45-year-old woman had been well until she developed increasing shortness of breath two days ago.

**Q** What is your differential diagnosis?

## A

There is widespread ground-glass opacification throughout both lungs, with some patchy consolidation in the right perihilar region. There is a small right pleural effusion. The differential diagnosis for this includes pulmonary oedema, atypical infection (including viral and *Pneumocystis jiroveci*), pulmonary haemorrhage and hypersensitivity pneumonitis.

In addition, there are multiple enlarged mediastinal lymph nodes.

These could be reactive to infection or caused by sarcoidosis, lymphoma or metastatic disease. The combination of the ground-glass opacities and the lymphadenopathy would favour infection.

On the DVD images, some of the lymph nodes have calcification within them.

## LEARNING POINT

The significance of ground-glass opacification depends on the clinical scenario, the distribution of the opacification on the CT and the presence or absence of other findings on the CT.

## PROBLEM 1.63

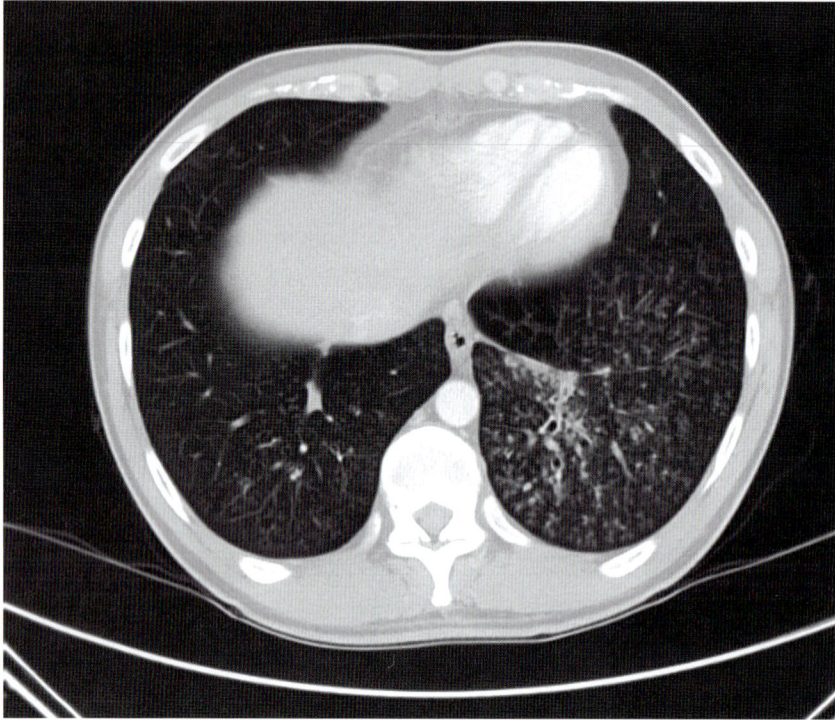

This 27-year-old man presented with a five-day history of productive cough and increasing shortness of breath.

**Q**
1. Outline your findings on the CT.
2. Suggest a diagnosis.

## A

1. There are centrilobular nodules in both lower lobes. In the left lower lobe, a classic "tree-in-bud" pattern is seen. In both lungs, there are areas where the diameter of the lobular bronchus is larger than that of the accompanying lobular artery, suggesting bronchiectasis.

2. Bronchiectasis with concomitant infection.

## LEARNING POINT

Lung nodules are discrete opacities ranging in size from 2 to 30 mm. Depending on their distribution relative to the secondary pulmonary lobule, they are subdivided by their appearance on chest CT scan into (Gotway, 2005):

- centrilobular with or without tree-in-bud configuration: causes include infective diseases, aspiration, hypersensitivity pneumonitis and vasculitis. These nodules are less defined than the perilymphatic and random ones
- perilymphatic: causes include sarcoidosis, lymphangitis carcinomatosis and lymphoproliferative diseases
- random: caused by haematogenously disseminated infections (tuberculosis, fungal or viral) and neoplasms

A tree-in-bud pattern is a form of centrilobular nodular pattern, almost always due to infection. It is caused by clogging of the bronchioles by inflammatory material. It has a branching pattern, likened to that of a budding tree (Gotway, 2005).

## PROBLEM 1.64

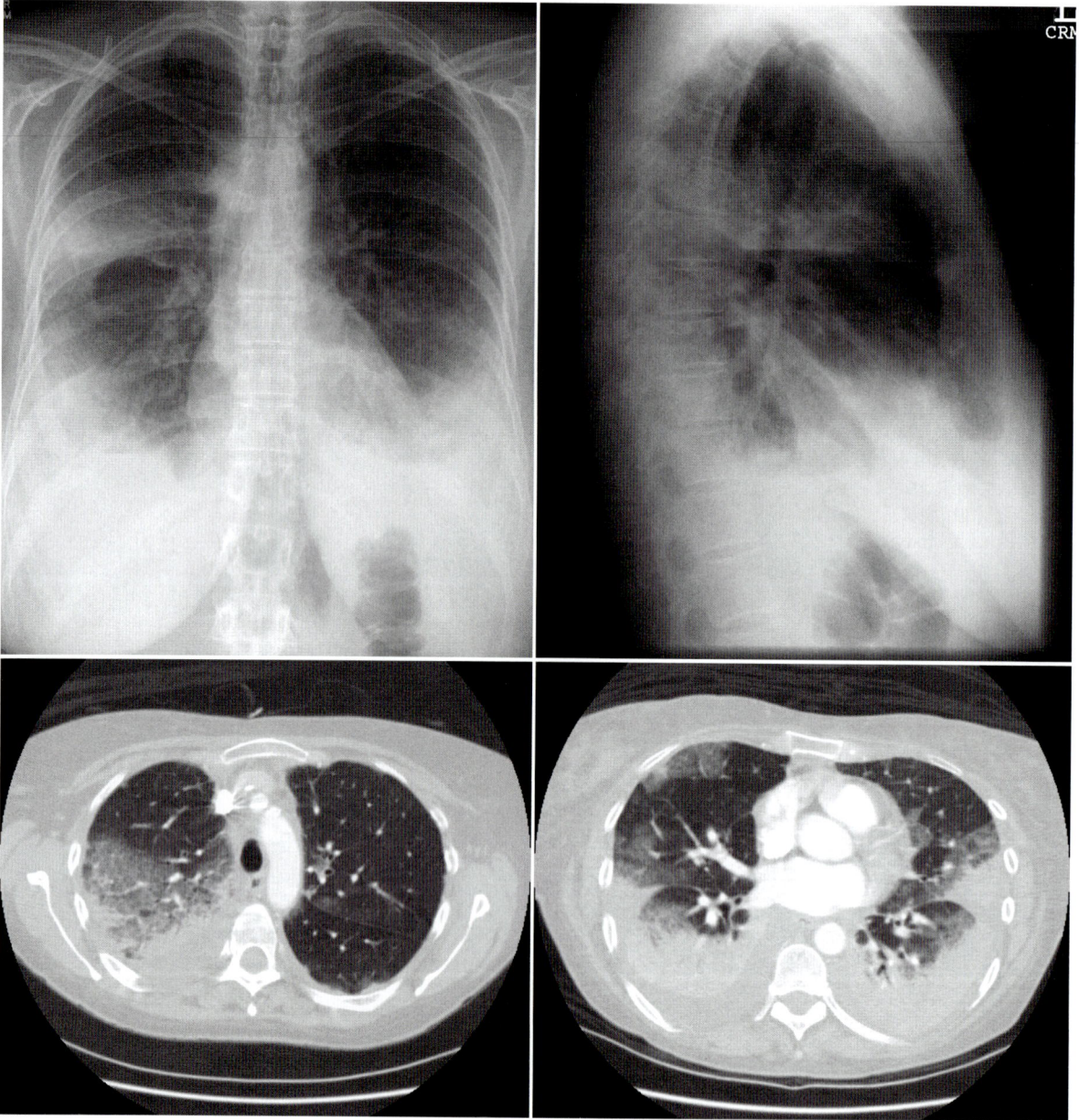

This 58-year-old woman presented with a non-productive cough, malaise and weight loss for eight weeks. She is becoming increasingly short of breath. There has been no improvement despite two courses of antibiotics appropriate for community acquired pneumonia.

**Q**

1. What are the findings on the images?
2. What is your differential diagnosis?

# A

1. The chest X-ray images show bilateral patchy consolidation and bilateral pleural effusions. The CT images show bilateral patchy consolidation and ground-glass opacification, mainly in the periphery of the lungs. There is no septal thickening or traction bronchiectasis. The CT confirms the presence of pleural effusions.

2. The differential diagnosis in this patient is broad and should include:
   • infections not covered by standard antibiotics for community-acquired pneumonia (e.g. *Mycobacterium tuberculosis*, *Coxiella burnetii* [causes Q fever], viruses)
   • bronchiolitis obliterans organising pneumonia (BOOP)
   • chronic eosinophilic pneumonia
   • hypersensitivity pneumonitis
   • drug reaction
   • vasculitis (Wegener's granulomatosis, systemic lupus erythematosus, Churg-Strauss syndrome)
   • sarcoidosis
   • thromboembolic disease, with multiple pulmonary infarcts
   • atypical pulmonary oedema
   • bronchoalveolar carcinoma

   This patient underwent open lung biopsy that demonstrated BOOP. There was a good response to steroid therapy.

## LEARNING POINT

The differential diagnosis for consolidation is extensive. Narrowing the differential diagnosis requires careful integration of the clinical history and imaging features. The distribution of the findings on the CT may be helpful. In particular, the finding of peripheral consolidation should trigger consideration of certain specific diagnoses: BOOP, chronic eosinophilic pneumonia, atypical pulmonary oedema, Churg-Strauss syndrome, drug reactions, pulmonary contusion, pulmonary infarct and sarcoidosis (Gotway, 2005). Several of these conditions are steroid responsive, so recognising this pattern of peripheral consolidation is important.

The terms BOOP and cryptogenic organising pneumonia are used interchangeably. For definitive diagnosis, a lung biopsy is required, preferably via video-assisted thoracoscopy. BOOP is usually steroid responsive, but may relapse when steroids are stopped.

## PROBLEM 1.65

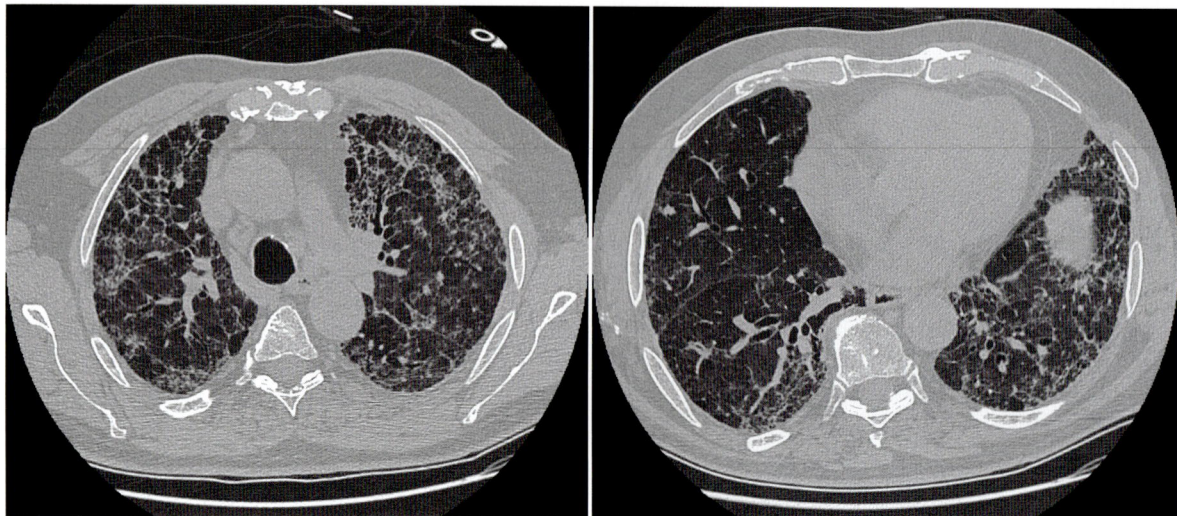

This 55-year-old man complained of increasing shortness of breath for several months. Recently, he developed hypoxaemic respiratory failure requiring urgent admission to the ICU.

**Q** What disease process is suggested by these HRCT scans?

## A

There are multiple cystic areas within the lung, typical of "honeycomb" lung cysts. There is extensive thickening of intralobular and interlobular septae, architectural distortion and traction bronchiectasis. The traction bronciectasis is most prominent at the bases. These features are strongly suggestive of usual interstitial pneumonia (UIP). Dilated corrugated bronchi with absence of peripheral tapering are seen. This is typical of traction bronchiectasis, which is common in fibrotic lung disease. No ground-glass opacification or consolidation is seen.

## LEARNING POINT

In a patient with interstitial pneumonia, the presence of ground-glass opacification often reflects active inflammation (alveolitis) and some reversibility.

Interlobular septae border the secondary pulmonary lobules. They are best identified in the lung apices and bases along the subpleural regions. They are 1–2.5 cm long, often in a polyhedral arrangement. One feature that distinguishes them from blood vessels is that they may reach the pleural surface, whereas blood vessels do not. Intralobular septae lie within the secondary pulmonary lobule and appear as ground-glass opacity; individual intralobular septae cannot be seen on HRCT (Gotway, 2005).

High Resolution CT (HRCT) obtains very thin (1 mm) axial sections of the chest. The sections are spaced 10–20 mm apart. In this way, approximately 10% of the lung is sampled (Gotway, 2005). The sections are processed using a sharp or "bone" algorithm to enhance the detection of edges. No intravenous contrast is administered.

HRCT is indicated when interstitial lung disease is suspected, as it visualises the lung interstitium better than conventional CT. There are limitations to the technique, as mediastinal and hilar structures are poorly visualised and small lung nodules are readily missed.

Conventional CT requires the administration of contrast to highlight mediastinal structures. The entire thorax is imaged with no skip areas and slices are 5–10 mm thick. It is indicated in trauma, neoplasia and complicated infections.

## PROBLEM 1.66

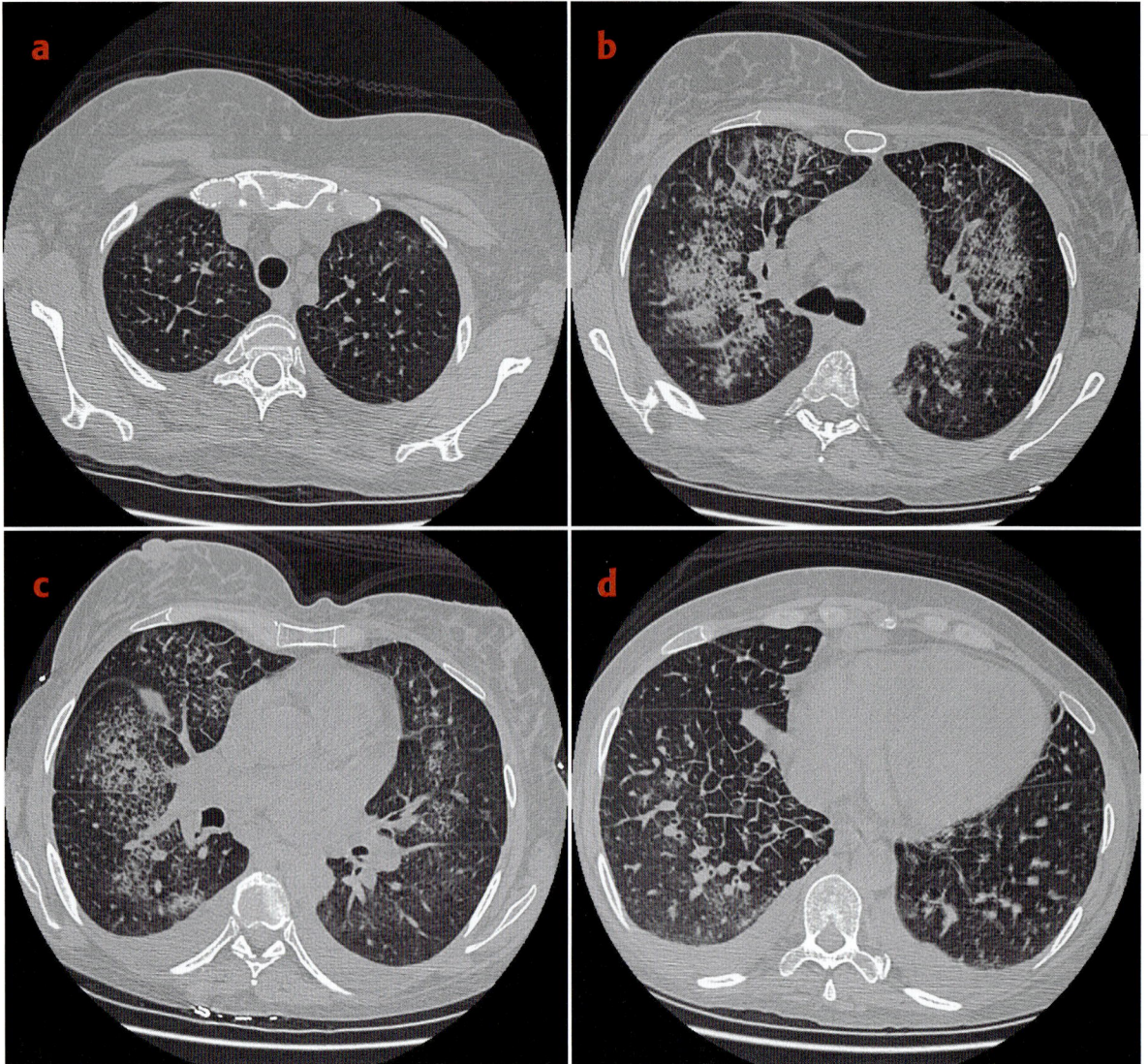

This 48-year-old woman developed chest tightness and shortness of breath earlier today.

Q

1. Outline your findings on the HRCT.
2. What is the most likely diagnosis?

# A

1. There is interlobular interstitial septal thickening in the apices (image a) and bases (image d) and intralobular interstitial thickening in a perihilar distribution (images b and c). There are patches of ground-glass opacification and bilateral pleural effusions. Peribronchial cuffing is present. No honeycombing or traction bronchiectasis is seen to suggest a chronic process.

2. In this clinical context, the most likely diagnosis is cardiogenic pulmonary oedema.

## LEARNING POINT

Intralobular and interlobular interstitial septal thickening is common in the idiopathic interstitial pneumonias. It may also occur in pulmonary infections, especially *Pneumocystis jiroveci*, pulmonary oedema and lymphangitis carcinomatosis.

The differential diagnosis for interlobular interstitial thickening includes the above conditions, but a broad range of other conditions should also be considered, including dust-related diseases, sarcoidosis, pulmonary haemorrhage, alveolar proteinosis and chronic hypersensitivity pneumonitis (Webb, 2006).

Peribronchial cuffing implies fluid is present in the peribronchovascular interstitium. This sign may be seen on plain X-ray or CT scan.

## PROBLEM 1.67

a — Parasternal long axis
85 bpm

b — Parasternal short axis
86 bpm

c — Subcostal 4 chamber
86 bpm

d — 2.78 cm — IVC
2.78 cm
84bpm

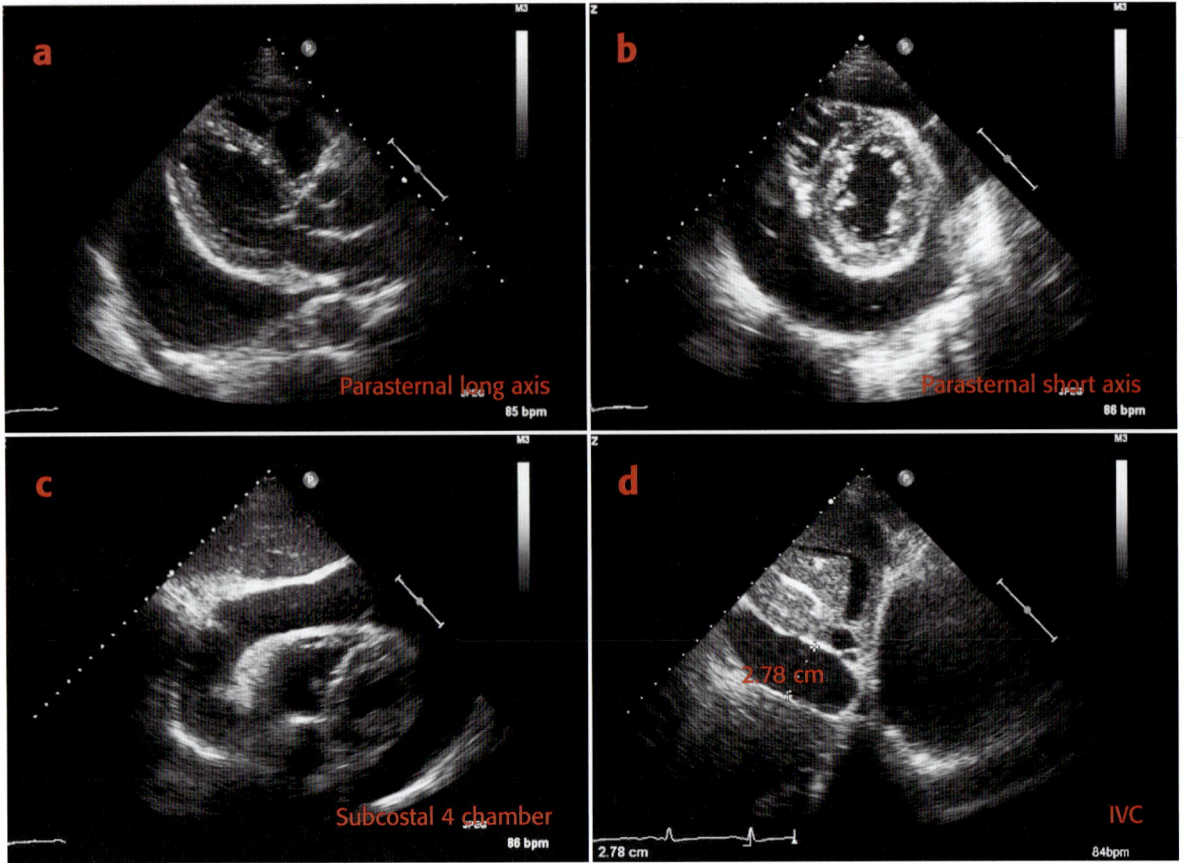

This 38-year-old man has been unwell for the last six weeks with malaise and lethargy. He now presents with hypotension, requiring vasopressor therapy.

**Q**

Is the cause of the hypotension apparent on these images from a transthoracic echocardiogram?

## A

These images demonstrate a large pericardial effusion. The inferior vena cava is dilated (>2.0 cm; image d), consistent with pericardial tamponade. No obvious chamber compression is apparent, even on the dynamic images shown on the DVD. Further information is required to fully assess for tamponade physiology.

## LEARNING POINT

Distinguishing between pericardial and pleural fluid can be difficult on echocardiographic images. The pericardium and pericardial space lie between the descending aorta and the left atrium in the parasternal long axis view, while the pleural space does not. Fluid separating the aorta and left atrium must lie in the pericardial space (see image a).

Pericardial tamponade is a clinical diagnosis. The echocardiogram is helpful to confirm the presence of a pericardial effusion and may suggest tamponade physiology, but the imaging features must be put into the clinical context.

Echocardiographic features of tamponade physiology include (Otto, 2004):
- dilated inferior vena cava that does not collapse with respiration
- right ventricular diastolic collapse
- reciprocal variation in right and left ventricular volumes with respiration
- respiratory variation in right and left ventricular diastolic filling

These features have only been validated in the spontaneously breathing patient and are less useful during mechanical ventilation.

## PROBLEM 1.68

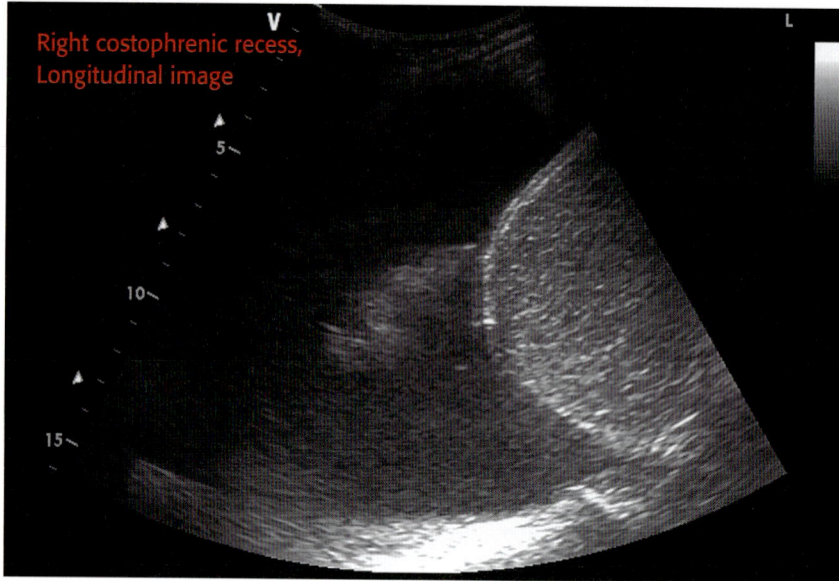

Right costophrenic recess,
Longitudinal image

This 52-year-old man was admitted to the ICU following severe abdominal trauma. Two weeks later he has been slow to wean from mechanical ventilation. Chest X-ray shows changes at the right lower zone, but it is uncertain whether the main problem is effusion or collapse.

**Q** Describe the findings on this ultrasound image.

## A

The liver is located on the right of the image and is of normal texture. To the left of the liver is an echo-free space up to 14 cm deep, consistent with a large pleural effusion. Within the echo-free space an echogenic mass is seen, consistent with atelectatic lung.

## LEARNING POINT

A plain chest X-ray does not always answer the clinical question of whether there is sufficient pleural fluid present to warrant drainage. Ultrasound can rapidly and non-invasively assess the size of a pleural effusion and whether loculations are present or not. It can be performed at the bedside, which is a significant advantage over CT for the critically ill patient.

## REFERENCES

Clarke GM. Chest injuries. In Oh TE, ed. Intensive care manual. 4th edn. Oxford: Butterworth-Heinemann; 1997

Dahnert W, ed. Radiology review manual. 6th edn. Philadelphia: Lippincott Williams and Wilkins; 2007

Foot CL, Coucher J, Stickley M, Mundy J, Venkatesh B. The imaginary line method is not reliable for identification of prosthetic heart valves on AP chest radiographs. Crit Care Resusc 2006; 8: 15–18

Golledge J, Eagle KA. Acute aortic dissection. Lancet 2008; 372: 55–66

Gotway MB, Reddy GP, Webb WR, Elicker BM, Leung JW. High-resolution CT of the lung: patterns of disease and differential diagnoses. Radiol Clin North Am 2005; 43: 513–42

Losanoff JE, Richman BW, Jones JW. Disruption and infection of median sternotomy: a comprehensive review. Eur J Cardiothorac Surg 2002; 21: 831–9

Minniti S, Visentini S, Procacci C. Congenital anomalies of the venae cavae: embryological origin, imaging features and report of three new variants. Eur Radiol 2002; 12: 2040–55

Ng CJ, Chen JC, Wang, LJ, et al. Diagnostic value of the helical CT scan for traumatic aortic injury: correlation with mortality and early rupture. J Emerg Med 2006; 30: 277–82

Otto CM. Textbook of clinical echocardiography. 3rd edn. Philadelphia: Saunders; 2004

Webb WR. Thin-section CT of the secondary pulmonary lobule: anatomy and the image – the 2004 Fleischner lecture. Radiology 2006; 239: 322–38

Ziter FM, Westcott JL. Supine subpulmonary pneumothorax. Am J Roentgenol 1981; 137: 699–701

# CHAPTER 2

# ABDOMEN AND PELVIS

# APPLIED ANATOMY

## Free fluid and gas (Figure 2.1)

Free fluid accumulates in the dependent parts of the peritoneal cavity, where it may be seen on CT or ultrasound. Dependent areas in the supine patient include the pelvis, the paracolic gutters, the hepatorenal recess (Morrison's pouch) and the perisplenic space. Within the pelvis, fluid tends to accumulate in the rectouterine pouch (of Douglas) in females, the rectovesical pouch in males or laterally in the paravesical space in both genders.

In contrast, free intraperitoneal gas rises to the least dependent part of the abdomen. This is usually in the midline anteriorly, or anterior to the liver. Free gas may be better appreciated on lung windows.

## Retroperitoneal structures in the upper abdomen (Figure 2.2)

The coeliac axis (CA) and the superior mesenteric artery (SMA) are the first two anterior branches of the abdominal aorta. To help identify the pancreas, duodenum, blood vessels and other structures, the origin of these vessels should be identified. As they arise from the aorta in close proximity to each other, they should be followed distally to ensure they have been correctly identified.

### Identifying the duodenum

The duodenum is a C-shaped tube passing from the stomach to the duodenojejunal flexure. Once the stomach is identified on the CT, the course of the duodenum can be followed by scrolling through the images. This is helped by positive identification

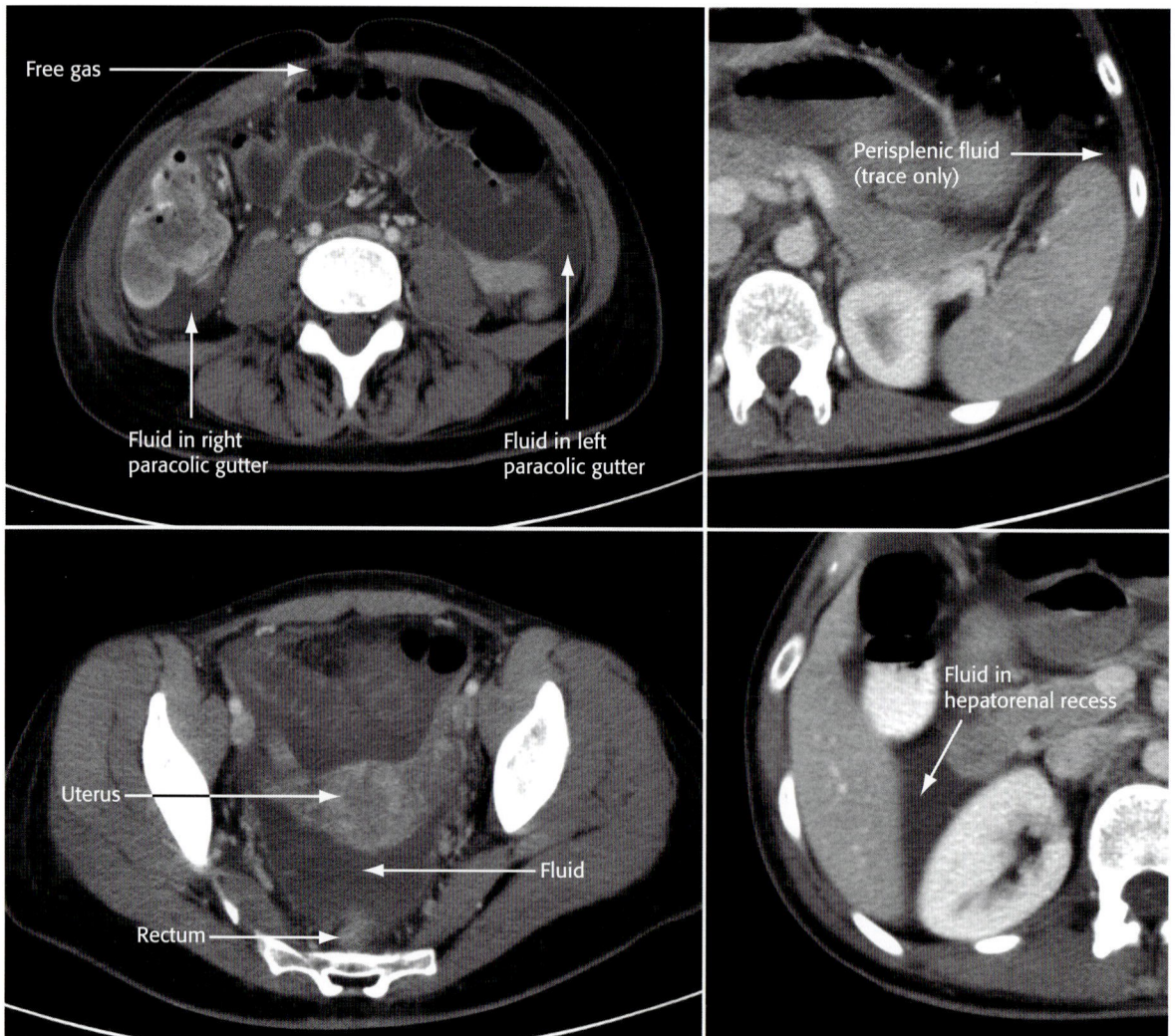

**FIGURE 2.1** Free fluid and gas.

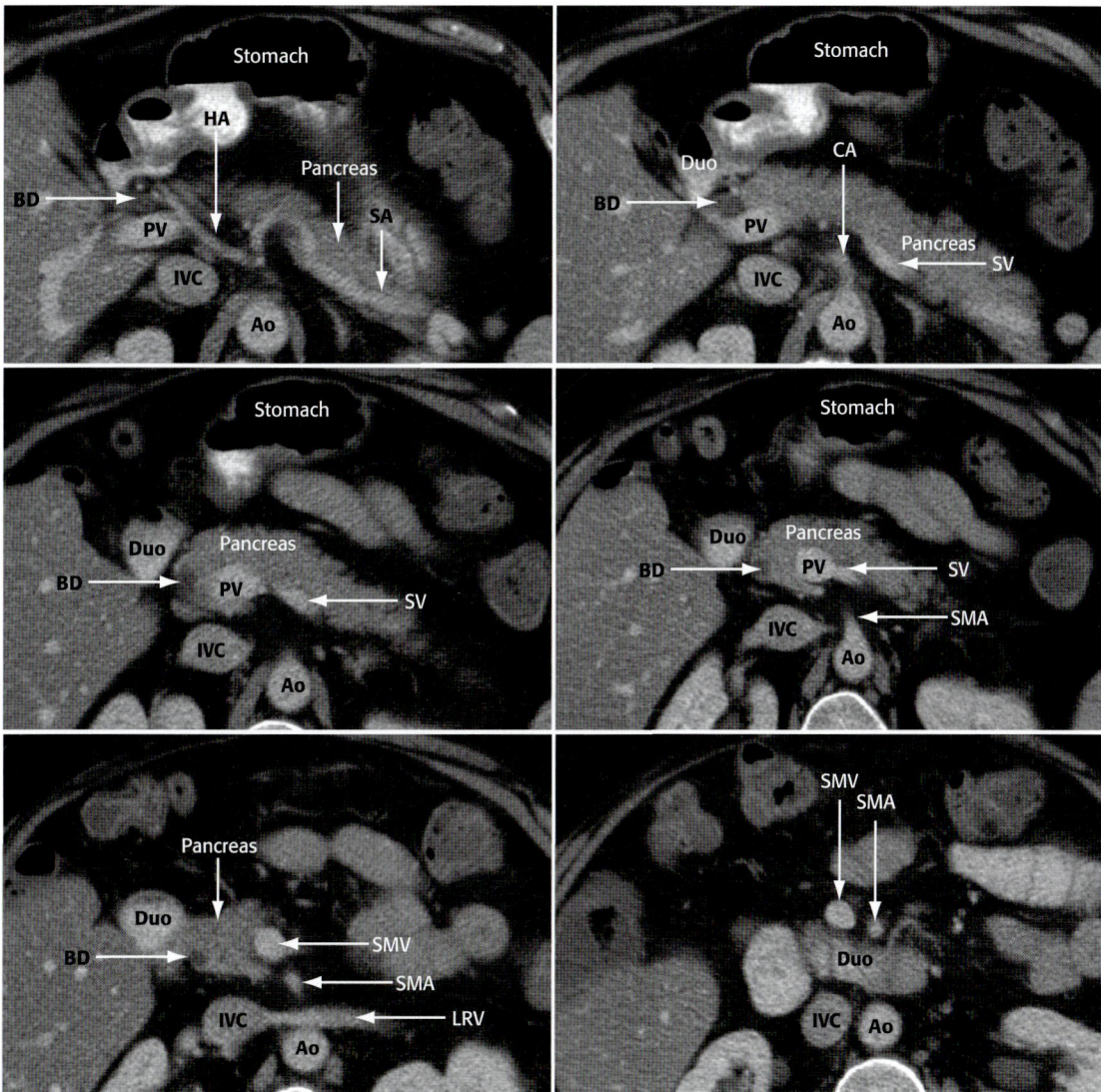

**FIGURE 2.2** Retroperitoneal structures in the upper abdomen.
BD = Bile duct; PV = Portal vein; HA = Hepatic artery; IVC = Inferior vena cava; Ao = Aorta; SV = Splenic vein; SA = Splenic artery; SMV = Superior mesenteric vein; LRV = Left renal vein; SMA = Superior mesenteric artery; IMA = Inferior mesenteric artery; Duo = Duodenum. This patient has had a cholecystectomy.

of the third part of the duodenum. Firstly, find the origin of the SMA. Next identify the left renal vein, which lies between the aorta and the SMA as it passes from the left kidney to the IVC. The third part of the duodenum is inferior to this, between the aorta and the SMA. The inferior border of the duodenum is adjacent to the origin of the inferior mesenteric artery (IMA). The IMA is not always visible on venous-phase CT.

### Identifying the pancreas
Between the origin of the CA and the SMA, the aorta is crossed by the pancreas and the splenic vein (SV). The SV runs posterior to the pancreas,

passing from the spleen to join with the superior mesenteric vein (SMV) behind the neck of the pancreas, forming the portal vein. The splenic artery follows the superior border of the pancreas from the CA to the spleen. The pancreatic head lies in the concavity of the duodenum. The pancreas is obliquely oriented in the retroperitoneum, with its head lower than its tail. The tail is seen first close to the splenic hilum. Following it inferiorly will help identify the neck, head and uncinate process.

## Structures passing to the porta hepatis (Figure 2.3)
The right and left hepatic ducts join to form the

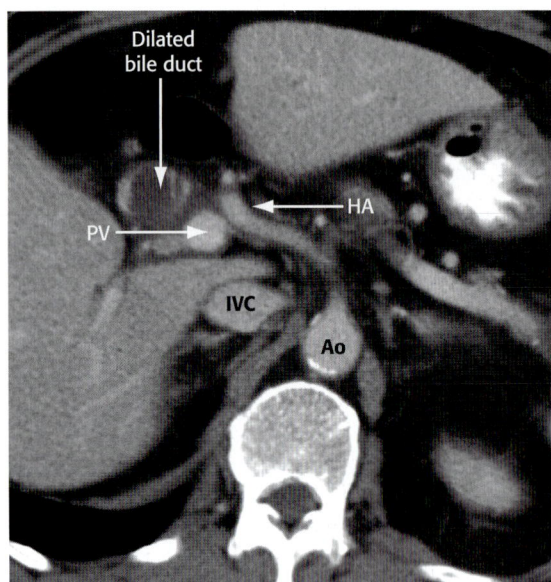

**FIGURE 2.3** Structures passing to the porta hepatis. PV = Portal vein; IVC = Inferior vena cava; Ao = Aorta; HA = Hepatic artery.

common hepatic duct, which in turn joins with the cystic duct to form the bile duct. The bile duct passes down the free edge of the lesser omentum where it is accompanied by the portal vein and hepatic artery. It then passes behind the first part of the duodenum, between the second part of the duodenum and the pancreas, to join with the pancreatic duct at the ampulla of Vater and enter the posteromedial aspect of the second part of the duodenum. Unless it is dilated, the entire course of the bile duct may not be seen on CT scan.

The portal vein forms behind the neck of the pancreas, and the hepatic artery is a branch of the coeliac axis. They both pass up the free edge of the lesser omentum with the bile duct, then divide into branches for the left and right lobes of the liver. The relations in the free border of the lesser omentum are portal vein behind, bile duct in front and to the right, and hepatic artery in front and to the left.

## Adrenal glands (Figure 2.4)

The adrenal glands lie anterosuperior to the upper part of each kidney. On the right side, the gland lies posterolateral to the IVC and posteromedial to the liver. On the left side, the gland lies lateral to the left crus of the diaphragm, and posterior to the pancreas and splenic vessels.

## Arterial supply of the gut

The coeliac axis supplies the gut from the lower oesophagus to the entry point of the bile duct into the duodenum, the liver (with the portal vein), the pancreas and the spleen. The SMA supplies the gut from the entry point of the bile duct into the duodenum to the splenic flexure. The IMA supplies the gut from the splenic flexure to the anal canal.

## Lateral recess of peritoneal cavity and retroperitoneal spaces (Figure 2.5)

The peritoneum of the lateral abdominal wall reflects at the lateral recess of the peritoneal cavity (paracolic gutter), then passes over the front of the descending (or ascending) colon and kidney. The depth of the lateral recess is variable and it may extend behind the colon, or even posterolateral to the kidney.

The anterior and posterior layers of the renal (Gerota's) fascia fuse laterally to form the lateroconal fascia, which blends in the flank with the peritoneal reflection of the lateral recess of the peritoneal cavity. The retroperitoneum is divided into three spaces by the renal fascia. The perirenal space is bounded anteriorly by the anterior renal fascia and posteriorly by the posterior renal fascia. It contains the kidney and adrenal gland.

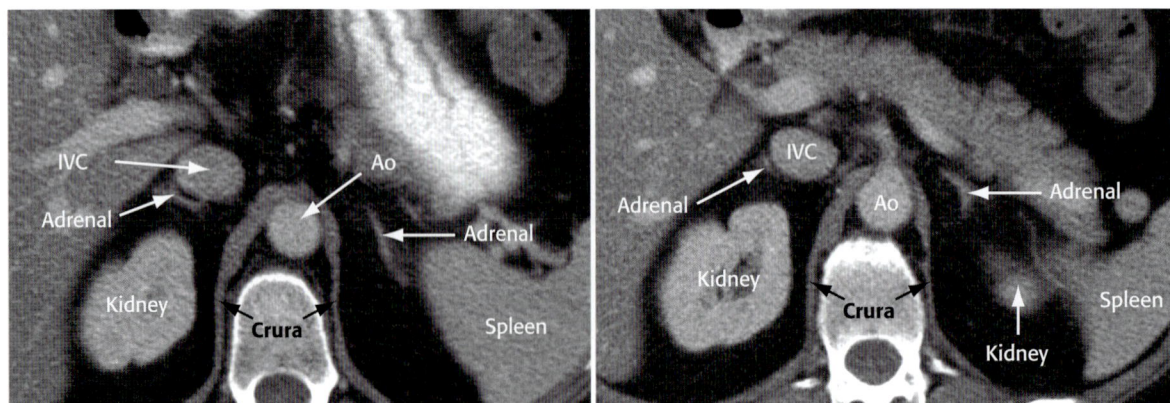

**FIGURE 2.4** The adrenal glands. IVC = Inferior vena cava; Ao = Aorta.

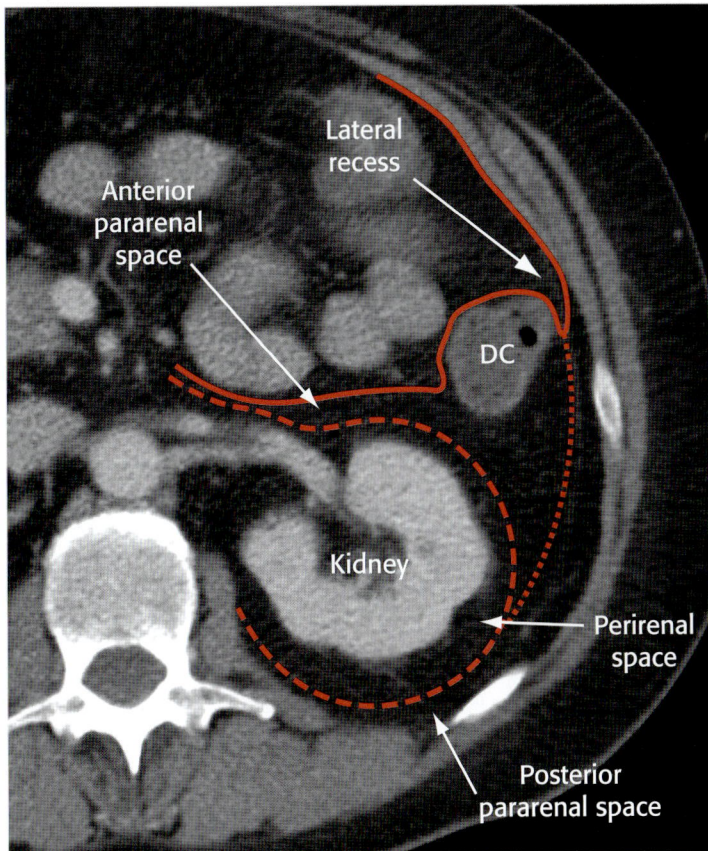

DC = Descending Colon

——— Peritoneum

······· Lateroconal Fascia

– – – Renal Fascia

**FIGURE 2.5** Lateral recess of the peritoneal cavity and retroperitoneal spaces.

The anterior pararenal space is bounded by the peritoneum anteriorly, the anterior renal fascia posteriorly and the lateroconal fascial laterally. It contains the retroperitoneal portions of the duodenum and colon, and the pancreas. The posterior pararenal space lies behind the posterior renal fascia and the lateroconal fascia. It contains no organs (Dodds, 1986).

## Pelvic organs (Figure 2.6)

Assessment of the abdominal scan should include the soft tissues of the pelvis. It is not uncommon for inexperienced doctors to interpret a CT scan as showing a pathological mass when the appearance is actually that of a normal uterus.

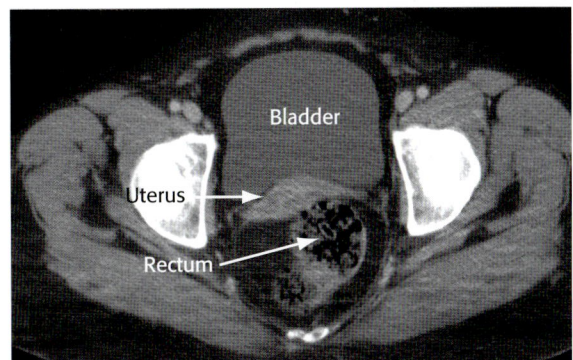

**FIGURE 2.6** Pelvic organs.

## PROBLEM 2.01

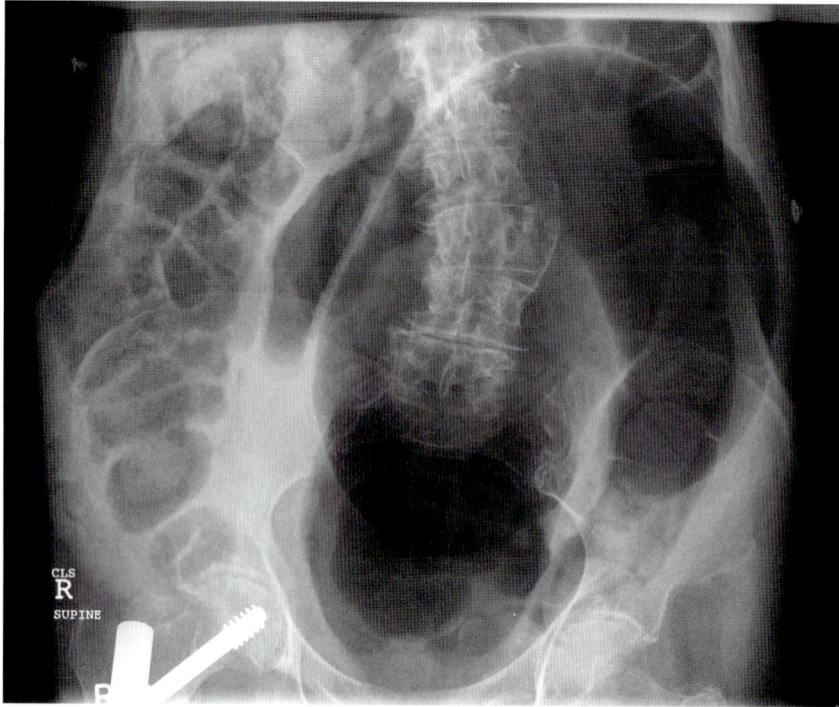

This 79-year-old woman presented with genera-lised abdominal pain and vomiting.

**Q**

What is the likely problem?

# A

A markedly distended loop of bowel extends from the pelvis to the upper abdomen, tapering inferiorly. No haustra are visible in this segment of bowel. It has the appearances of a "bent inner tube" or a "coffee bean". The rest of the large bowel is also distended, though less markedly, and the haustral pattern is retained. These features are typical of a sigmoid volvulus.

# Learning point

The vast majority of cases of volvulus involve either the caecum or the sigmoid colon (Matsumoto, 2004). Abdominal X-ray is diagnostic in the majority of cases of sigmoid volvulus, though CT may be required if the diagnosis is uncertain.

## PROBLEM 2.02

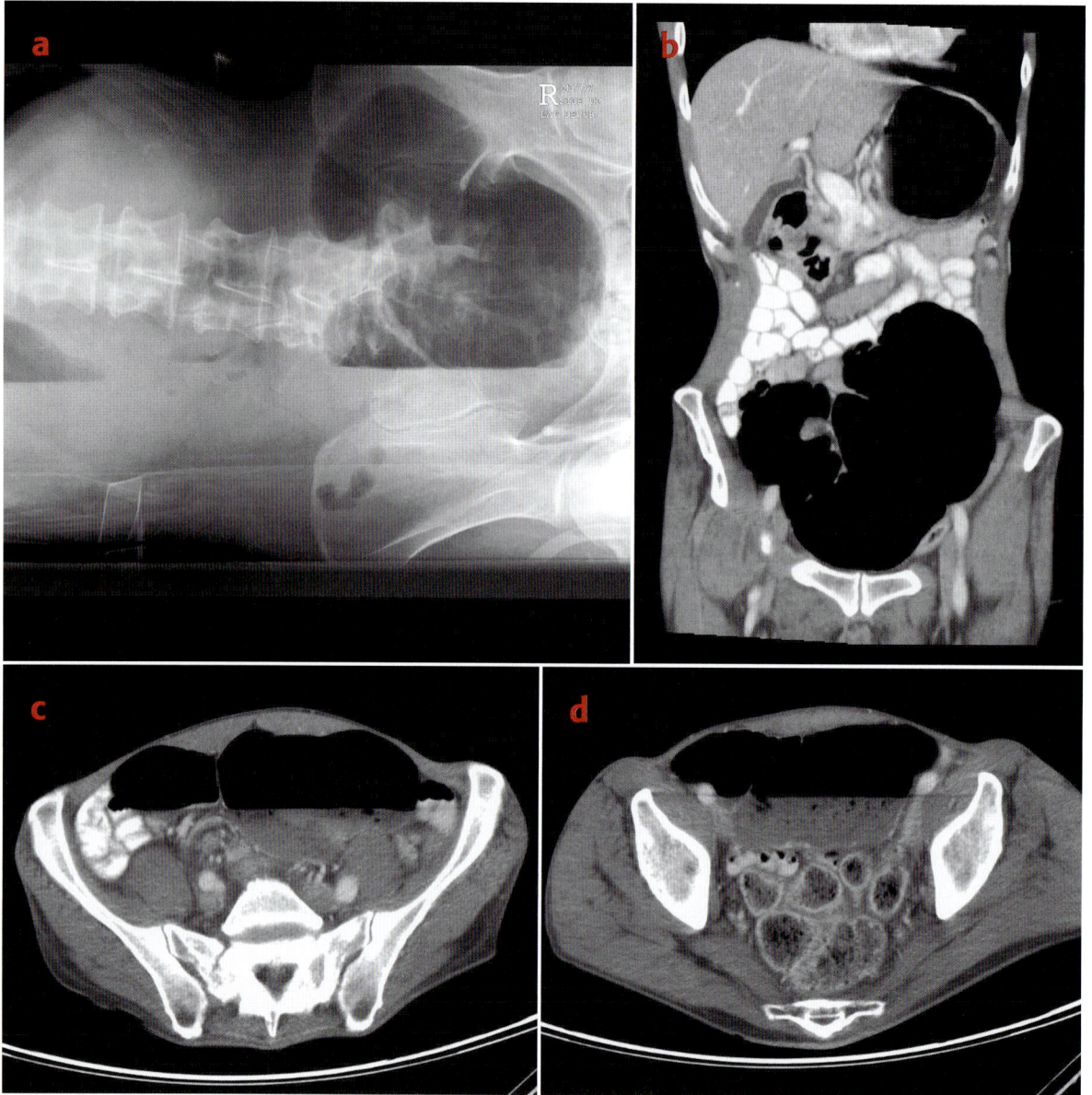

This 54-year-old man presented with vomiting and abdominal pain. Soon after these images were acquired, he vomited, aspirated and required intubation and ventilation.

**Q**

What diagnosis is suggested by these images?

# A

The plain film shows a large bowel loop in the pelvis, with haustral creases and an air fluid level. It has the appearance of a "coffee bean", on both the plain film and the coronal image of the CT. No other distended loops of large bowel are visible. The CT scans confirm this, but also show multiple loops of normal sigmoid colon in the pelvis (image d), excluding a sigmoid volvulus. Image c demonstrates the "whirl sign" just anterior to the iliac vessels. This sign is the direct visualisation of the twisted segment of bowel. The coronal view demonstrates the origin of the distended loop from the right iliac fossa adjacent to the proximal ascending colon. These findings are typical of caecal volvulus.

## LEARNING POINT

The vast majority of cases of volvulus occur either in the caecum or the sigmoid colon. Both are characterised on CT by (Matsumoto, 2004; Moore, 2001):

- a very distended segment of large bowel folded back on itself so that the twisted loop forms two compartments with a central double wall ending at the apex of the twist. This is the "coffee bean" sign, and is well demonstrated on the plain film example of a sigmoid volvulus (Problem 2.01)
- progressive tapering of the bowel leading up to the volvulus, both from above and below. When this tapered bowel is filled with contrast, it has the appearance of a bird's beak (not seen in the images from this problem)
- spiralling of collapsed loops of bowel and vessels at the site of the twist (known as the whirl sign)

In the case of sigmoid volvulus, the proximal large bowel is distended, while small bowel distension may or may not occur. With caecal volvulus, there is no proximal large bowel to distend.

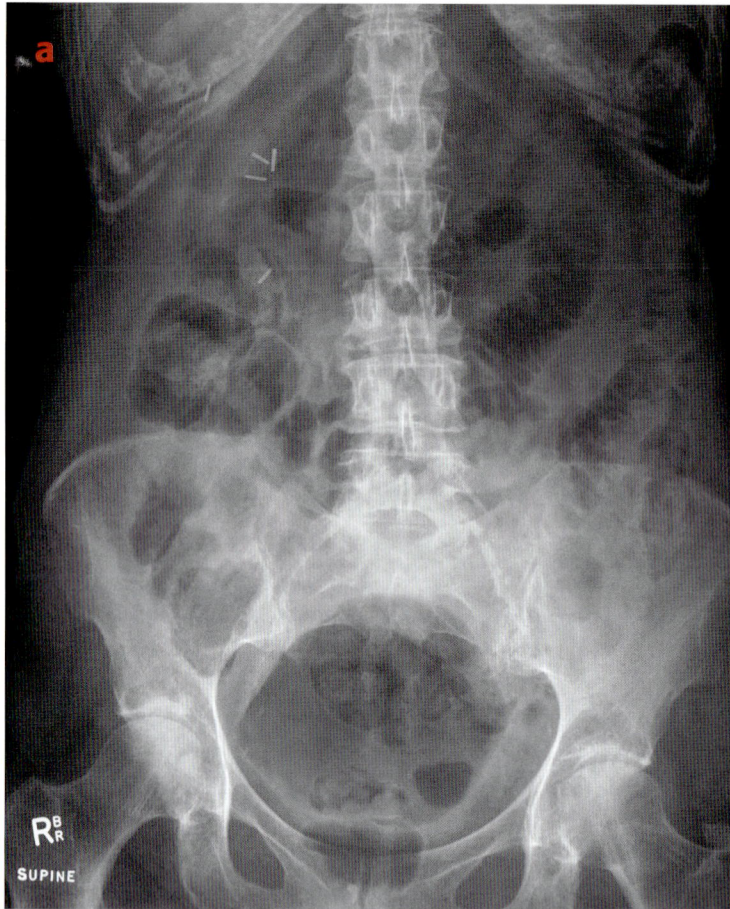

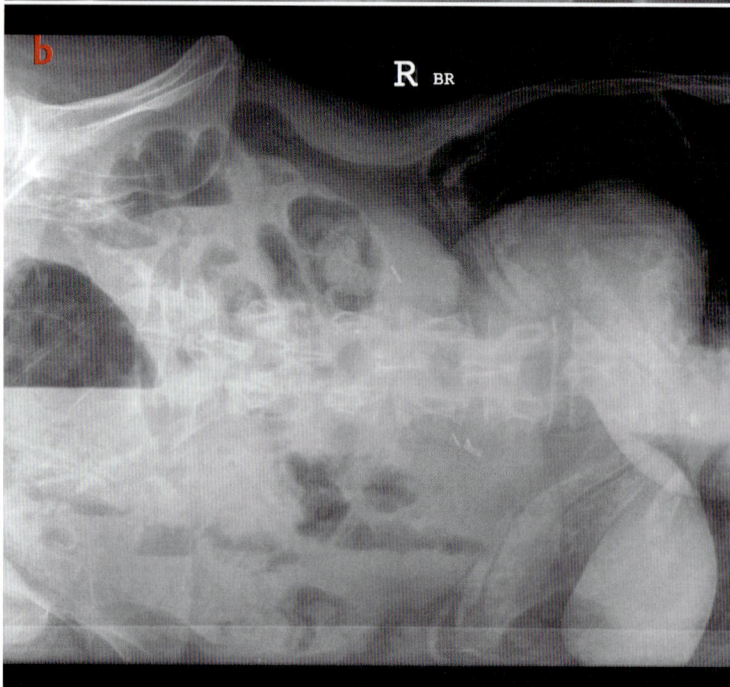

This 69-year-old woman was receiving mechanical ventilation for community acquired pneumonia when she developed generalised abdominal pain and hypotension.

**Q**

What problem do these images suggest?

**A**

The supine film (image a) shows surgical clips in the right upper quadrant and multiple gas-filled loops of small and large bowel. In some of the bowel loops, both inner and outer aspects of the bowel wall can be seen (Rigler's sign). This suggests a visceral perforation, unless there has been a recent laparotomy. In this case, the appearances of pneumoperitoneum are relatively subtle and could easily be missed on the supine film.

The left lateral decubitus film (image b) clearly demonstrates a moderate-sized pneumoperitoneum. Free gas is seen lateral to the liver, extending caudally to the iliac crest.

**LEARNING POINT**

Often it is impractical to perform erect chest and abdominal films in critically unwell patients. Left lateral decubitus abdominal X-rays are much more sensitive than supine abdominal films for detecting pneumoperitoneum. Gas rises to the non-dependent part of the abdomen and, in the left lateral position, this is lateral to the liver.

Gas may persist in the peritoneal cavity for up to a week following laparotomy.

## PROBLEM 2.04

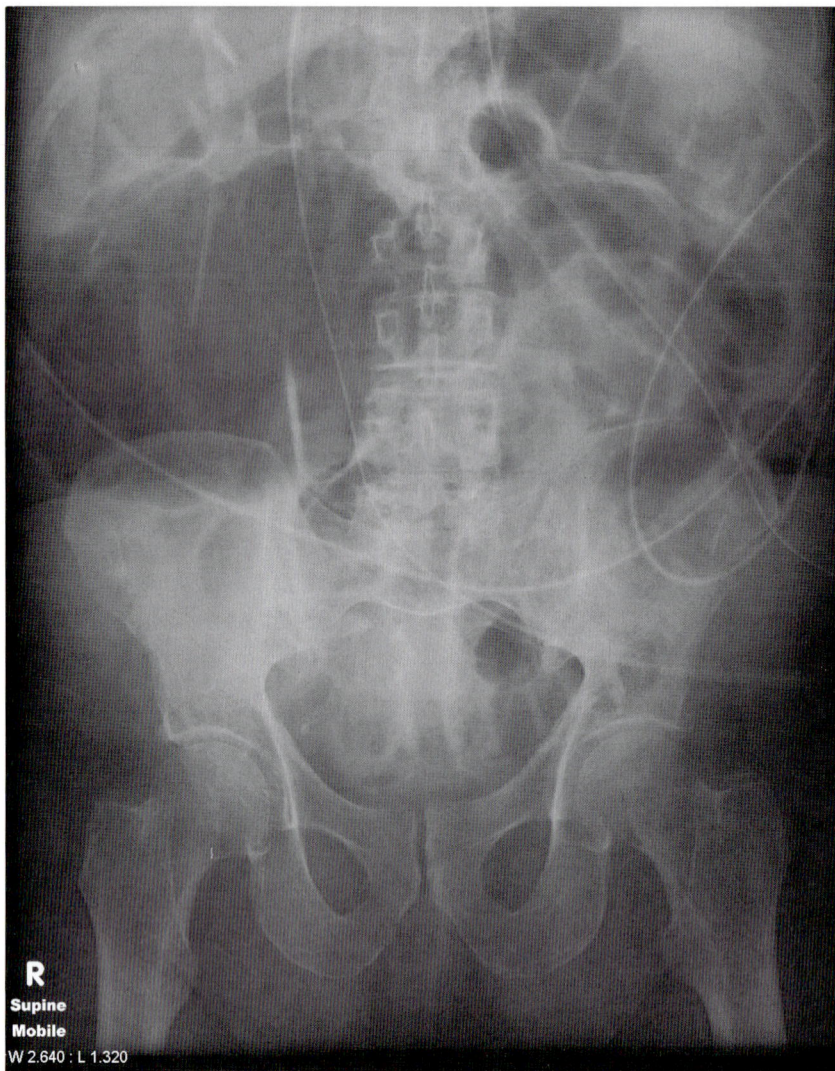

R
Supine
Mobile
W 2.640 : L 1.320

This 77-year-old man has been ventilated since undergoing cardiac surgery two weeks ago. He has had increasing abdominal distension and has not yet passed a bowel motion.

**Q**

What problem does this image suggest?

## A

There are multiple distended loops of small and large bowel. The caecum is grossly dilated. Air is seen in the rectum. There is a high risk of perforation with this degree of caecal dilatation, but there is no direct evidence of perforation on this image.

The caecal dilatation would be in keeping with caecal volvulus, but the distal large bowel distension and presence of gas in the rectum make this unlikely. In this clinical context, the most likely diagnosis is pseudo-obstruction.

## LEARNING POINT

Acute intestinal pseudo-obstruction presents with a similar clinical and radiological picture to large bowel obstruction. Characteristically, the caecum, ascending colon and transverse colon are dilated, but the dilatation may extend as far distally as the sigmoid colon. The presence of air in the rectum is common with pseudo-obstruction, but rare with complete mechanical obstruction (Batke, 2008).

Distinguishing pseudo-obstruction from mechanical large bowel obstruction may be difficult. Flexible colonoscopy and sometimes a barium enema may be required if the diagnosis is unclear on imaging.

If the diameter of the caecum exceeds 12 cm, there is a high risk of perforation and decompression should be considered (Batke, 2008).

# PROBLEM 2.05

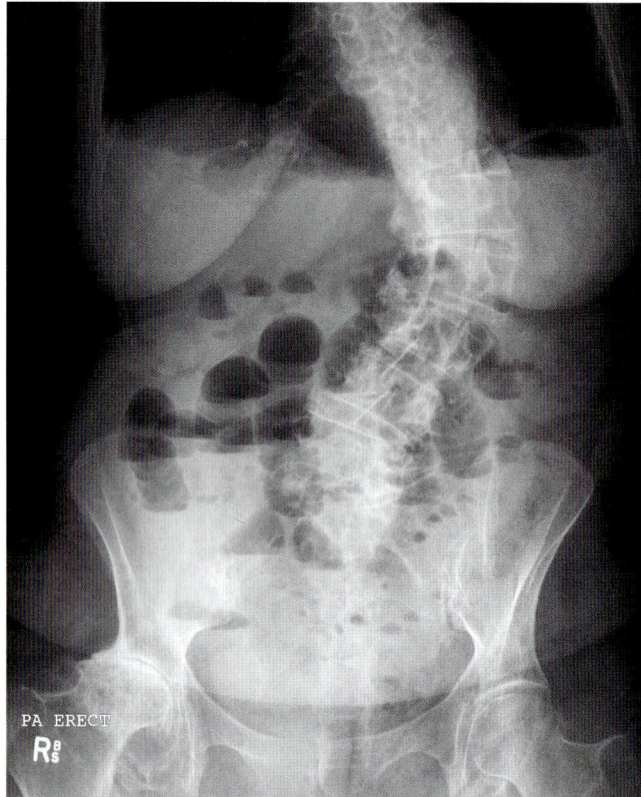

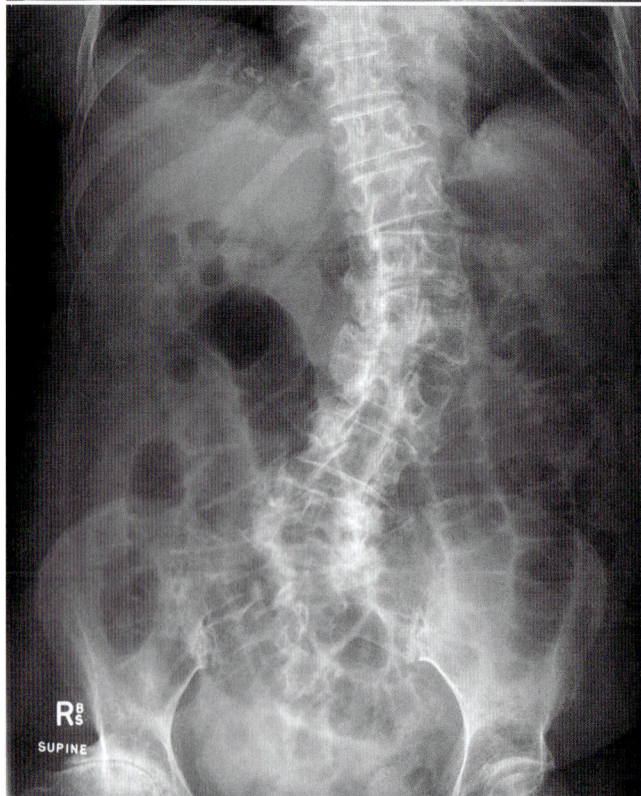

This 76-year-old woman presented with abdominal pain and vomiting.

**Q**

What problem do these images suggest?

**A**

There are dilated loops of small bowel, with multiple air–fluid levels. A "string of pearls" sign is present on the erect projection (see the Learning point below for a description of this sign). A small amount of gas is seen in the hepatic flexure and descending colon, which are not dilated. These findings denote an early, or partial, distal small bowel obstruction. No evidence of bowel infarction or perforation is seen.

Incidentally, there is also marked scoliosis of the spine.

## LEARNING POINT

Characteristic features of small bowel obstruction include distended (> 3 cm) loops of small bowel, multiple air fluid levels, thickening of the small bowel wall and collapse of the colon. There may be small bubbles of gas contained within the plicae circulares, giving the appearance of a "string of pearls", which is accentuated when a large volume of fluid residue is present in the small bowel (Nicolaou, 2005).

Small bowel may be distinguished from large bowel by two features. Firstly, large bowel is at the periphery of the abdomen, while small bowel is more central. Secondly, the mucosal folds have a different appearance. Specifically, the plicae circulares (valvulae conniventes) of the small bowel extend across the full diameter of the bowel while the haustra of the colon do not.

When the imaging suggests small or large bowel obstruction, features of perforation (free gas) or gut infarction (pneumatosis intestinalis and/or gas in the portal vein) should be looked for (Nicolaou, 2005). Hernial orifices should also be assessed for incarcerated bowel, both clinically and radiologically.

## PROBLEM 2.06

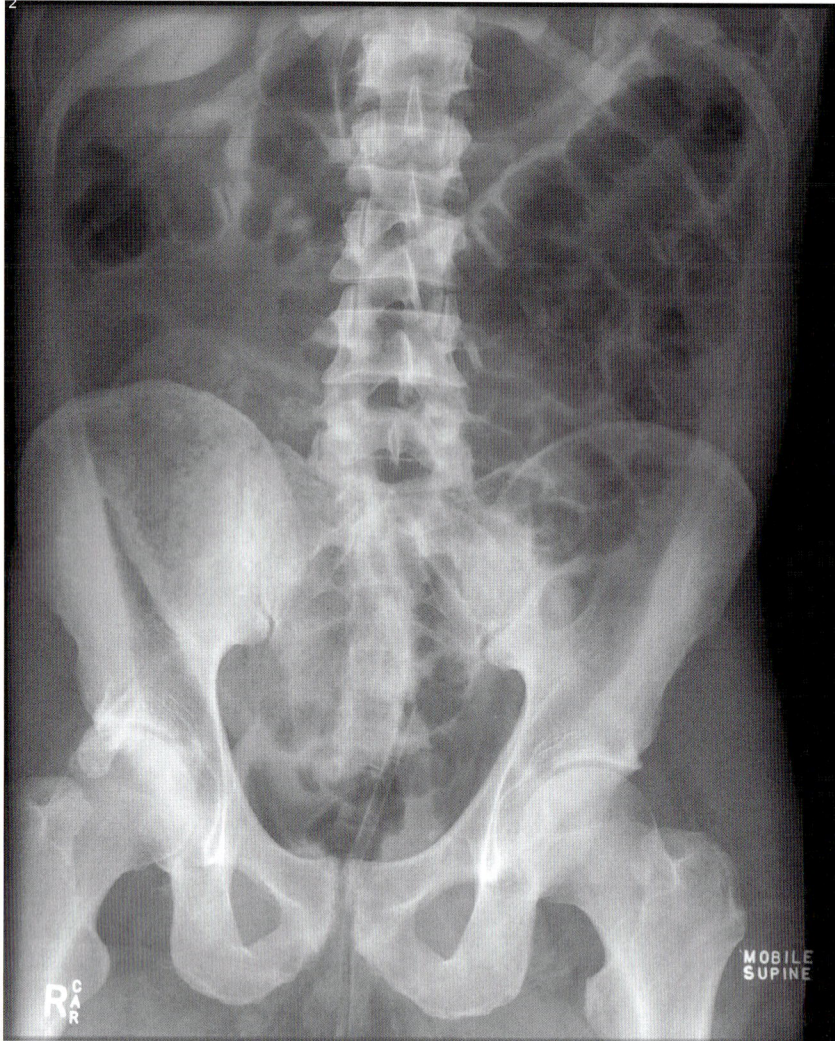

This 32-year-old man presented to the emergency department with severe abdominal pain and shock.

**Q**
What cause of shock does this image suggest?

# A

This image has multiple features of a large pneumoperitoneum, including the "football sign", Rigler's sign, interloop triangular lucency (just above the tip of the 12th left rib), air in the subhepatic space and outlining of the falciform ligament by air. Visceral perforation with sepsis is the likely cause of this patient's shock state.

## LEARNING POINT

Many signs of pneumoperitoneum have been described on the supine abdominal X-ray. Some of the more useful ones are (Khan, 2008):

- Rigler's sign: both inner and outer borders of the bowel are well defined. This is caused by the normal interface between the inner aspect of bowel wall and luminal gas, and the abnormal interface between the outer aspect of bowel wall and gas in the peritoneal cavity.
- football sign: in which air seems to outline the entire peritoneal cavity with a football shape. This represents a large air collection within the greater sac.
- interloop triangular lucency: this is a triangular collection of gas between two loops of bowel and the abdominal wall.
- subhepatic air: gas in the right upper quadrant outlines the inferior border of the liver. It may also be seen as an inverted V in the ligamentum teres notch between the left and right lobes of the liver.
- falciform ligament outlined by air: the falciform ligament may be outlined by air and visible as a vertical soft tissue density between the umbilicus and the notch between the left and right lobes of the liver.

## PROBLEM 2.07

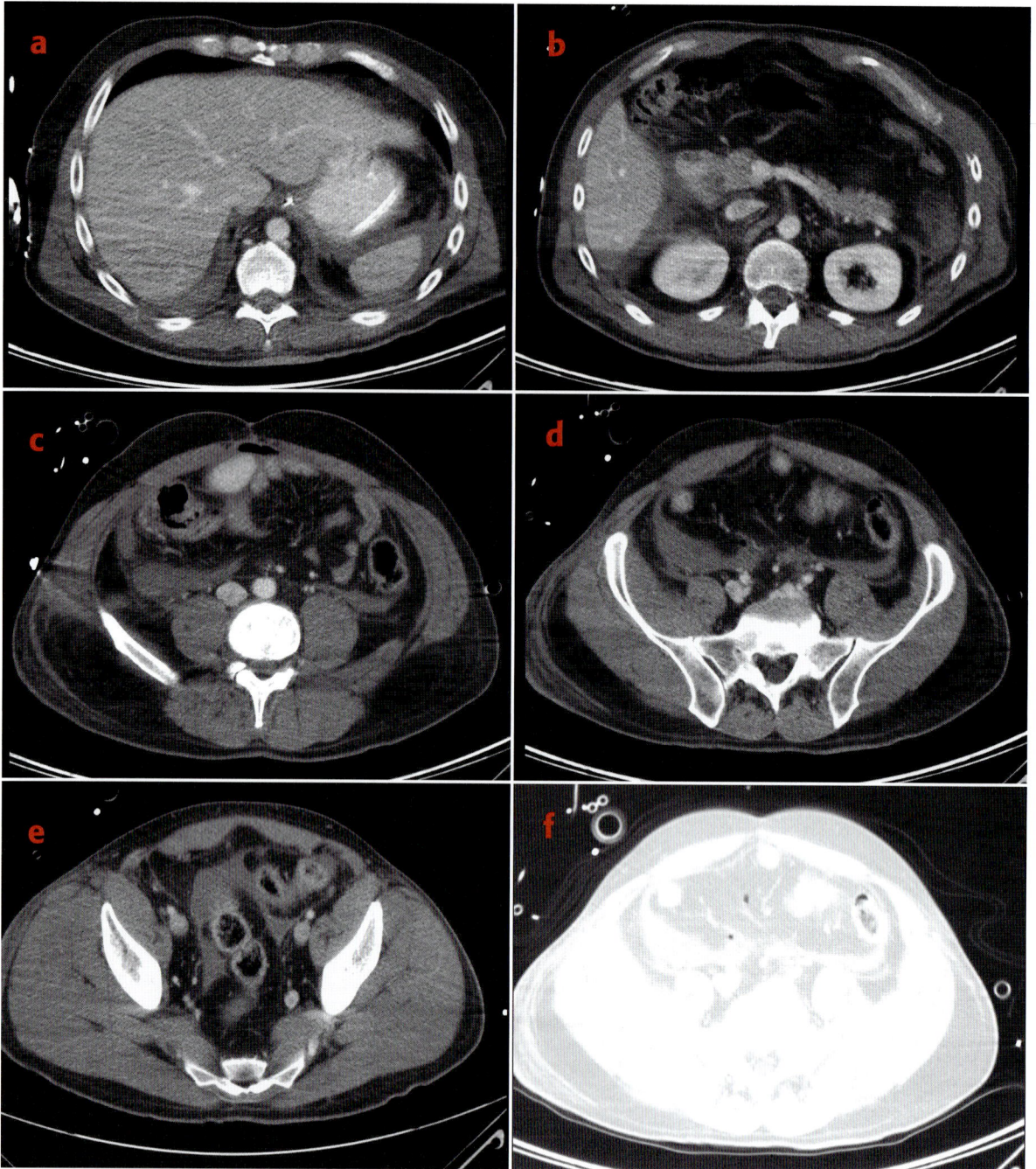

This 28-year-old-man developed lower abdominal pain following a car crash earlier today.

**Q** What injury is suggested by these images?

# A

Within the peritoneal cavity, there is a moderate amount of free fluid, and free gas is seen anteriorly. In the absence of a recent laparotomy, these findings are strongly suggestive of hollow visceral perforation. The wall of the sigmoid colon and the descending colon is thickened and there is gas within the mesentery (well seen on the lung windows, image f), suggesting a colonic injury. There is fluid around the spleen, but there is no splenic injury identified on these images. The perisplenic fluid could indicate a splenic injury that is below the resolution of CT scan to detect or it could be part of the free peritoneal fluid, which is seen in multiple locations throughout the abdomen. On the DVD images, there is an incidental right adrenal lesion.

## LEARNING POINT

Lung windows may help to demonstrate subtle evidence of intra-abdominal free gas.

## PROBLEM 2.08

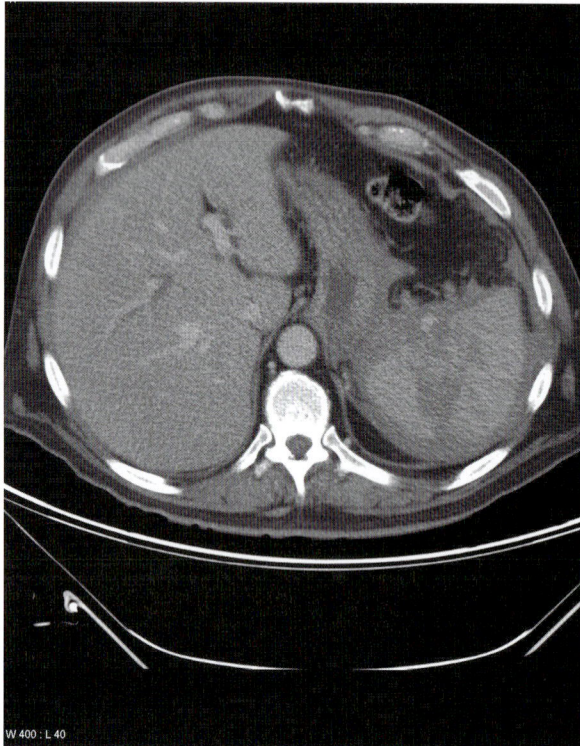

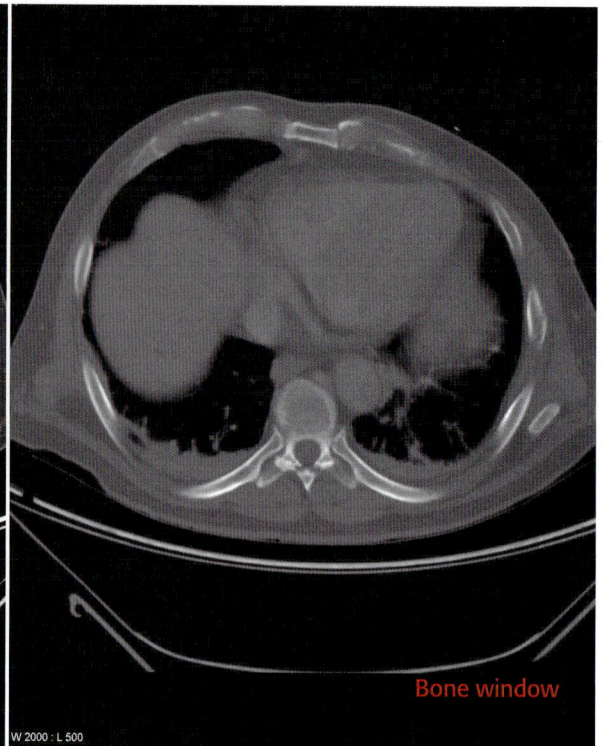

This 65-year-old man fell while crossing the road earlier today. He complains of left upper quadrant abdominal pain, with tenderness over the adjacent chest wall.

**Q** What injuries are demonstrated on these images?

## A

There is a laceration through the spleen with a surrounding haemorrhage. A small area of contrast extravasation is noted at the splenic hilum. These features are consistent with a grade IV splenic injury. Two ribs on the left have minimally displaced anterior fractures. More rib fractures are demonstrated on the DVD images.

## LEARNING POINT

The organ injury scale of the American Association for the Surgery of Trauma is used to grade injury to individual organs (Tinkoff, 2008). It may be used for a range of organs, including liver, spleen and kidneys. Grades I to V represent increasingly severe injuries in salvageable patients, while grade VI represents an unsurvivable injury.

Splenic injuries may include subcapsular or parenchymal haematomas, lacerations and injury to the vessels supplying the spleen, with or without devascularisation. As the spleen is not necessary for survival, splenic injuries are graded from I to V (see Appendix 1 for details).

Splenic injuries are often associated with lower rib fractures on the left side.

## PROBLEM 2.09

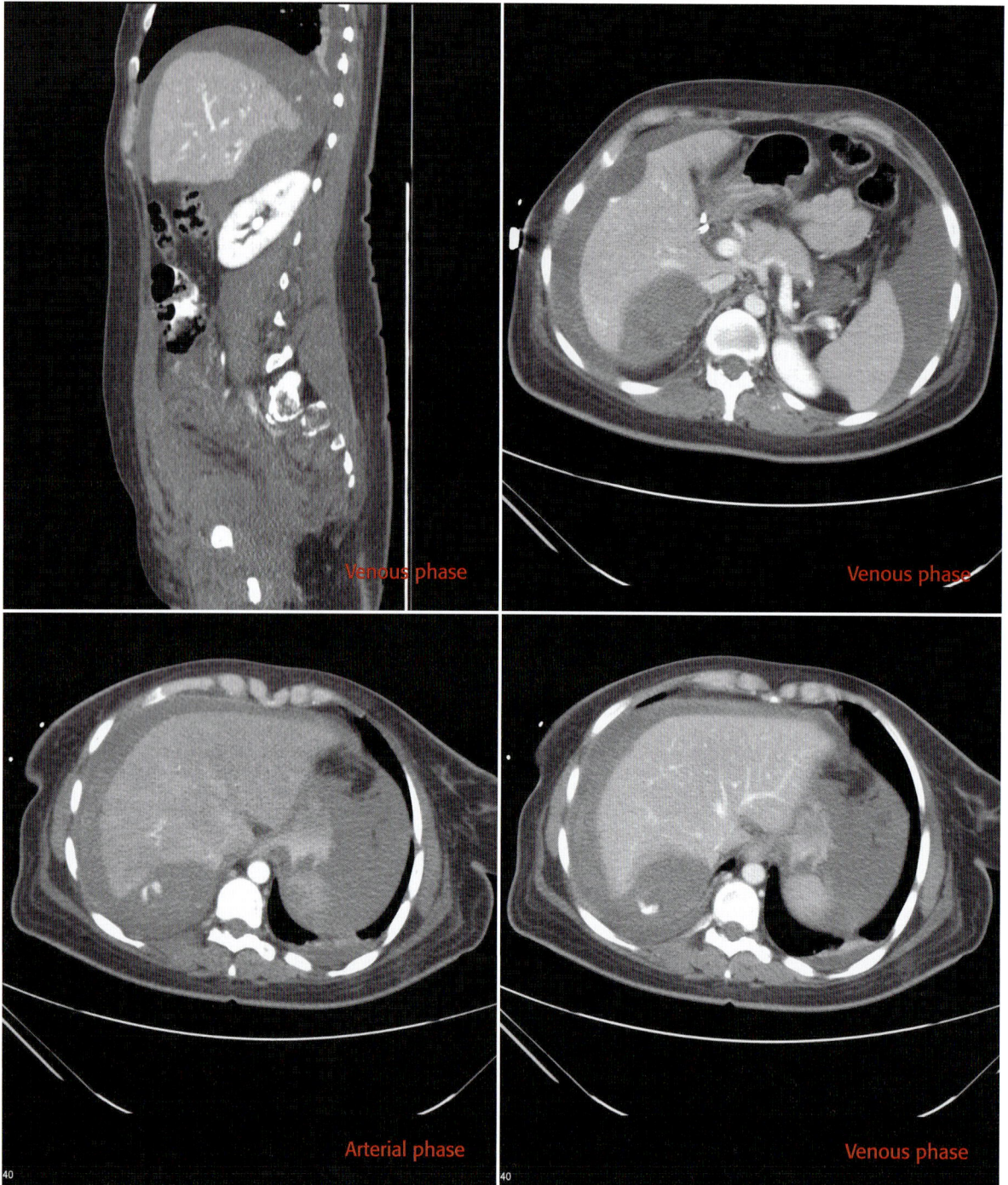

Venous phase

Venous phase

Arterial phase

Venous phase

This 29-year-old woman was involved in a high-speed car crash two hours ago. She was hypotensive on presentation and initially responded to intravenous fluid resuscitation. She has now become hypotensive again, and is confused and agitated.

**Q**

Describe the injuries.

# A

There are two large subcapsular haematomas of the liver, seen best on the axial images. On the parasagittal image, a relatively small laceration of the posterior aspect of the liver is seen. Contrast extravasation is seen on the arterial phase image, suggesting active bleeding. This is consistent with a grade III liver injury. There is also a large haemoperitoneum and, on the parasagittal images, a retroperitoneal haematoma inferior to the kidney can be seen. On the DVD images, there is a vertical shear injury to the pelvis with extensive retroperitoneal haematoma.

## LEARNING POINT

Subcapsular haematomas appear as elliptical collections of low attenuation between the liver capsule and the enhancing liver parenchyma. They can be differentiated from free peritoneal blood in the perihepatic space because they indent or flatten the underlying liver margin. Parenchymal haematomas or contusions are irregular, focal, low-attenuation areas in the parenchyma of the liver. Lacerations appear as linear or branching low-attenuation areas in the parenchyma. Contrast extravasation on arterial phase images indicates active haemorrhage (Yoon, 2005). Liver injuries are graded from I to VI (see Appendix 1 for details) (Tinkoff, 2008).

## PROBLEM 2.10

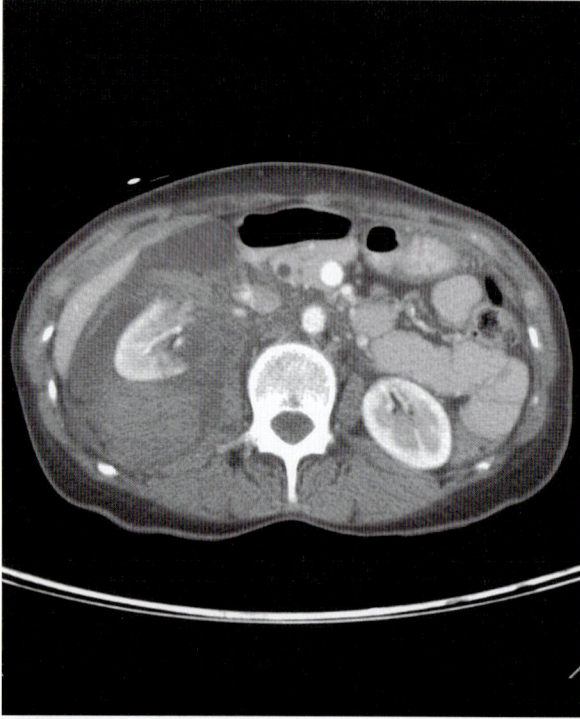
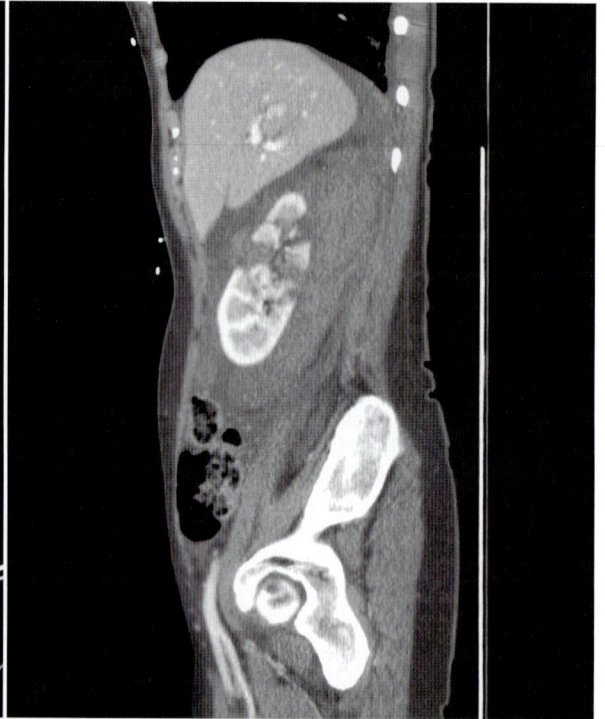
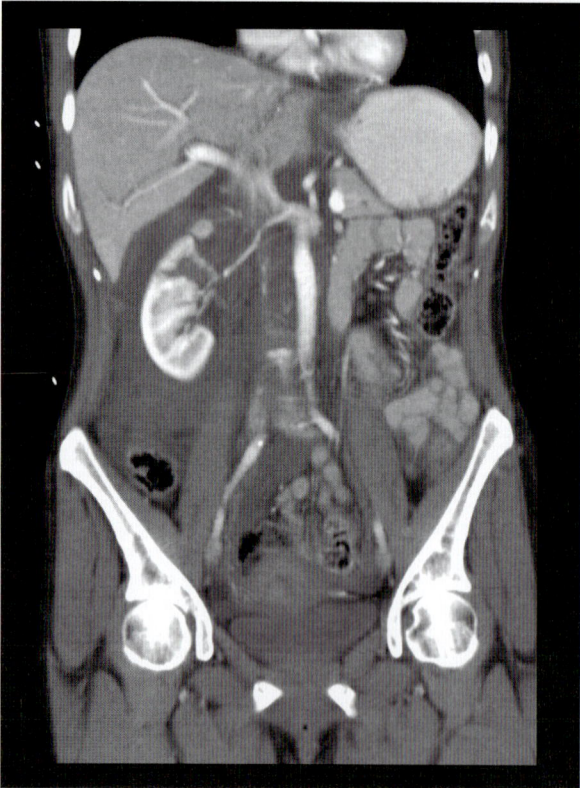
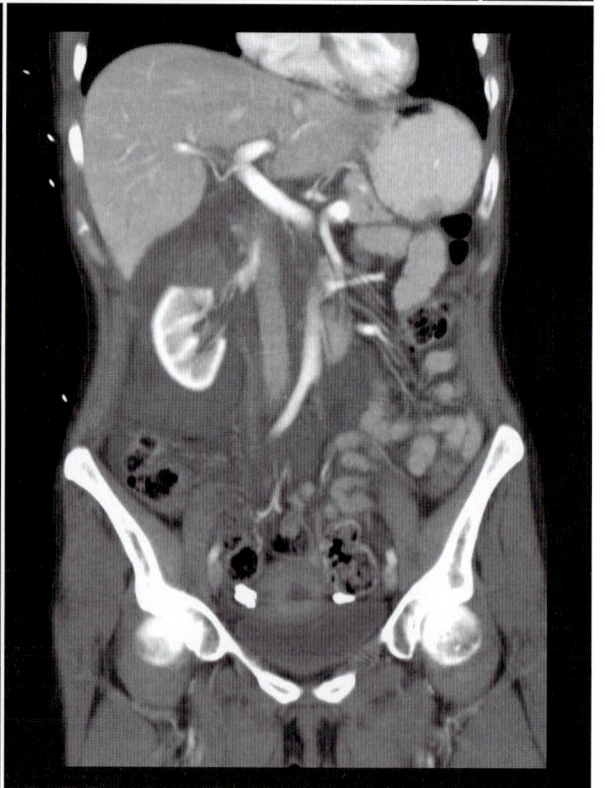

This 64-year-old woman was in a high-speed car crash earlier today. She complains of abdominal and back pain. Macroscopic haematuria was noted when a urinary catheter was inserted.

# Q

What injury is demonstrated by these venous phase images?

# A

The upper half of the right kidney has multiple deep lacerations, extending through the corticomedullary junction into the collecting system. The renal artery and vein are well opacified with contrast and the renal parenchyma is enhancing with contrast. There is a large haematoma in the retroperitoneum surrounding the right kidney, in the perinephric space. On the images in the DVD, free fluid is seen within the peritoneal cavity in the pelvis. These findings are consistent with a grade IV renal injury. The venous phase images shown in the book cannot exclude urine extravasation, but the delayed phase (pyelographic) images on the DVD show no evidence of this.

# LEARNING POINT

Renal injuries may include contusions, lacerations and injury to the renal vasculature. Renal injuries are graded from I to V (see Appendix 1 for details) (Tinkoff, 2008).

For full assessment of a renal injury by CT, a contrast study with both early phase (to assess the renal vasculature and parenchyma) and delayed phase images (to assess the collecting system) should be obtained. This allows any extravasation of urine to be identified.

## PROBLEM 2.11

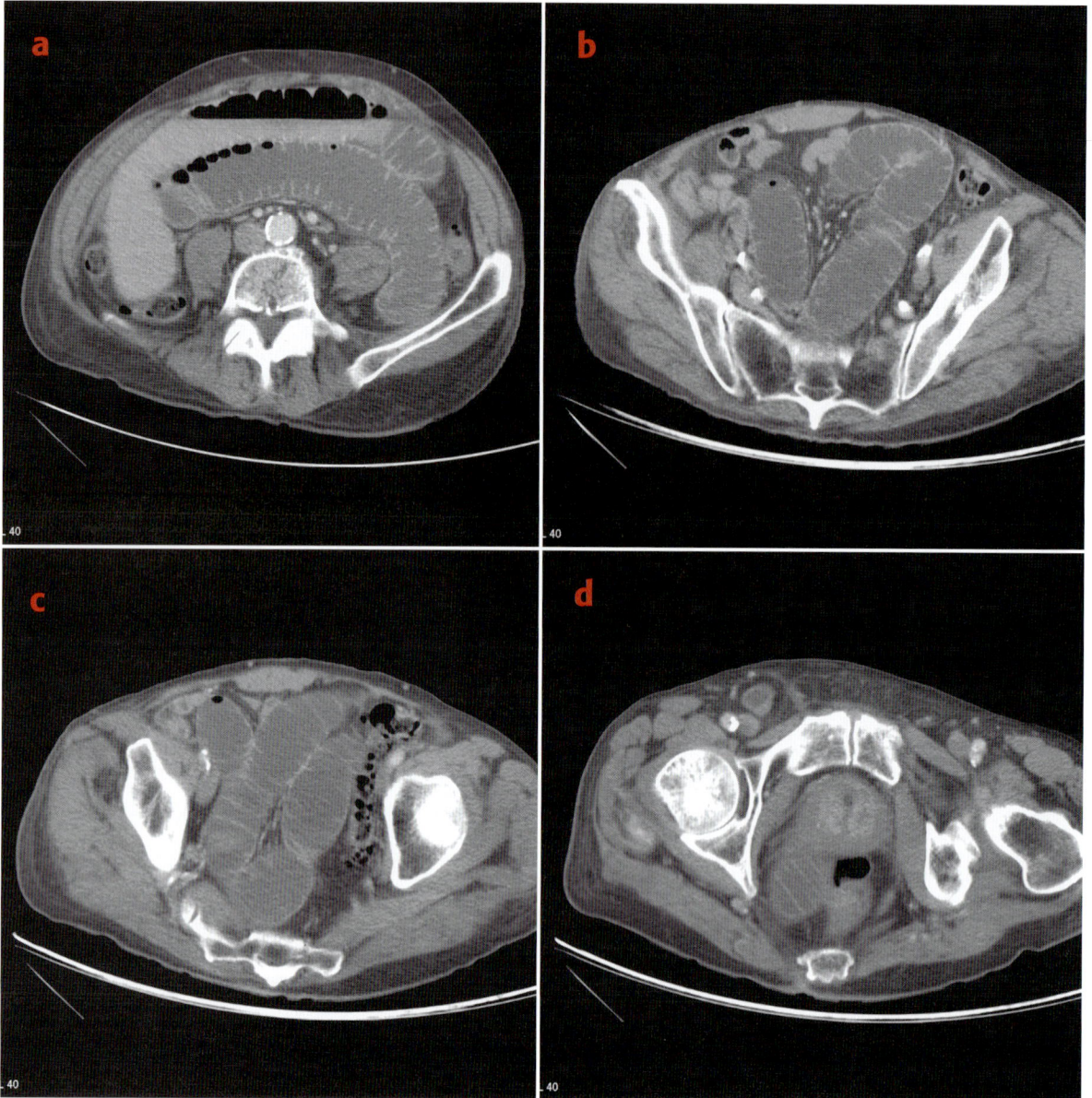

This 72-year-old man complained of vomiting and abdominal pain. His abdomen was markedly distended.

**Q**

What cause of this patient's abdominal symptoms do these images suggest?

# A

There are multiple distended loops of small bowel. The large bowel is not dilated. There are also non-distended collapsed loops of small bowel in the right iliac fossa (image b), with a transition from dilated to collapsed small bowel seen in image c. This transition is adjacent to the right inguinal region and bowel is seen in a femoral hernia adjacent to the femoral vessels in image d. This patient has an incarcerated femoral hernia causing a small bowel obstruction.

# LEARNING POINT

A transition point between dilated and collapsed bowel confirms the presence of a mechanical bowel obstruction and defines the site of obstruction (Nicolaou, 2005).

Whenever distended bowel is present, such a transition point should be sought. This requires a systematic process of following the bowel up from the rectum, examining in turn the sigmoid, descending, transverse and ascending colon, then finally the small bowel.

## PROBLEM 2.12

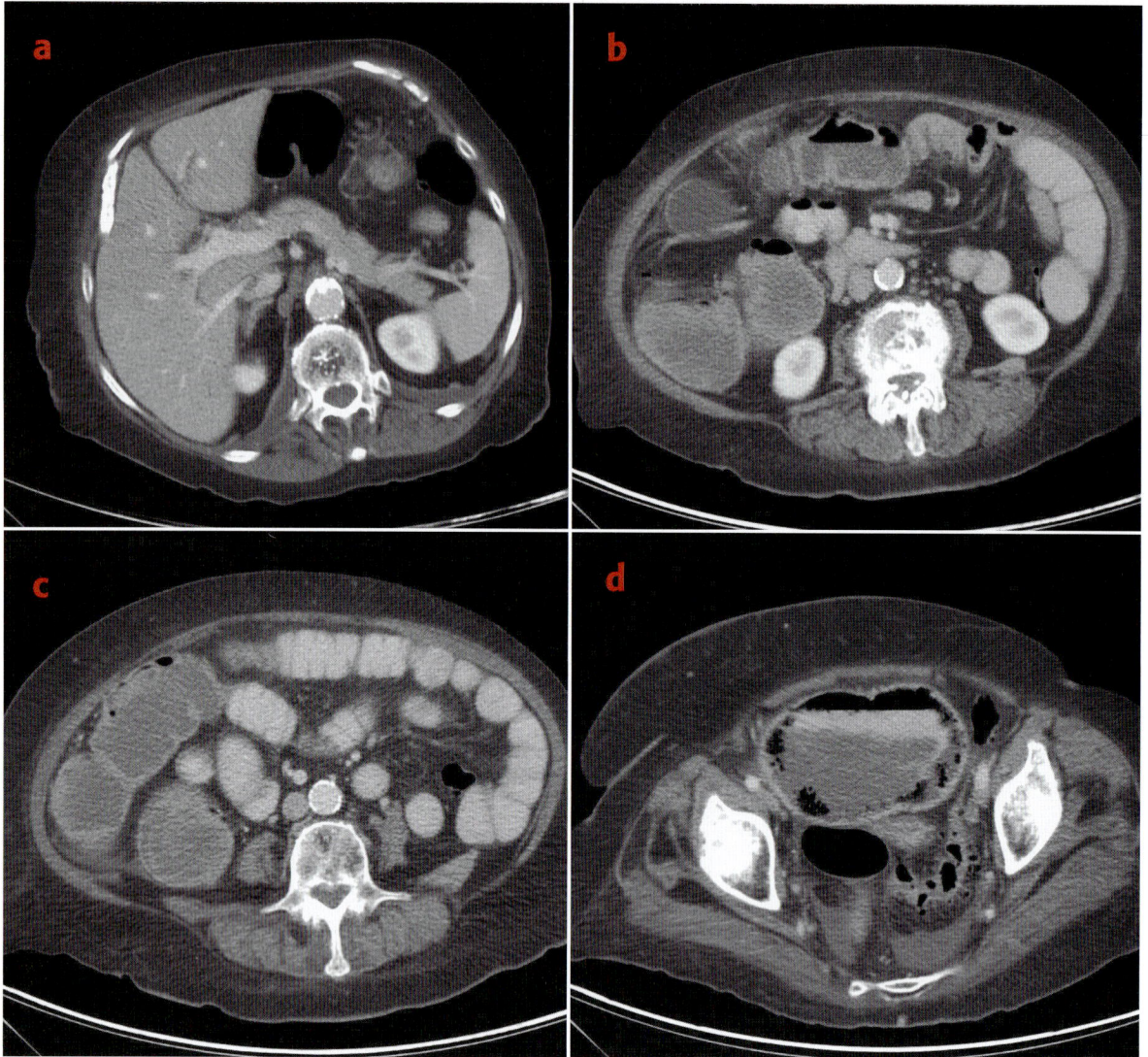

This 76-year-old woman required admission to ICU for management of acute renal failure from dehydration. The history revealed several days of abdominal pain and vomiting.

**Q**

What problem do these images suggest?

## A

The caecum, ascending colon and transverse colon are all dilated, while the descending and sigmoid colon are collapsed. A transition from dilated to collapsed large bowel is seen in image a, in the distal transverse colon near the splenic flexure (best appreciated on the DVD images, which allow the large bowel to be followed along its entire length). There is mural thickening at this transition point. The small bowel is also mildly dilated. There are no obvious liver metastases or lymphadenopathy and there is no evidence of ischaemia or perforation.

The problem suggested by these images is a large bowel obstruction. The most likely cause is bowel cancer.

## LEARNING POINT

The small bowel may or may not be dilated in large bowel obstruction, depending on the competence of the ileocaecal valve.

The upper limit of normal colon size is 6 cm, though the caecum may be up to 9 cm (Dahnert, 2007).

# PROBLEM 2.13

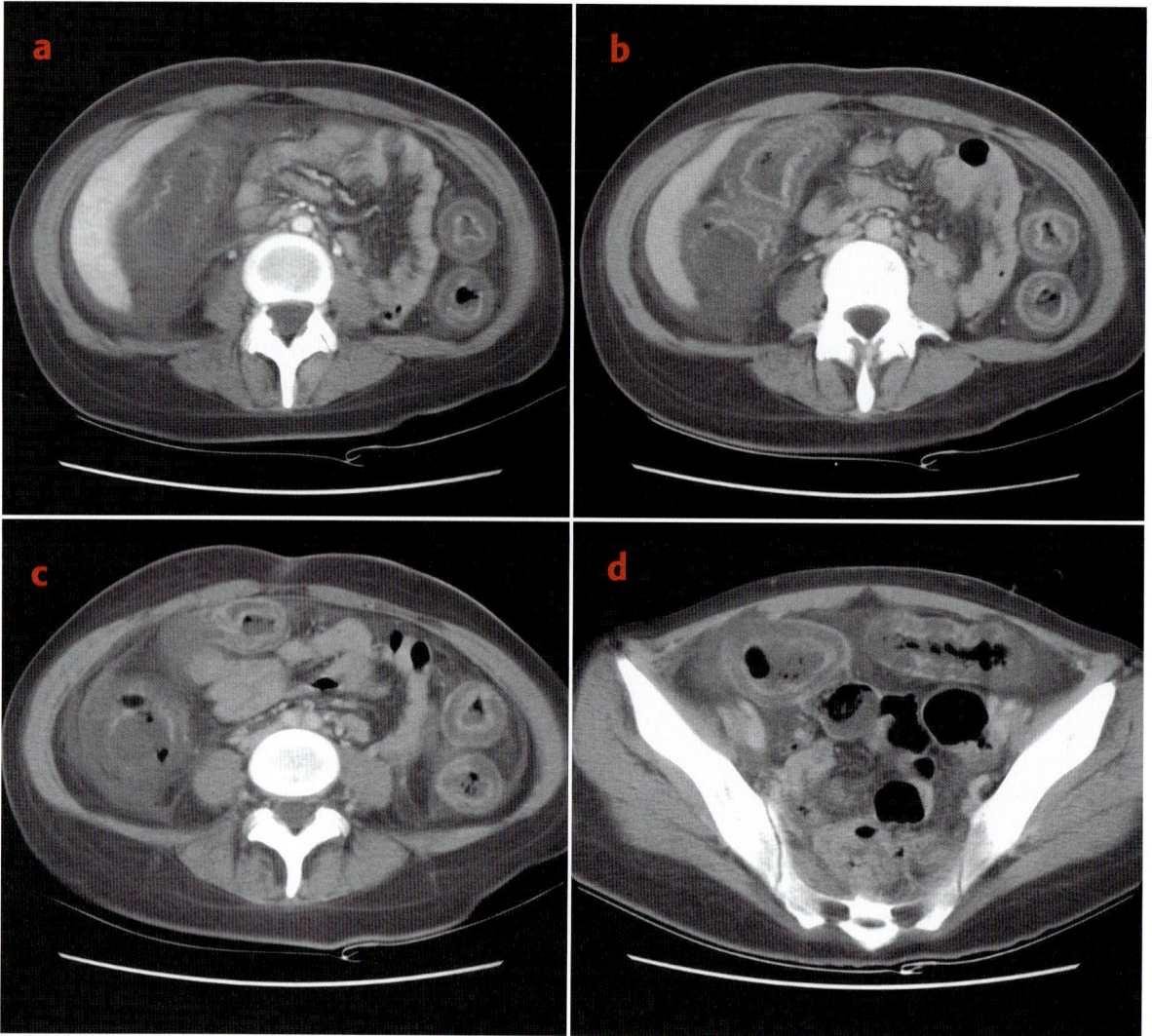

This 24-year-old woman received chemotherapy for leukaemia one week ago. She is now profoundly leucopenic and febrile with abdominal pain and distension.

Q
What problem is suggested by these images?

## A

There is marked thickening of the large bowel wall, involving the descending, ascending and transverse colon and the caecum. The small bowel is normal distally and slightly distended proximally (seen on DVD images). These appearances suggest that the main problem is colitis, with typhlitis (inflammation of the caecum). In this clinical context, neutropenic typhlitis/colitis is likely, but pseudomembranous colitis should be considered.

Of concern, there is gas in the bowel wall (image c), and the enhancing mucosa of the ascending colon is discontinuous (image b) with surrounding fluid. This is suspicious of a perforation but, as no free gas is seen on these images, the presence of a perforation is uncertain.

## LEARNING POINT

In patients with neutropaenic typhlitis, CT is helpful to confirm the diagnosis and identify problems that may need surgical management. Such problems include perforation leading to peritonitis or abscesses.

Uncomplicated typhlitis is treated with antibiotics and supportive management.

## PROBLEM 2.14

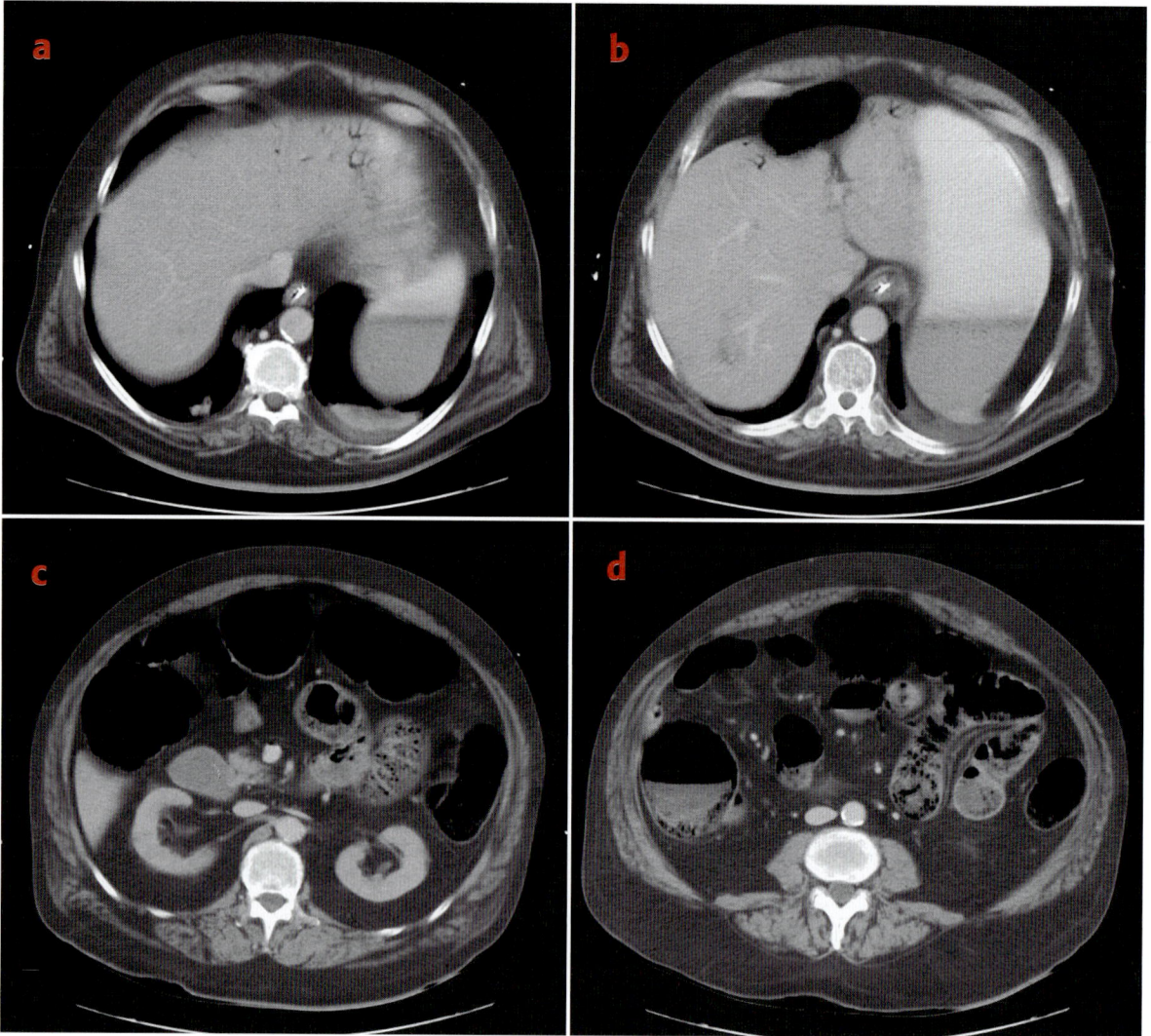

This 66-year-old man developed central abdominal pain two days ago. The pain has become progressively worse and he has now developed septic shock with severe lactic acidosis.

**Q**
What problem do these images suggest?

# A

There is gas in the substance of the liver. It has a branching linear pattern and is seen peripherally in the liver, consistent with portal venous gas. Gas is also seen within the superior mesenteric vein. In addition, there is an area of low attenuation in the posterior aspect of the right hepatic lobe (image b), which may represent early abscess formation. There is extensive air within the wall of both small and large bowel, most prominent in the ascending colon. It is seen both in the dependent and non-dependent parts of the bowel wall, suggesting that it is submucosal rather than luminal. In this clinical context, these findings would be consistent with necrotising enterocolitis or mesenteric vascular occlusion causing infarcted gut. The relative sparing of the transverse and descending colon would favour gut infarction.

## LEARNING POINT

The differential diagnosis for gas with a branching linear pattern within the liver includes portal venous gas and pneumobilia. The flow of portal venous blood is from the hilum outwards, and portal venous gas is seen branching to within 2 cm of the periphery of the liver. In cases where it is more centrally distributed, the continuity of the gas filled branches with the contrast-containing branches of the portal vein may be apparent. The flow of bile is from the periphery to the porta hepatis and, with pneumobilia, gas tends to accumulate in the large central bile ducts near the hilum.

Pneumatosis intestinalis (gas in the bowel wall) may be primary (which is both idiopathic and benign) or secondary. Secondary causes include bowel necrosis, a range of non-necrotising bowel diseases (bowel obstruction, Crohn's disease, ulcerative colitis), immunosuppression, abdominal trauma and pulmonary barotrauma (Dahnert, 2007; Knechtle, 1990).

# PROBLEM 2.15

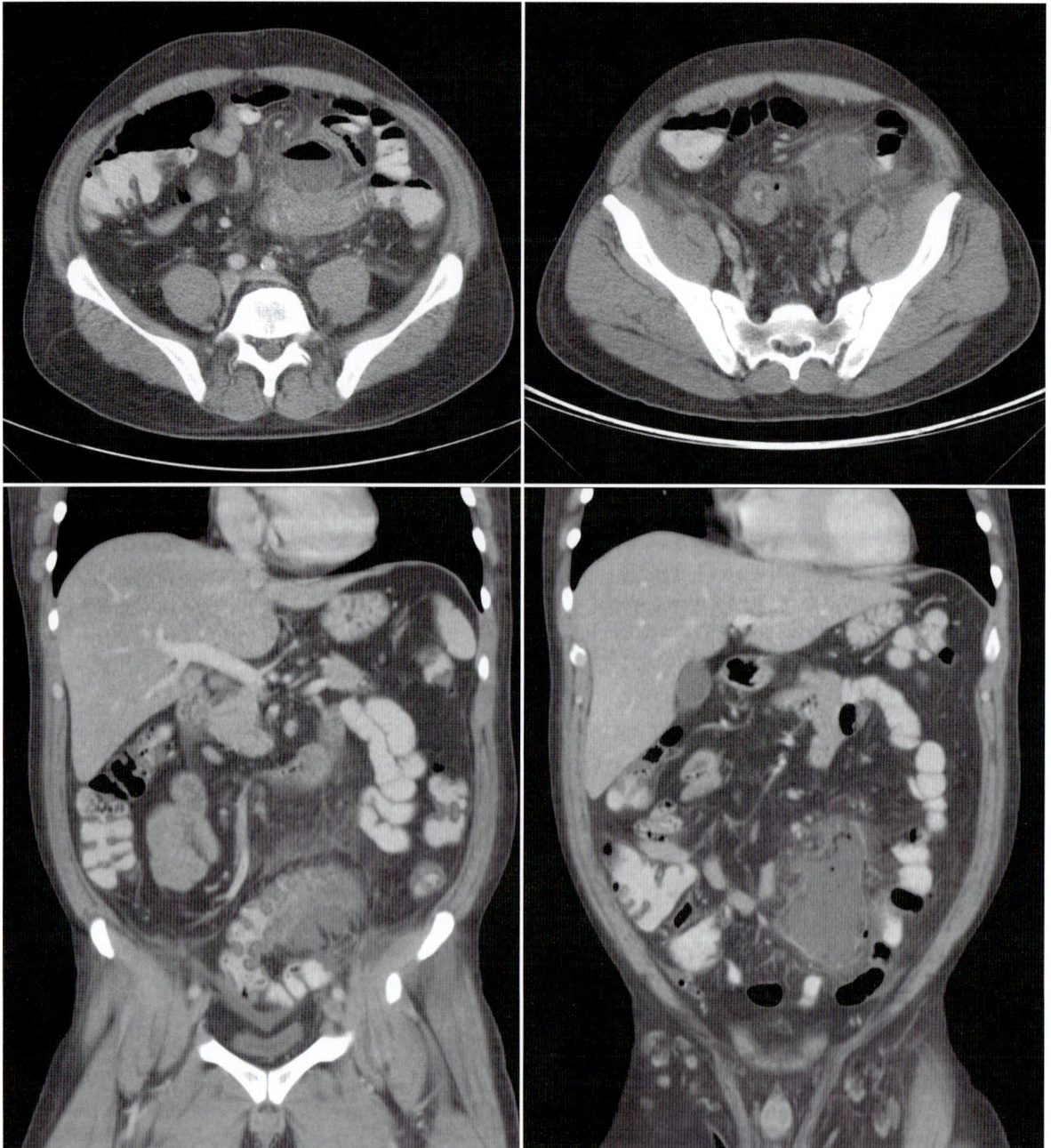

This 44-year-old man presented with three days of lower abdominal pain and is now in septic shock.

**Q** What pathological process is suggested by these images?

## A

The wall of the sigmoid colon is thickened and at least one diverticulum is seen. Adjacent to the thickened area of colon is a collection containing fluid and gas with some rim enhancement. The most likely cause of these findings is diverticulitis with localised perforation and abscess formation.

## LEARNING POINT

When a collection suggestive of an abscess is identified on a CT scan, the rest of the scan should be reviewed for possible causes of intra-abdominal abscess. Common causes include appendicitis, diverticulitis, gangrenous cholecystitis, pancreatitis, mesenteric ischaemia with gut infarction and other gastrointestinal tract perforations.

# PROBLEM 2.16

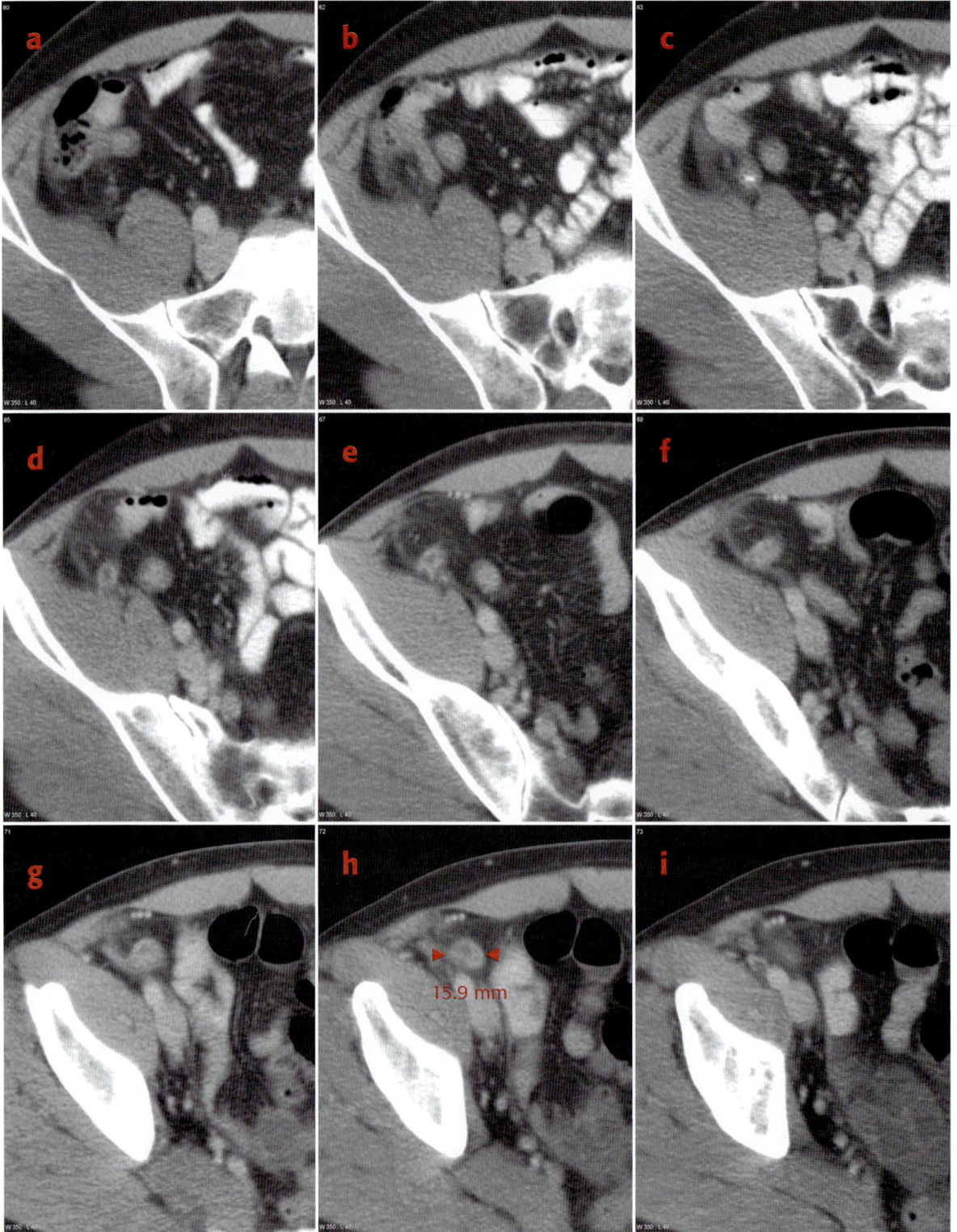

This 44-year-old man presented with right lower quadrant abdominal pain and is now waiting for surgery. He is known to have C1 esterase inhibitor deficiency and an ICU bed has been requested for postoperative monitoring.

## Q

What diagnosis do these images suggest?

## A

The appendix is markedly enlarged (15.9 mm) and contains a calcified appendicolith. There is periappendiceal fat stranding, suggesting inflammation. There is contrast enhancement of the appendiceal wall, which is best appreciated in image d, where it may be compared with the adjacent terminal ileum. These findings are strongly suggestive of appendicitis. There is no evidence of perforation.

## LEARNING POINT

The CT findings of appendicitis include (Curtin, 1995; Jain, 2006):

- circumferential and symmetric wall thickening with a "two wall" diameter > 6 mm. If the lumen is filled with fluid, the walls may not be distinguishable from the luminal contents; in this circumstance, a diameter of up to 10 mm may be normal.
- enhancement of the appendiceal wall with IV contrast
- periappendiceal inflammation with fat stranding
- presence of a calcified appendicolith
- perforation suggested by the presence of a peri-caecal phlegmon or abscess formation

Other findings that may be found with perforation include extraluminal air and thickening of the adjacent caecum or terminal ileum. A conglomerate of inflamed and adherent bowel loops may obscure the inflamed appendix in some cases.

## PROBLEM 2.17

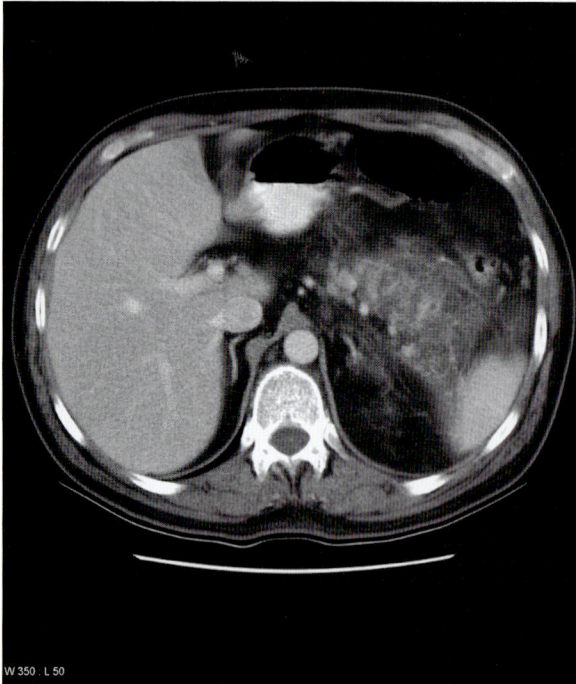

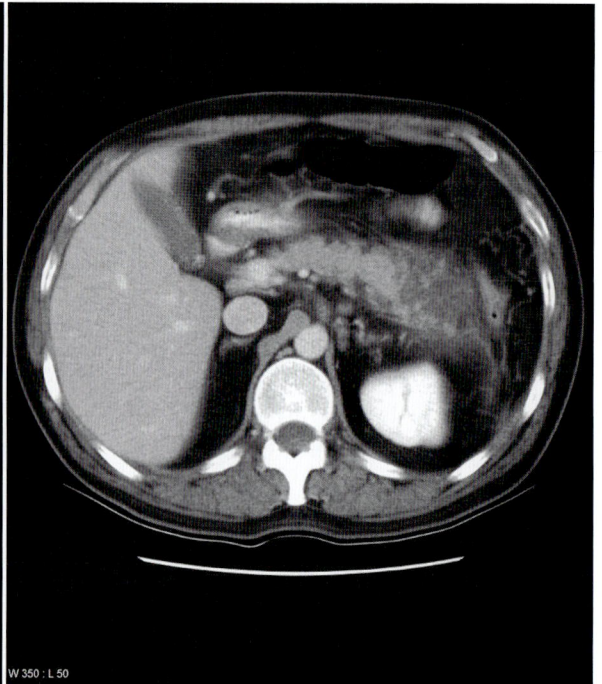

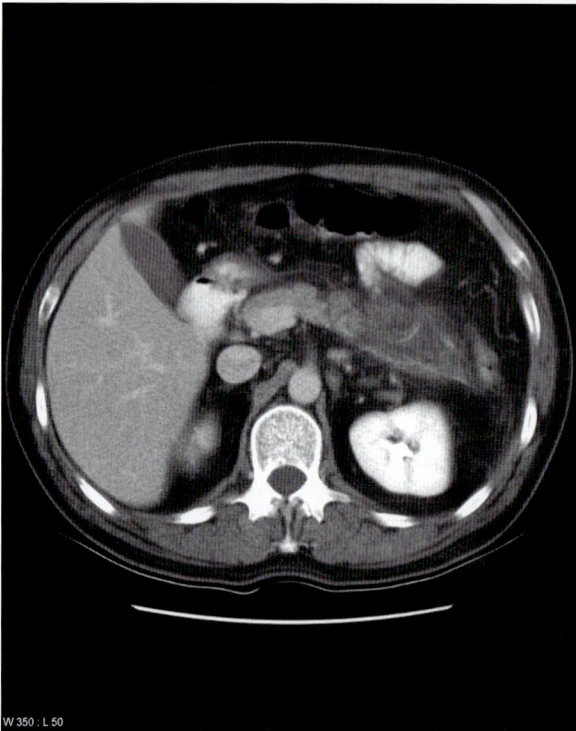

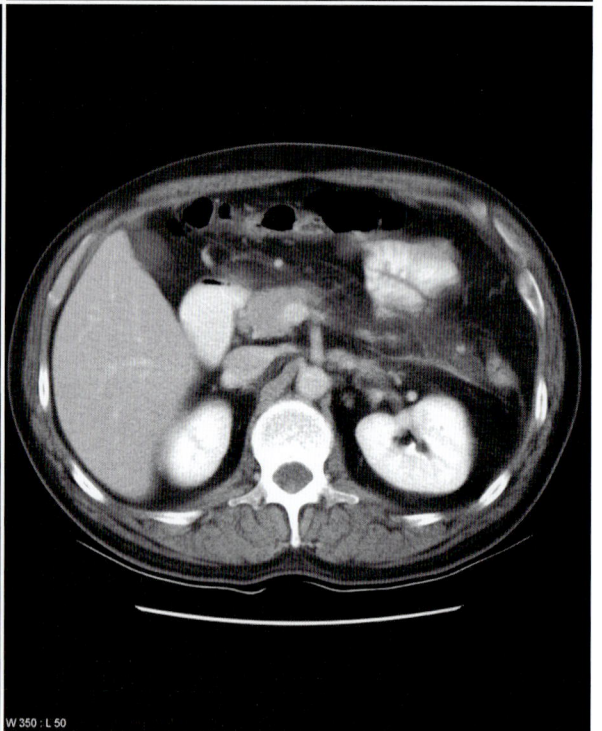

This 50-year-old alcoholic man was admitted to the ICU with severe abdominal pain, tachycardia and hypotension.

**Q** What pathological process is suggested by these images?

## A

The head of the pancreas appears normal. There is an inflammatory mass (phlegmon) centred on the body and tail of the pancreas. Most of the pancreas enhances well, but the tail does not enhance normally, suggesting pancreatic necrosis. There are inflammatory changes in the surrounding fat (fat stranding) with associated thickening of the perirenal (Gerota's) fascia.

There is no evidence of local complications of pancreatitis, such as fluid collections, pseudocysts, abscesses, pseudoaneurysm or haemorrhage. There are no gallstones seen on these images and the bile ducts are not obviously dilated.

## LEARNING POINT

The role of CT in acute pancreatitis is:
- diagnostic
- grading of severity
- identification of complications

The severity of pancreatitis may be graded on CT. The Balthazar Severity Index (Balthazar, 1990) has two components, which are combined to give a total score:
1. the findings on unenhanced CT (inflammation, fluid collections and gas in the tissues, both pancreatic and peripancreatic)
2. the amount of necrosis on contrast enhanced CT

Gallstones are a common cause of pancreatitis. A large proportion of gallbladder stones are not visible on CT. Ultrasound is a better modality for detecting gallstones.

## PROBLEM 2.18

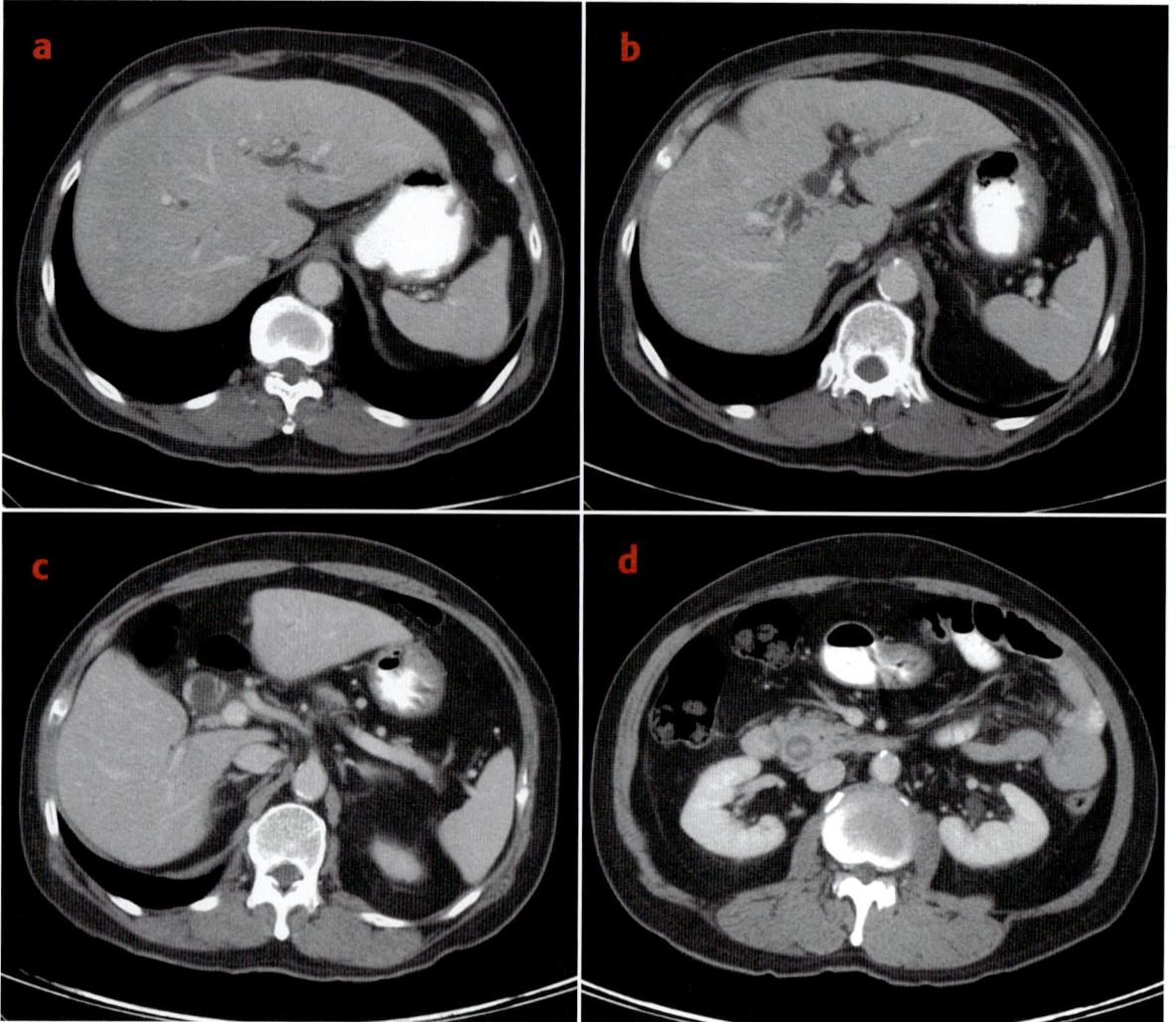

This 62-year-old man had a cholecystectomy three months ago. He now presents with jaundice and septic shock.

**Q** What problem do these images suggest?

## A

Within the liver there is a linear branching hypodensity, which lies adjacent to, but not within, the portal venous branches. This represents dilated intrahepatic bile ducts. The extrahepatic bile duct is markedly dilated and, at its distal end (image d), it contains a large calculus. The problem is obstruction of the common bile duct by a calculus that was not removed at the time of cholecystectomy. Biliary stones are often difficult to see on CT, as they may be poorly calcified or display a soft tissue density as in this case.

## LEARNING POINT

Biliary calculi may be missed at the time of cholecystectomy.

## PROBLEM 2.19

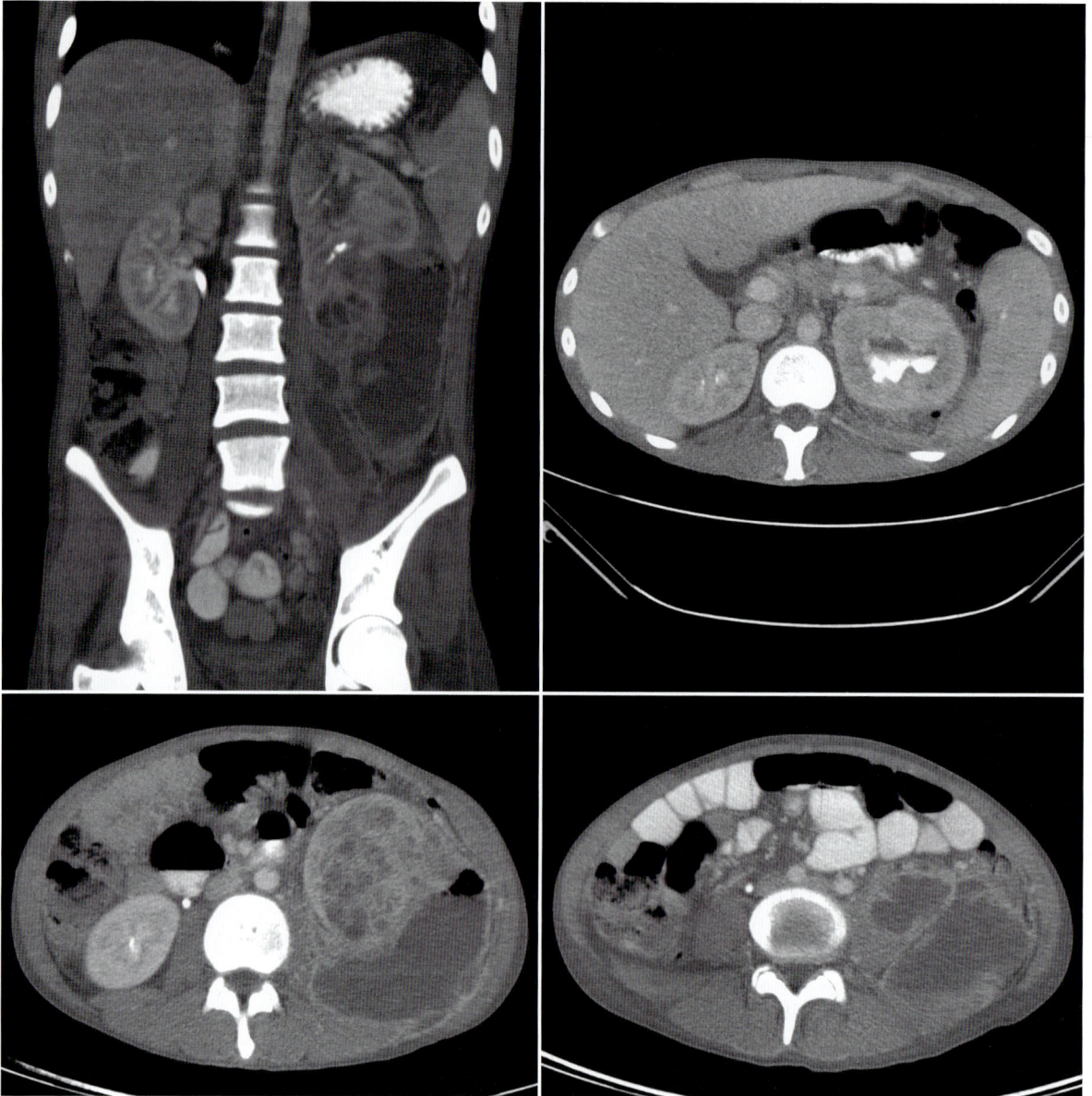

This 18-year-old man gave a one-week history of back pain, fevers and rigors. At presentation to the emergency department, he was in septic shock.

**Q** What problem is suggested by these images?

# A

There is a large multiloculated fluid collection in the retroperitoneum, involving the lower pole of the left kidney and extending down to the pelvis. There is rim enhancement and gas is seen within the collection. The left kidney is swollen and abnormal and there is calyceal dilatation consistent with obstruction. There is no parenchymal gas to suggest emphysematous pyelonephritis. The left psoas muscle is involved in the process. These findings are consistent with pyelonephritis complicated by intrarenal, perinephric and psoas abscess.

## LEARNING POINT

When a patient with acute pyelonephritis has severe sepsis, imaging should be performed to look for complications that require surgical treatment. These include emphysematous pyelonephritis (urgent nephrectomy), ureteric obstruction (stent or percutaneous nephrostomy) and perinephric abscess (percutaneous or surgical drainage).

The CT may be normal with uncomplicated pyelonephritis. Findings that suggest pyelonephritis include renal enlargement, focal swelling, thickening of Gerota's fascia and perinephric fat stranding. A patchy or striated nephrogram with wedge areas of decreased attenuation is also suggestive of the diagnosis in the correct clinical context (Dahnert, 2007).

## PROBLEM 2.20

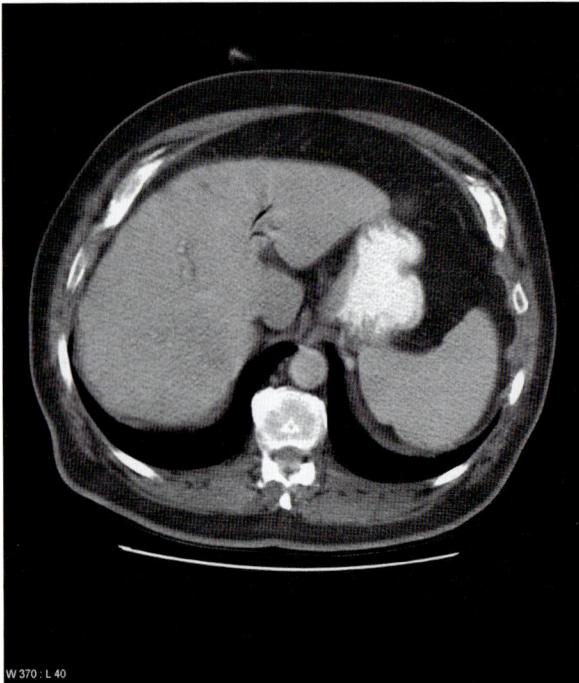

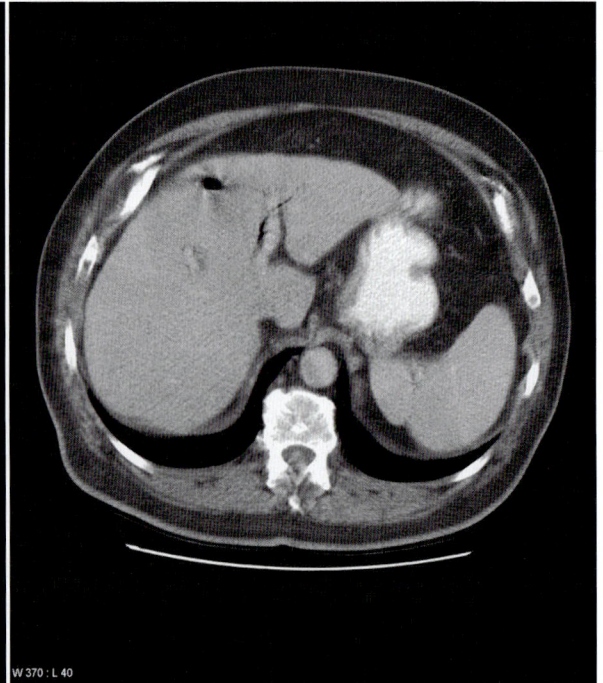

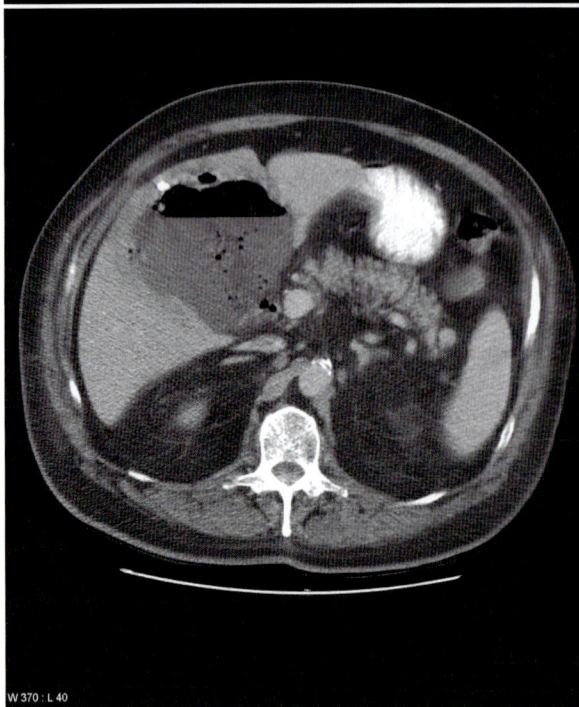

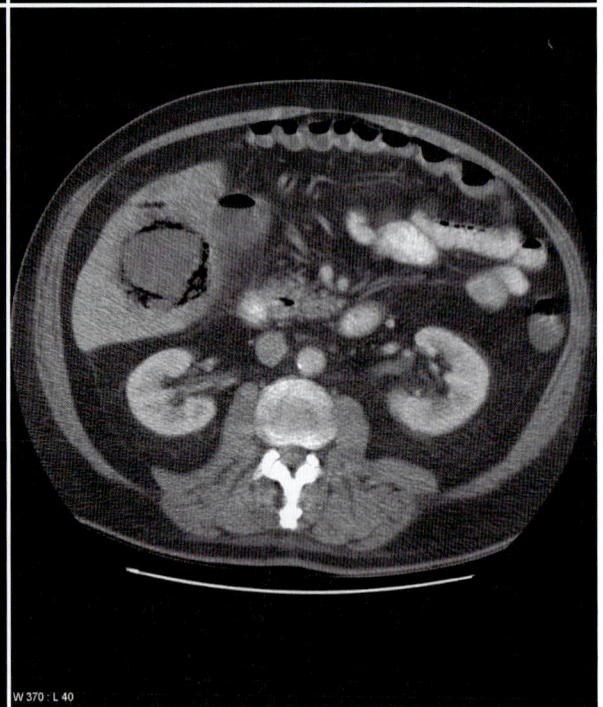

This 65-year-old man gave a one-week history of right upper quadrant pain. On presentation, he was jaundiced and rapidly developed septic shock.

**Q**
What problem do these images suggest?

# A

There is a large lesion in the liver, which contains gas and an air–fluid level. The gas in the liver substance has a branching linear pattern and does not extend to within 2 cm of the periphery of the liver. It is separate from the adjacent branch of the portal vein and consistent with pneumobilia.

There is also gas within the gallbladder.

These findings suggest a liver abscess and biliary sepsis with emphysematous cholecystitis. The liver lesion could be a tumour but, given the other findings, this is less likely.

## LEARNING POINT

Gas in the biliary tree is most commonly due to surgery or instrumentation of the biliary tree. Other causes include an incompetent sphincter of Oddi (sphincterotomy or passage of a gallstone), trauma, gallstone ileus, duodenal ulcer perforating into the bile duct, and severe biliary sepsis with emphysematous cholecystitis (Dahnert, 2007).

Common causes of pyogenic liver abscess include biliary tract disease, infection of organs with portal venous drainage (including appendicitis) and haematogenous spread during systemic bacteraemia. Non-pyogenic liver abscess may be due to amoebic or fungal infections. Abdominal CT and biliary tract ultrasound are helpful in delineating underlying causes of pyogenic liver abscesses (Dahnert, 2007).

## PROBLEM 2.21

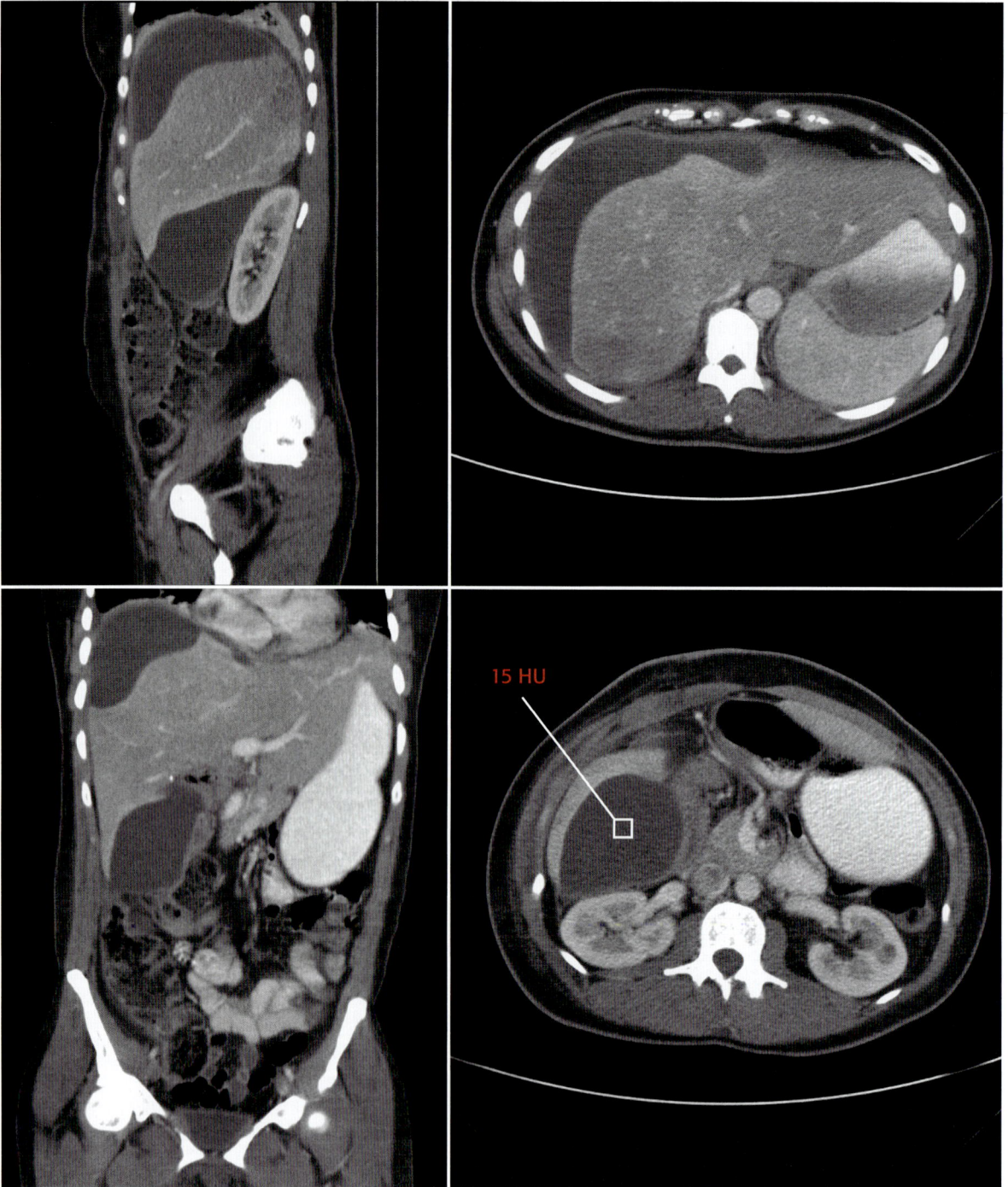

15 HU

This 36-year-old woman sustained an iatrogenic bile duct injury during cholecystectomy. This was managed with biliary reconstruction ten days ago. She now has abdominal pain and sepsis.

Q

What problem is suggested by these images?

**A**

There are large fluid collections in the right subphrenic and subhepatic spaces, with compression of the liver substance. Both demonstrate rim enhancement. The density of the collections is 10–15 Hounsfield units, consistent with fluid and most likely bile (see Chapter 6: Imaging modalities, p 374). In this clinical context, these findings are suggestive of a bile leak, with secondary subphrenic and subhepatic collections of infected bile.

**LEARNING POINT**

When a collection is seen on CT, measuring its density in Hounsfield units may help determine its composition (see Chapter 6: Imaging modalities, p 374 for more details).

## PROBLEM 2.22

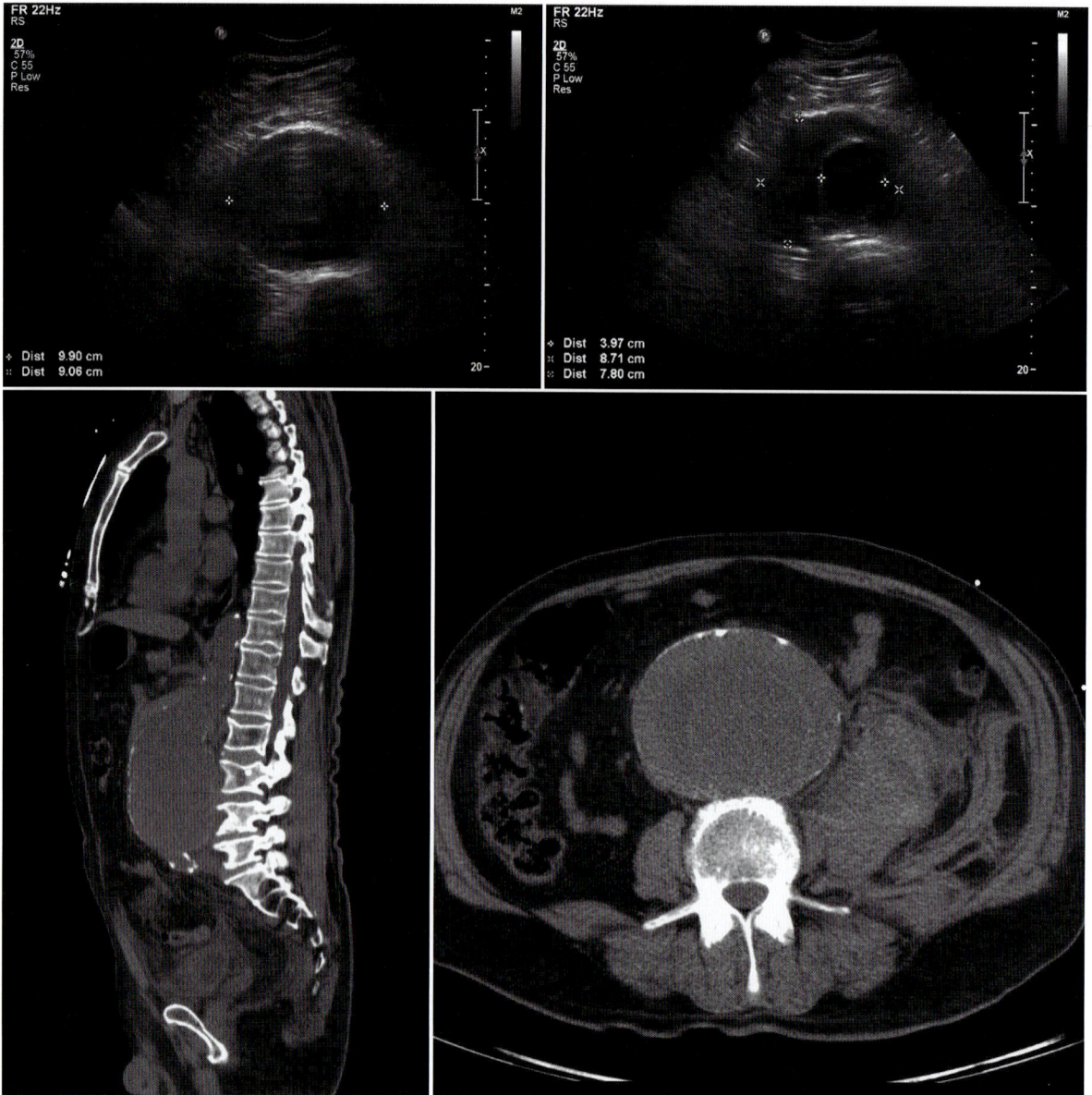

This 70-year-old man had a new onset of back pain. The blood pressure and heart rate were normal. A non-tender pulsatile mass was palpable in the abdomen, consistent with a known abdominal aortic aneurysm. This was being monitored with serial imaging by the vascular surgeons.

**Q** Does this patient need an urgent operation?

# A

There is a large (9.9 cm transverse diameter) abdominal aortic aneurysm seen on both the ultrasound and CT images. On the ultrasound images, there is a cresentic hypoechoic area adjacent to the patent lumen. It is uncertain on these images whether this represents a rupture of the aneurysm or thrombus within its lumen.

On the CT images, the aneurysm extends up to the level of the renal arteries and there is calcification in its wall. There is retroperitoneal haemorrhage adjacent to, and partly involving, the left psoas muscle. There is a crescentic luminal thrombus, corresponding to the hypoechoic area on the ultrasound. No free intraperitoneal blood is seen on the images in the book, though a small amount of pelvic fluid is seen on the DVD images. These findings suggest retroperitoneal rupture of the aneurysm and urgent surgery is indicated.

# LEARNING POINT

When the diagnosis of ruptured abdominal aortic aneurysm is suspected, an abdominal ultrasound can be performed rapidly by the bedside without delaying emergency surgery. If the patient is stable, CT is preferred as it will provide more information about the anatomy and pathological process, even in the absence of IV contrast administration.

## PROBLEM 2.23

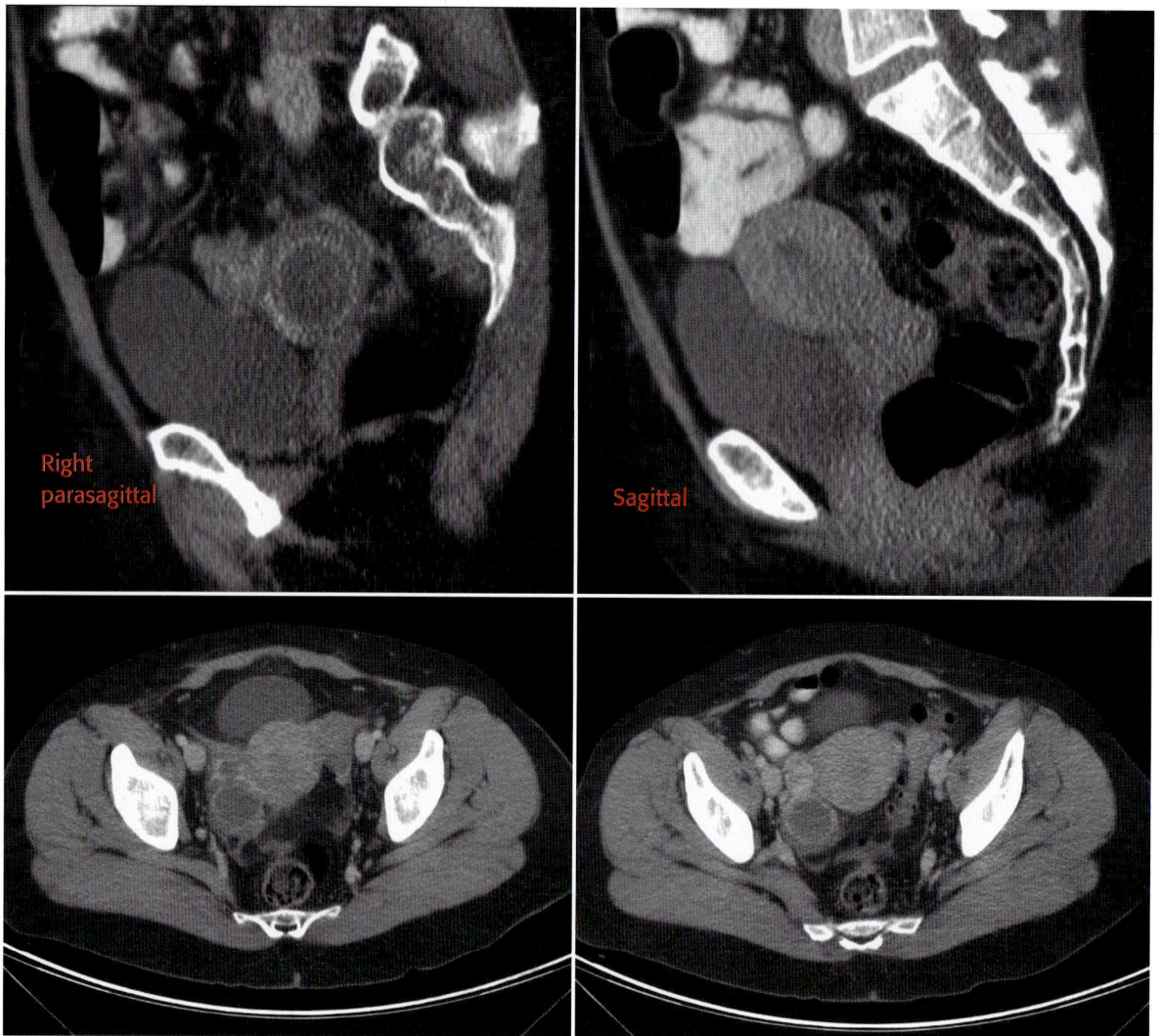

This 35-year-old woman had lower abdominal pain for two weeks and subsequently developed severe sepsis.

**Q**

What cause for her symptoms do these images suggest?

# A

A multilocular cystic lesion is seen within the right side of the pelvic cavity, with a thin enhancing wall. Inflammatory change and fat stranding is seen adjacent to this mass. It is intimately related to the right fallopian tube and ovary.

The differential diagnosis for the CT findings would include tubo-ovarian abscess, pyosalpinx, or acute haemorrhage/infection in a pre-existing ovarian cyst. Ovarian carcinoma would be less likely, particularly in this clinical context.

# LEARNING POINT

Gynaecological infection should be considered in the differential diagnosis of severe sepsis in a woman of reproductive age. Pelvic examination is mandatory when the clinical presentation is one of sepsis with no obvious site.

# PROBLEM 2.24

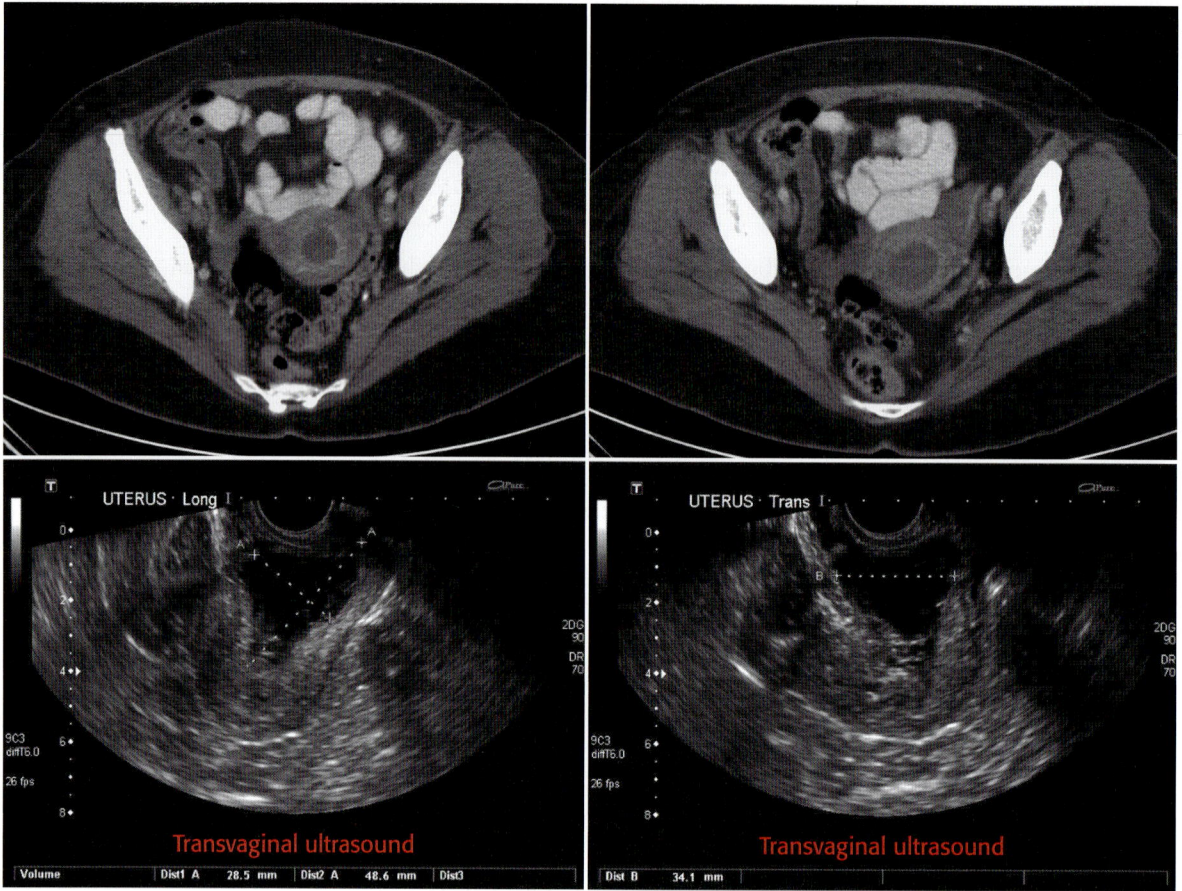

Transvaginal ultrasound

Transvaginal ultrasound

This 39-year-old woman delivered a healthy baby by caesarean section five weeks ago. She has been admitted to the ICU with septic shock.

**Q** What cause for her sepsis is suggested by these images?

# A

On the CT, the uterine cavity is enlarged and fluid filled. While this would be normal in the early postpartum period, by five weeks postpartum the size of the cavity should be almost normal. The endometrium is thickened and has enhanced with contrast.

On the transvaginal ultrasound, the uterine cavity is enlarged and contains hypoechoic fluid.

There are low-level internal echoes, consistent with complex fluid. The outline of the cavity is irregular, as is the interface between the endometrium and myometrium. In this clinical scenario, the findings of both the ultrasound and the CT are strongly suggestive of retained products of conception.

## LEARNING POINT

Sepsis from retained products of conception can occur following caesarean section and these are best imaged with ultrasound.

## PROBLEM 2.25

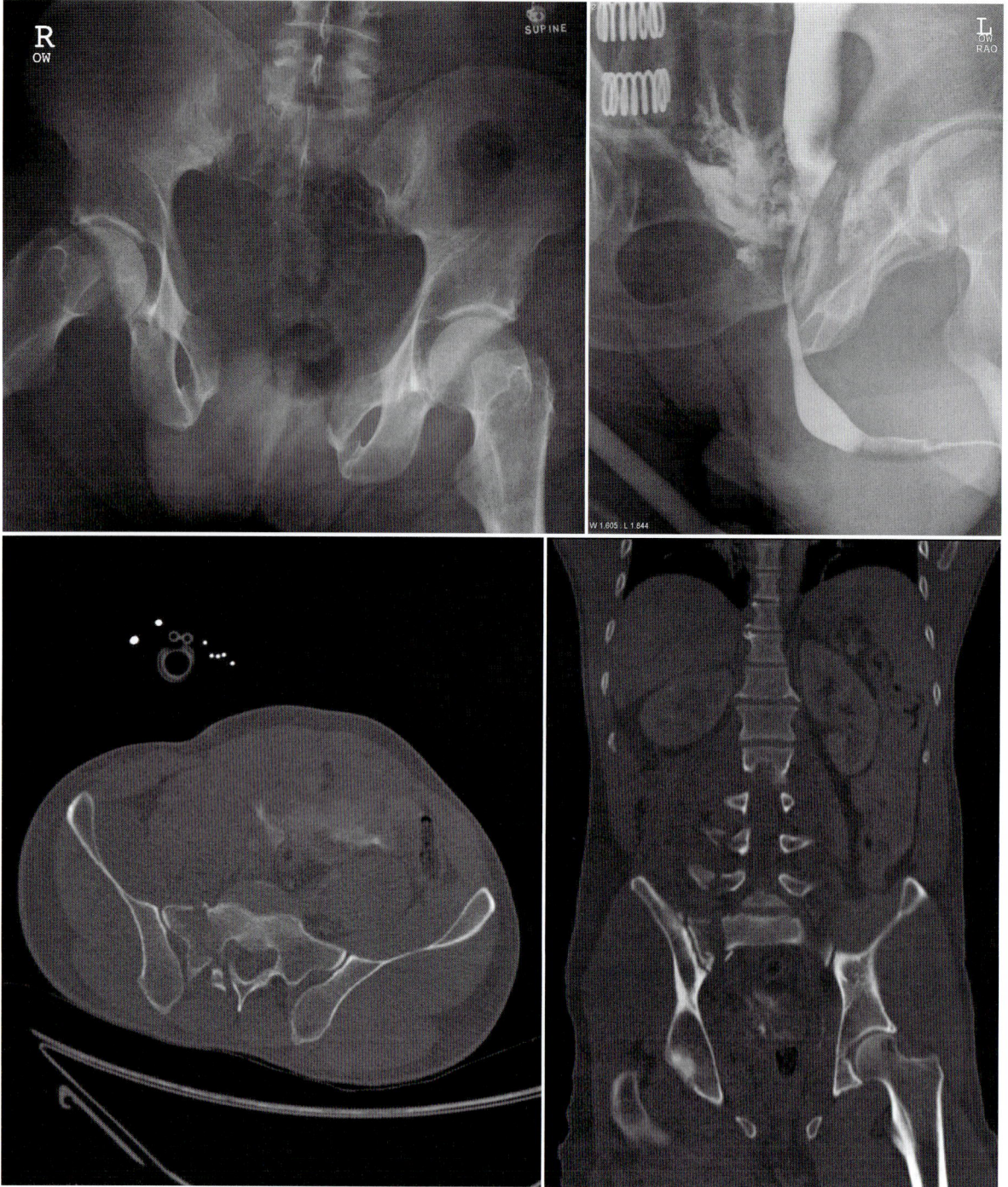

This 46-year-old man fell from a six metre high scaffold. A pelvis X-ray and retrograde urethrogram were performed in the emergency department with a subsequent CT scan.

**Q**

What injuries do the images demonstrate?

## A

There are fractures of the right L4 and L5 transverse processes. There is a vertical shear fracture of the right sacral ala and marked diastasis of the symphysis pubis. The sacroiliac joints are intact with no diastasis. Extravasation of contrast from the urinary system is seen from the urethra (on the retrograde urethrogram), but there is also contrast in the peritoneal cavity indicating a bladder rupture. On the DVD (not seen on images in the book), there is also a left L2 transverse process fracture and a minimally displaced fracture of the left superior pubic ramus.

These features suggest a vertical shear injury to the pelvis with associated bladder and urethral injury.

## LEARNING POINT

Pelvic fractures are classified according to the patterns of force creating the injury, into four categories: anteroposterior (AP) compression (characterised by external rotation of the hemipelvis), lateral compression (characterised by internal rotation of the hemipelvis), vertical shear and complex (a combination of more than one pattern of force) (Young, 1986; 1990).

Vertical shear injuries usually result from a fall. The sacrum is driven down between the iliac wings. Typical findings include vertical (sagittal) fractures through the sacrum and pubic rami. There may be fractures of the acetabular roof, symphysis pubis diastasis and vertical iliac wing fractures. Displacement of the hemipelvis is in a vertical direction (Young, 1990).

Bladder and urethral injury is common with major pelvic injury. Bladder rupture may be either into the peritoneal cavity or extraperitoneal. The commonest site of traumatic urethral rupture is in the membranous urethra, as this is a relatively fixed site.

## PROBLEM 2.26

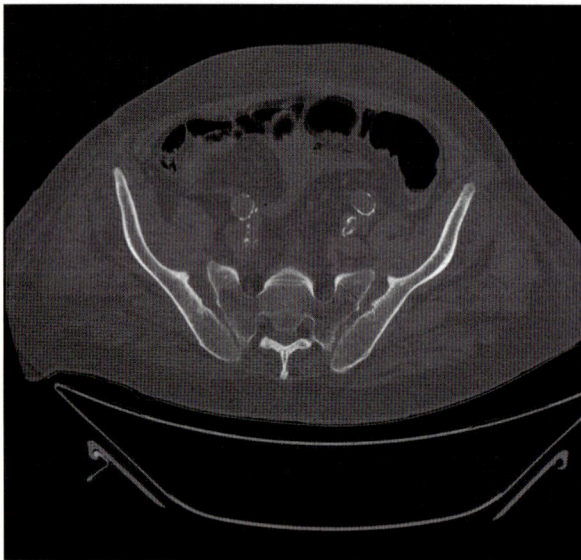

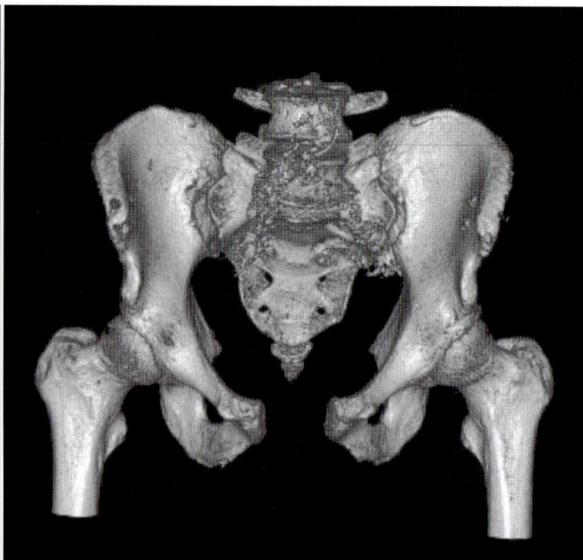

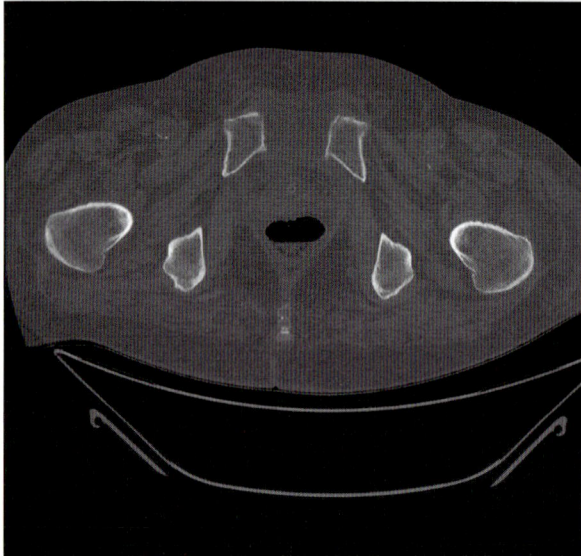

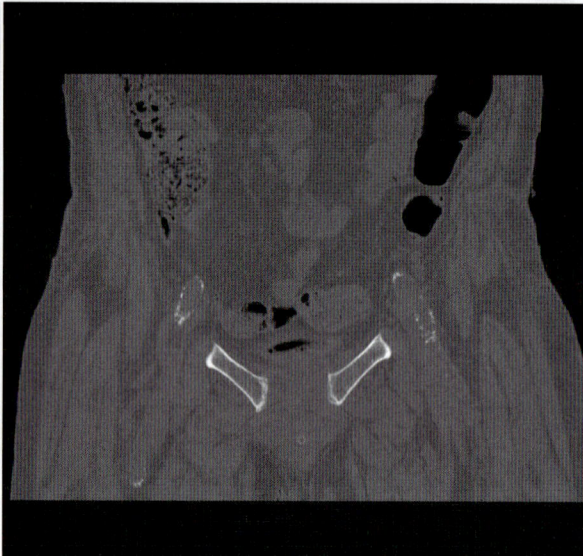

This 74-year-old man was injured in a high-speed car crash earlier today. His pelvis feels unstable on clinical examination.

**Q**

Describe the pelvic injury.

## A

There is wide diastasis of the symphysis pubis, well in excess of 2.5 cm. Both sacroiliac joints are widened anteriorly. No bony fractures are seen. These findings are in keeping with an AP compression injury.

There is incidental calcification in the iliac arteries. On the DVD, the astute reader may note pin tracts in the ilium from previous instrumentation, a lytic lesion in the left ilium, which may be a cyst or enchondroma, and bilateral hip osteoarthritis.

## LEARNING POINT

AP compression injury commonly occurs in a motor vehicle crash. Typically, the anterior pelvis is disrupted, which causes either symphysis diastasis or vertical (sagittal) fractures of the pubic rami. When the trauma is more severe, there is splaying of the anterior pelvis, with external rotation of one or both hemipelvises. If this occurs, the sacroiliac joint on the side of the rotated hemipelvis is disrupted, with the posterior part of the sacroiliac joint acting as a hinge. Sacral fractures are rare and iliac wing fractures are not part of this injury pattern. Fractures of the posterior acetabulum are common (often due to posteriorly directed forces from the flexed femur impacting on the dashboard), though anterior acetabular fractures may occur (Young, 1990).

If the ligaments of the symphysis pubis are completely divided, but this is the only injury, the amount of diastasis is limited to 2.5 cm because of the posterior ligamentous structures. Symphysis pubis diastasis of greater than 2.5 cm implies additional injury to the posterior ligaments of the pelvis (Young, 1990).

An important feature distinguishing AP from lateral compression injury is that the pubic rami fractures are vertical (sagittal) in an AP compression injury but horizontal (coronal) in a lateral compression injury (Young, 1990).

## PROBLEM 2.27

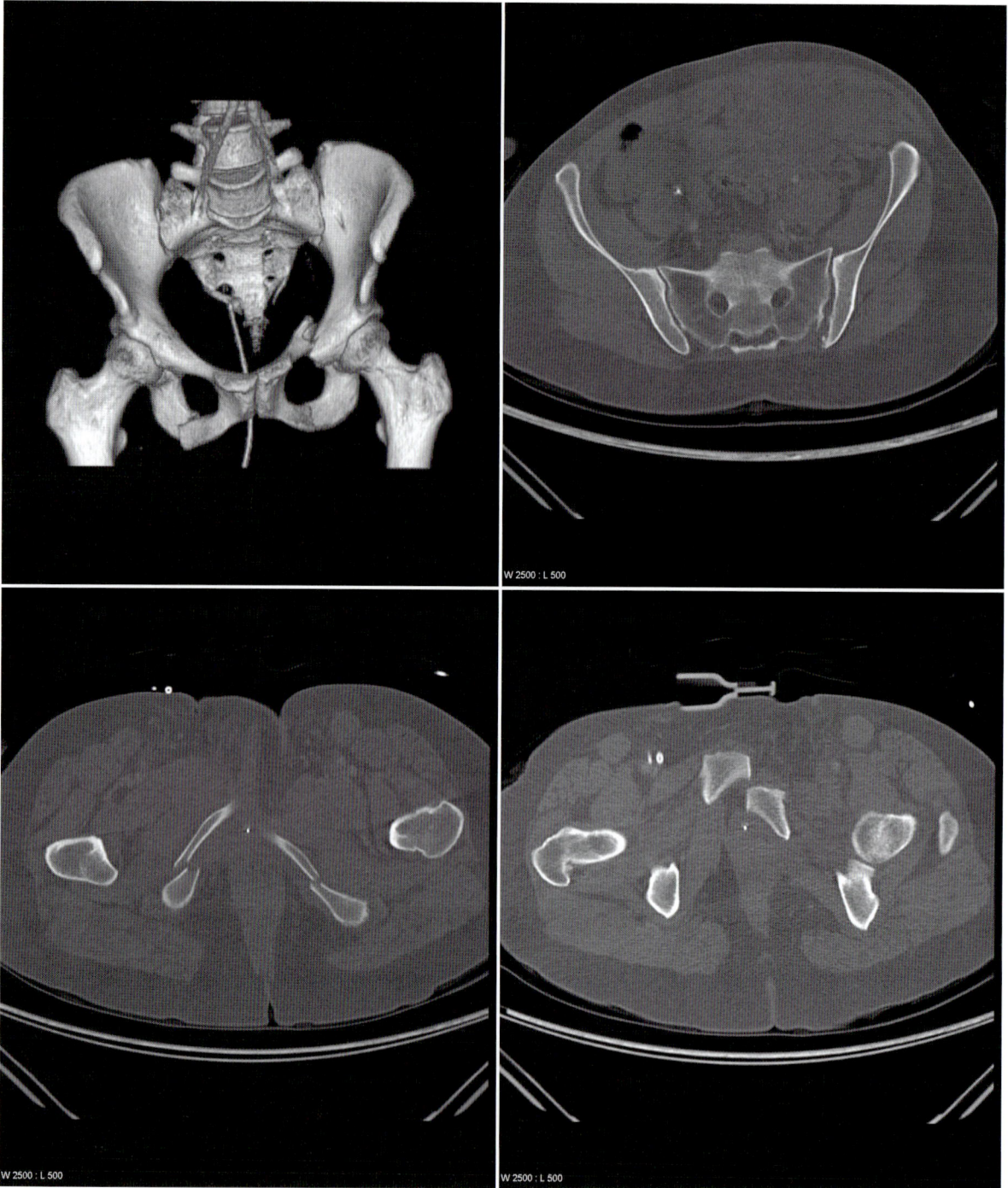

This 36-year-old woman survived a single vehicle rollover car crash, in which two people died. She is complaining of severe pain in her lower abdomen and groin.

## Q
What mechanism of injury do these images suggest?

## A

There are horizontal (coronal) fractures of both inferior pubic rami. There is also a fracture of the superior ramus on the left. The symphysis pubis is disrupted such that the right pubic bone lies in front of the left, with slight overlap. The left sacroiliac joint is disrupted, with predominantly posterior widening. The left hemipelvis is rotated internally, hinging on the anterior aspect of the sacroiliac joint. These features are in keeping with a lateral compression injury.

## LEARNING POINT

Lateral compression injuries typically cause horizontal (coronal) fractures of the pubic rami and impacted fractures of the sacrum may occur. When the trauma is more severe the affected hemipelvis rotates internally, either disrupting the ipsilateral sacroiliac joint with the anterior aspect of this joint acting as a pivot or obliquely fracturing the ipsilateral iliac wing. If enough force is applied the contralateral hemipelvis may rotate externally. There may be fractures of the medial acetabulum, with central hip dislocation (Young, 1990).

## PROBLEM 2.28

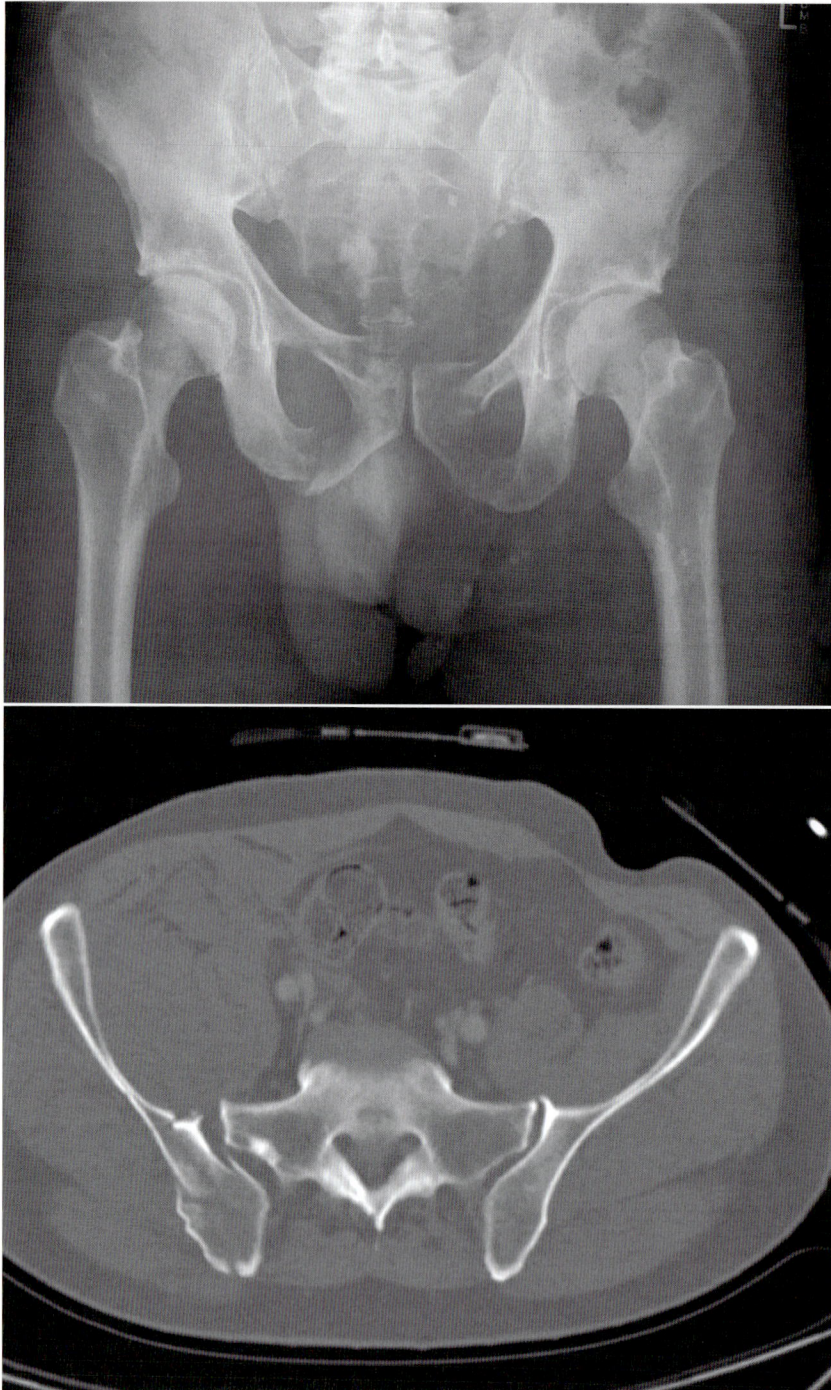

This 57-year-old man was in a high-speed car crash. He was intubated at the scene because of severe respiratory distress.

Q

What is the likely mechanism of injury to the pelvis?

## A

The right sacroiliac joint is disrupted, with both anterior and posterior widening. There is some posterior displacement of the hemipelvis, but minimal rotation. This pattern would be in keeping with an AP compression component to the injury. However, there is also an oblique fracture of the iliac wing, which is not typical of an AP compression injury and more in keeping with a lateral compression injury.

There are fractures of all four pubic rami. On the DVD, it can be seen that the inferior rami fractures are horizontal (coronal), in keeping with lateral compression. The superior ramus fracture on the left is vertical (parasagittal), in keeping with AP compression. On the other hand, the fracture on the right is in the axial plane.

Features of more than one injury pattern are present (AP compression and lateral compression), so this is classified as a "complex pattern" injury.

There is also a large retroperitoneal haematoma in the region of the right iliacus muscle, adjacent to the sacroiliac joint injury.

## LEARNING POINT

Not all pelvic injuries fit into the simple classification of AP compression, lateral compression and vertical shear. One in four pelvic injuries has elements of more than one of these patterns (Young, 1990).

## PROBLEM 2.29

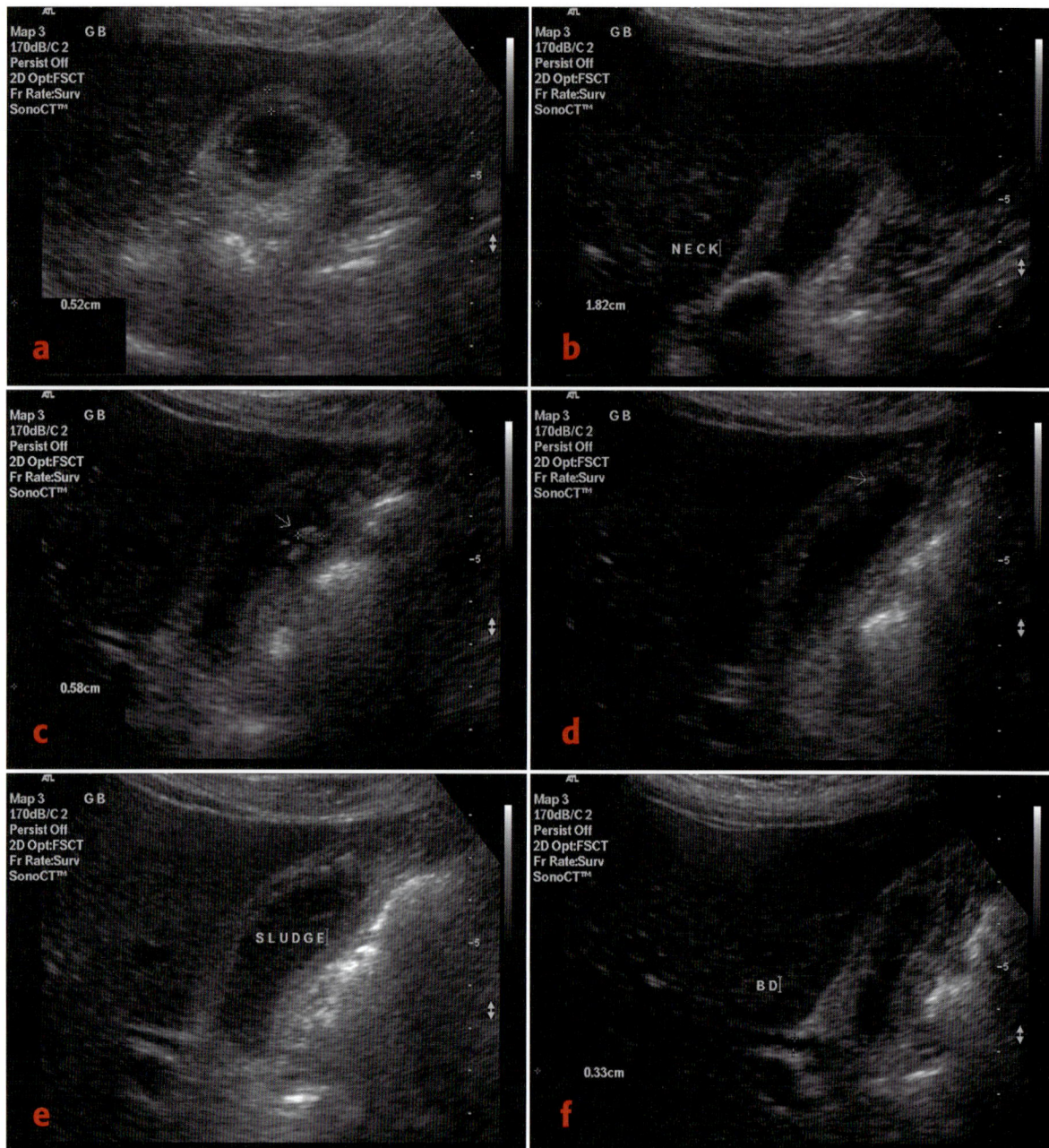

This 40-year-old woman presented with right upper quadrant abdominal pain and was admitted to the ICU with septic shock.

**Q** What pathological process do these ultrasound images of the gallbladder suggest?

# A

There is marked thickening of the gallbladder wall, which is hypoechoic between its inner and outer aspects indicating oedema. There is a large calculus at the neck of the gallbladder and also several smaller calculi in the dependent aspect of the body of the gallbladder. There is also sludge seen within the gallbladder. These findings are strongly suggestive of acute calculous cholecystitis. Pericholecystic fluid is commonly seen with cholecystitis, but is not demonstrated in these images.

In image d, there are small echogenic foci in the non-dependent gallbladder wall. While the appearance could be confused with gallstones, gallstones move with gravity and should be dependent. This finding suggests adenomyomatosis, which can also cause thickening of the gallbladder wall.

There is no extra-hepatic biliary duct dilatation (upper limit of normal 5 mm with gallbladder present, 8 mm following cholecystectomy) (Dahnert, 2007).

## LEARNING POINT

Ultrasound is a better investigation than CT for biliary disease. It has the added advantage that the images can be acquired at the bedside, avoiding transport of the critically ill patient. If ultrasound is equivocal, HIDA radioisotope scan is an alternative investigation, though its role in the critically ill patient is not well established.

Features of acute cholecystitis on ultrasound include (Dahnert, 2007):
- thickening of the gallbladder wall (upper limit of normal 3 mm)
- distension of the gallbladder (diameter > 4 cm, length > 10 cm)
- pericholecystic fluid
- sonographic Murphy sign (pain when probe is pushed onto the gallbladder)
- air in the gallbladder wall (suggests emphysematous cholecystitis)

Interpretation of ultrasounds for assessing biliary disease may be complex in critically ill patients; patients that are starved or on TPN often have sludge in the gallbladder.

When patients with cholecystitis have no gallstones in the gallbladder, they have acalculous cholecystitis. This condition accounts for around 10% of cases of cholecystitis and has a higher morbidity and mortality than calculous cholecystitis. The incidence is higher in critically ill patients (Kimura, 2007; Yasuda, 2007).

# PROBLEM 2.30

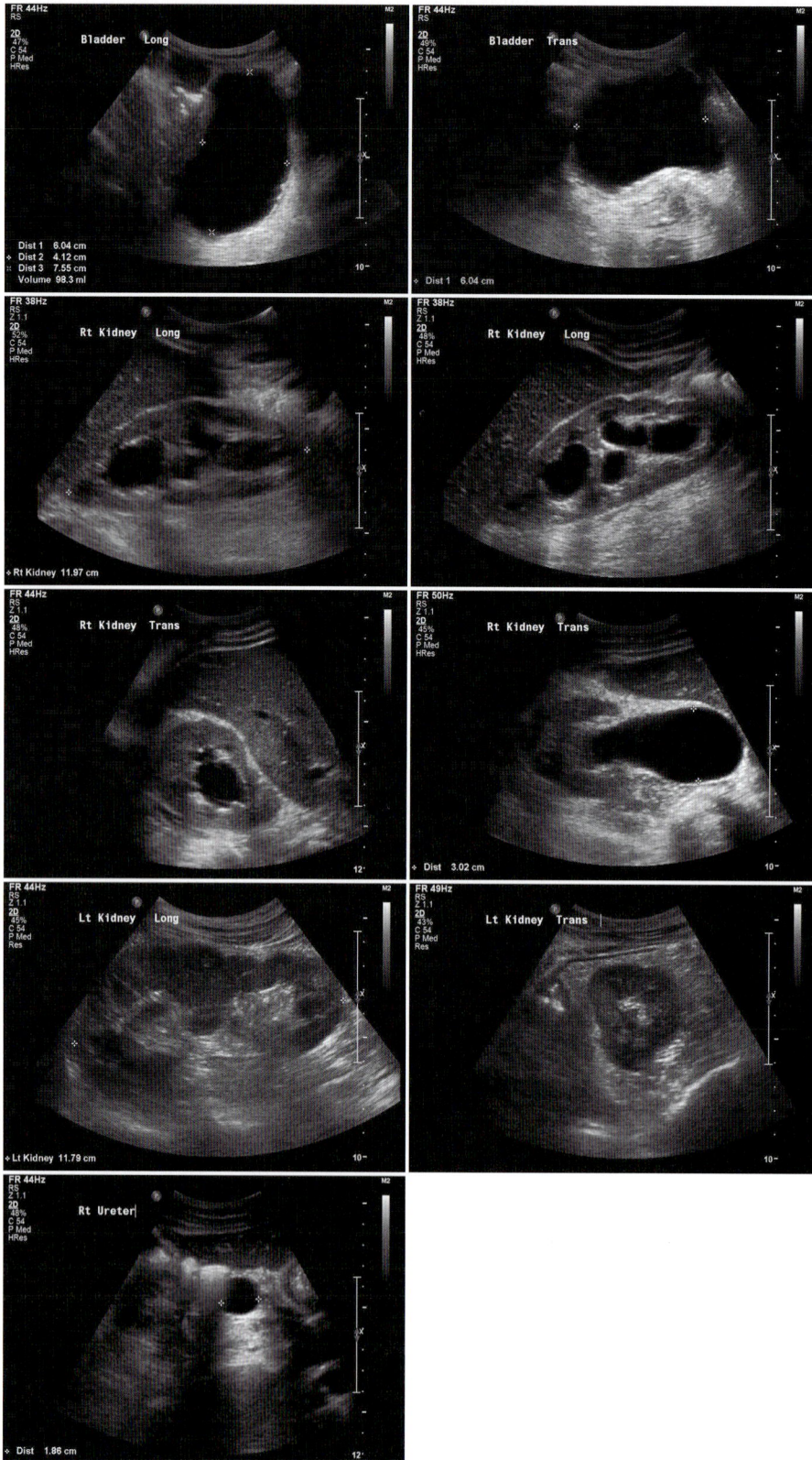

This 69-year-old man presented with lethargy and malaise and was found to be in acute renal failure. An ultrasound of the renal tract was performed.

## Q

What condition is demonstrated by these images?

## A

On the right side, there is significant calyceal dilatation and associated dilatation of the extrarenal pelvis and ureter. The kidneys are of normal size (9–12 cm in longitudinal axis) (Barozzi, 2007). The residual volume in the bladder is normal. The left kidney and ureter are normal. These findings are in keeping with right ureteric obstruction, though hydronephrosis may occur in the absence of obstruction. These findings alone cannot explain the acute renal failure, as renal failure should not develop with a normally functioning non-obstructed kidney on one side.

## LEARNING POINT

Obstruction must be excluded in patients with acute renal failure, as it is readily treatable. Ultrasound is the imaging modality of choice to assess for obstructive uropathy. Typically, it demonstrates dilation in the calyces or renal pelvis (Klahr, 2007).

Significant obstruction may occur without urinary system dilatation in some conditions. Examples of this include (Klahr, 2007; Kulkarni, 2005):

- acute obstruction, if the patient is volume depleted and has a low urinary output
- when the urinary system is encased in retroperitoneal tumour or fibrosis, although there is often dilated ureter proximal to the area of encasement

## PROBLEM 2.31

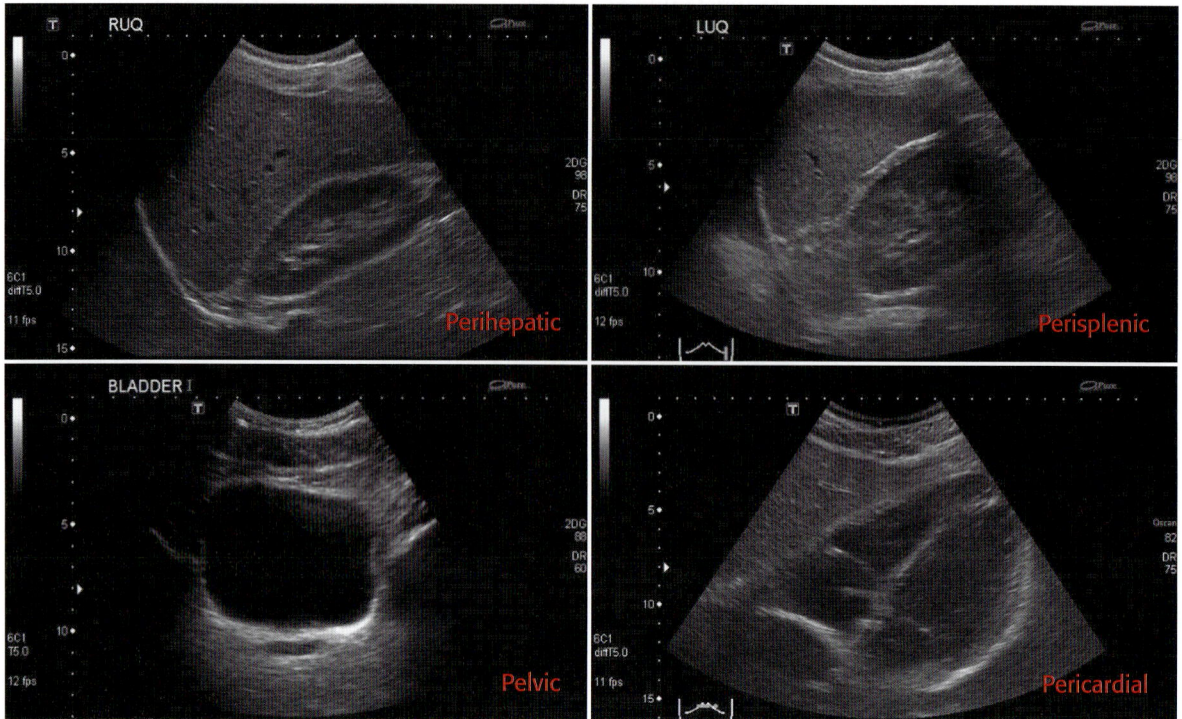

This 21-year-old man was a passenger in a high-speed car crash. This FAST scan was done 10 minutes after arrival in the emergency department because of hypotension. The hypotension responded to intravenous fluids, but 30 minutes after arrival the patient has become hypotensive again.

**Q**
1. What is your interpretation of these images?
2. Is there any point in repeating the FAST scan?

# A

1. This is a normal FAST scan.

2. Yes, the clinical scenario is highly suggestive of significant haemorrhage. If there has been ongoing haemorrhage into the abdomen, the volume of blood may have reached a point where it can be detected by FAST scan.

## Learning point

The Focussed Assessment with Sonography in Trauma (FAST) scan consists of perihepatic (including hepatorenal pouch), perisplenic, pelvic, and pericardial views. Depending on the expertise of the sonographer, these four "P" views may be supplemented by further views. Supplementary views allow more detailed assessment of organs and examination of other sites in which free fluid collects such as the paracolic gutters, but this takes longer in what may be a time-critical situation (Kirkpatrick, 2007).

FAST scans are good at detecting major intra-abdominal haemorrhage, but poor at detecting visceral perforation. A normal FAST scan at presentation does not rule out intra-abdominal bleeding, because early after injury the volume of blood in the peritoneal cavity may be too small to see. If there is continued bleeding, the volume of blood may increase to a point where it can be detected by sonography. Serial FAST scans have a higher sensitivity for intra-abdominal injury than a single scan (Kirkpatrick, 2007).

## REFERENCES

Balthazar EJ, Robinson DL, Megibow AJ, et al. Acute pancreatitis: Value of CT in establishing prognosis. Radiology 1990; 174(2): 331–6

Barozzi L, Valentino M, Santoro A, et al. Renal ultrasonography in critically ill patients. Crit Care Med 2007; 35(5 Suppl): S198–205

Batke M, Cappell MS. Adynamic ileus and acute colonic pseudo-obstruction. Med Clin North Am 2008; 92(3): 649–70

Curtin KR, Fitzgerald SW, Nemcek AA, et al. CT diagnosis of acute appendicitis: Imaging findings. Am J Roentgenol 1995; 164(4): 905–9

Dahnert W, ed. Radiology review manual. 6th edn. Philadelphia: Lippincott Williams and Wilkins; 2007

Dodds WJ, Darweesh RM, Lawson TL, et al. The retroperitoneal spaces revisited. Am J Roentgenol 1986; 147(6): 1155–61

Jain RK, Jain M, Rajak CL, et al. Imaging in acute appendicitis: a review. Indian J Radiol Imaging 2006; 16(4): 523–32

Khan AN, MacDonald S, Chandramohan M. Pneumoperitoneum. emedicine. In Lamki N, Coombs BD, Gay SB, Krasny EM, Lin EC. eds. WebMD: 2008. Available: http://emedicine.medscape.com/article/372053-overview; accessed 7 May 2009

Kimura Y, Takada T, Kawarada Y, et al. Definitions, pathophysiology, and epidemiology of acute cholangitis and cholecystitis: Tokyo guidelines. J Hepatobiliary Pancreat Surg 2007; 14(1): 15–26

Kirkpatrick AW. Clinician-performed focused sonography for the resuscitation of trauma. Crit Care Med 2007; 35(5 Suppl): S162–72

Klahr S. Chapter 25: Urinary tract obstruction. In: Schrier RW, ed. Diseases of the kidney & urinary tract. 8th edn. Philadelphia: Lippincott, Williams and Wilkins; 2007: 689–716

Knechtle SJ, Davidoff AM, Rice RP. Pneumatosis intestinalis: surgical management and clinical outcome. Ann Surg 1990; 212(2): 160–5

Kulkarni S, Jayachandran M, Davies A, et al. Non-dilated obstructed pelvicalyceal system. Int J Clin Pract 2005; 59(8): 992–4

Matsumoto S, Mori H, Okino Y, et al. Computed tomographic imaging of abdominal volvulus: pictorial essay. Can Assoc Radiol J 2004; 55(5): 297–303

Moore CJ, Corl FM, Fishman EK. CT of cecal volvulus: Unraveling the image. Am J Roentgenol 2001; 177(1): 95–8

Nicolaou S, Kai B, Ho S, et al. Imaging of acute small-bowel obstruction. Am J Roentgenol 2005; 185(4): 1036–44

Tinkoff G, Esposito TJ, Reed J, et al. American association for the surgery of trauma organ injury scale I: spleen, liver, and kidney, validation based on the national trauma data bank. J Am Coll Surg 2008; 207(5): 646–55

Yasuda H, Takada T, Kawarada Y, et al. Unusual cases of acute cholecystitis and cholangitis: Tokyo guidelines. J Hepatobiliary Pancreat Surg 2007; 14(1): 98–113

Yoon W, Jeong YY, Kim JK, et al. CT in blunt liver trauma. Radiographics 2005; 25(1): 87–104

Young JW, Resnik CS. Fracture of the pelvis: Current concepts of classification. Am J Roentgenol 1990; 155(6): 1169–75

Young JW, Burgess AR, Brumback RJ, et al. Pelvic fractures: Value of plain radiography in early assessment and management. Radiology 1986; 160(2): 445–51

# CHAPTER 3

# HEAD

# APPLIED ANATOMY

## Structures seen on cranial CT scan
(Figure 3.1)

### Brainstem
The brainstem consists of the medulla oblongata, pons and midbrain. The internal structure of the brainstem is poorly seen on CT because of the beam-hardening artefact (seen as linear streaks and bands) caused by the adjacent petrous bones. As the midbrain passes through the tentorial hiatus, it lies posteromedial to the uncinate process of the temporal lobe (uncus). With intracranial hypertension, the uncus may herniate, compressing the midbrain.

### CSF spaces
The basal cisterns are expansions of the subarachnoid space at the base of the brain and around the brainstem. The suprasellar cistern is superior to the pituitary gland and anterior to the midbrain. The quadrigeminal cistern lies posterior to the midbrain. The ambient cistern wraps around the pituitary gland and midbrain, connecting the suprasellar and quadrigeminal cisterns. The prepontine cistern lies directly anterior to the pons, and the paired cerebellopontine cisterns lie anterolateral to the pons and anterior to the adjacent part of the cerebellum. The premedullary and cerebellomedullary cisterns have a similar relationship to the medulla oblongata and adjacent cerebellum. The cisterna magna lies posterior to the medulla oblongata, anterior to the occipital bone, and inferior to the cerebellar vermis (Harnsberger, 2006).

Within the foramen magnum, the medulla oblongata is separated from the occipital bone by cerebrospinal fluid within the cisterna magna. The cerebellar tonsils are not normally seen at this level. If there is intracranial hypertension (or a Chiari malformation) the tonsils may herniate down into the foramen magnum and appear posterolateral to the medulla oblongata. Intracranial hypertension may also efface or obliterate the basal cisterns.

The ventricular system consists of the fourth ventricle, which lies between the pons/medulla oblongata and the cerebellum, the slit-like third ventricle, and the paired lateral ventricles. The third and fourth ventricles communicate via the cerebral aqueduct, while the third and the two lateral ventricles communicate by the Y-shaped interventricular foramen of Monro. Each lateral ventricle has a body, an anterior horn an occipital horn, and a temporal horn. Dilatation of the temporal horn is an early sign of hydrocephalus.

### Basal ganglia and thalamus
The components of the basal ganglia are the caudate nucleus and the lentiform nucleus (consisting of the putamen and globus pallidus). The caudate nucleus lies lateral to the anterior horn of the lateral ventricle and is separated from the lentiform nucleus by the anterior limb of the internal capsule. The lentiform nucleus is closely applied to the lateral aspect of the internal capsule.

The thalamus lies lateral to the third ventricle. It is separated from the lentiform nucleus by the posterior limb of the internal capsule (Harnsberger, 2006).

### White matter structures
Fibres pass between the brainstem and the cortex in the internal capsule and optic radiation. They diverge to form a radiating white matter mass, the corona radiata, which lies lateral to the lateral ventricles (Harnsberger, 2006).

In the centre of each cerebral hemisphere, above the level of the lateral ventricle, lies a mass of white matter known as the centrum semiovale. The corpus callosum connects the cerebral hemispheres. It forms the roof of the lateral ventricle and the anterior wall of the anterior horns of the lateral ventricles (Nakano, 1995).

## Lobes of the brain (Figure 3.2)
To identify the boundaries of the lobes, the central sulcus and the Sylvian fissure should be sought. The central sulcus is best identified on sagittal images, and on axial images it is identified in the superior cuts. It is the longest and most prominent sulcus and lies in the posterior half of the image. In older people with some cerebral atrophy, it is usually easily seen, but in young people, it may not be visible. The Sylvian fissure is usually easily seen in both age groups.

The frontal lobe is the anterior part of the cerebral hemisphere and rests in the anterior cranial fossa. It lies in front of the central sulcus and above the Sylvian fissure. The temporal lobe rests in the middle cranial fossa and lies below the Sylvian fissure, which separates it from the frontal lobe. Deep to the Sylvian fissure, adjacent to the frontal and temporal lobes is the insula. The occipital lobe is the posterior part of the cerebral hemisphere and rests on the tentorium cerebelli. The parietal lobe lies posterior to the central sulcus, which separates it from the frontal lobe, and anterior to the parietooccipital sulcus, which separates it from the occipital lobe.

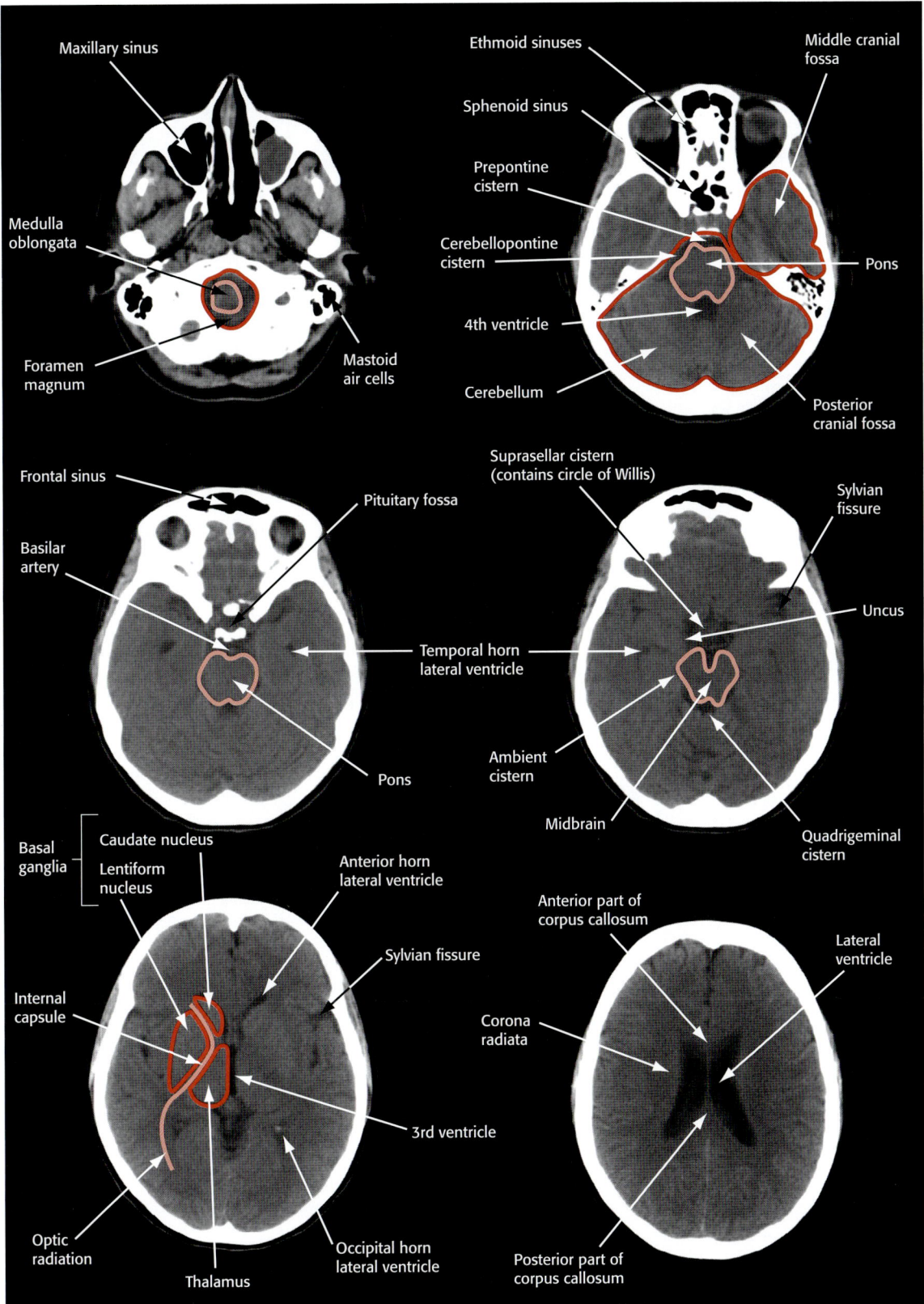

**FIGURE 3.1** Structures seen on cranial CT scan.

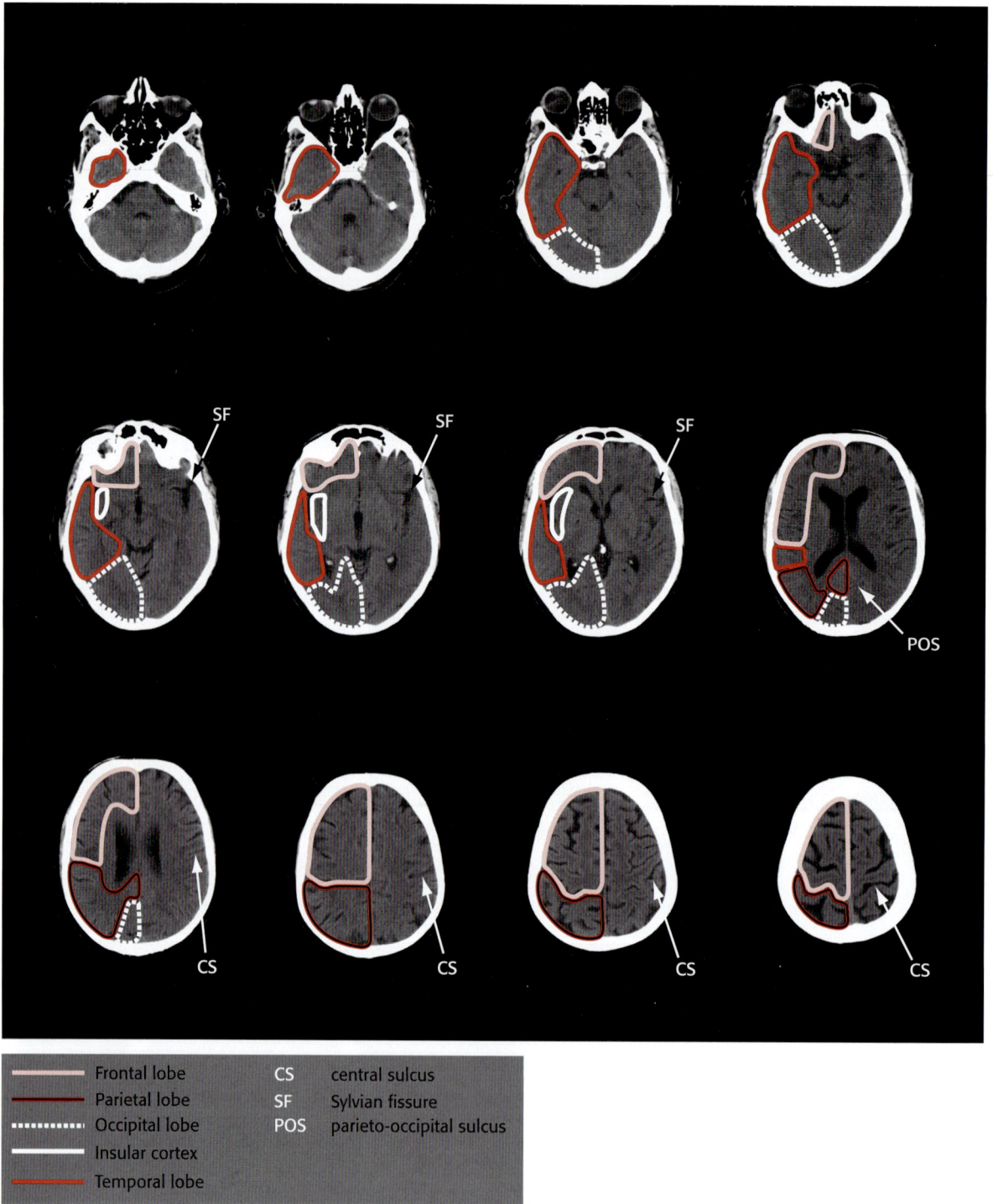

| | | | |
|---|---|---|---|
| —— | Frontal lobe | CS | central sulcus |
| —— | Parietal lobe | SF | Sylvian fissure |
| ········· | Occipital lobe | POS | parieto-occipital sulcus |
| —— | Insular cortex | | |
| —— | Temporal lobe | | |

**FIGURE 3.2** Lobes of the brain. Adapted from Moeller and Reif, 2000.

## Vascular territories (Figure 3.3)

The brain in entirely supplied by blood from branches of the two vertebral and two carotid arteries. The branches of the carotid artery give rise to the anterior circulation. The vertebral arteries join to form the basilar artery. The branches of the vertebral and basilar arteries give rise to the posterior circulation. The anterior and posterior circulations

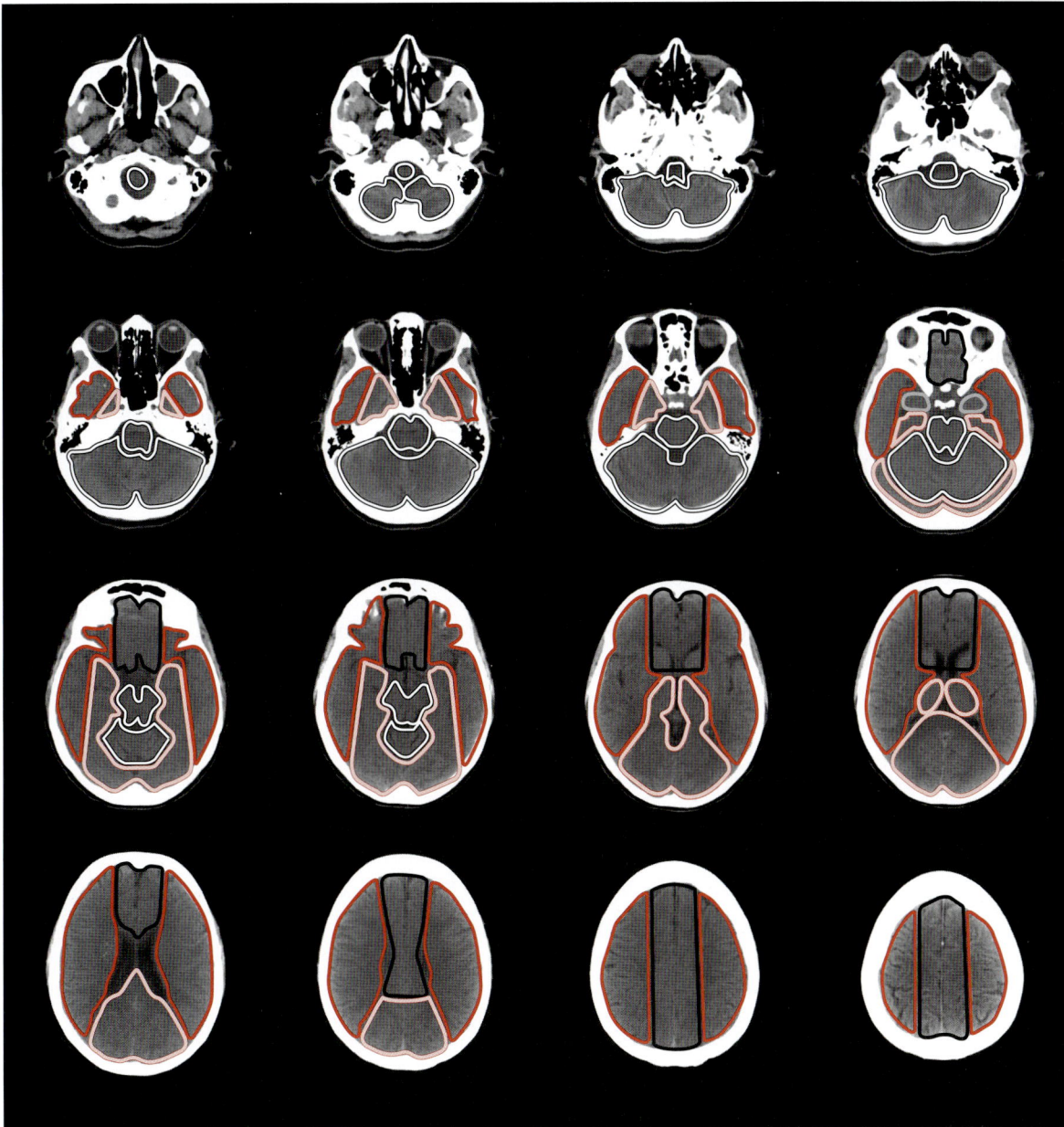

Anterior choroidal arteries
Anterior cerebral arteries
Middle cerebral arteries
Posterior cerebral arteries
Other areas supplied by the posterior circulation

**FIGURE 3.3** Vascular supply of the brain. Adapted from Moeller and Reif, 2000.

are joined by two posterior communicating arteries (PCOM), one of which passes from the carotid artery to the posterior cerebral artery on each side. The distribution of blood supply is highly variable.

The commonest distribution is described here (Carpenter, 1991; Berman, 1980; Hayman, 1981; Berman, 1984).

## Anterior circulation

The intracranial branches of the carotid artery that supply the brain are the posterior communicating artery, the anterior choroidal artery, and its two terminal branches: the middle cerebral artery (MCA) and the anterior cerebral artery (ACA).

The anterior choroidal artery supplies the amygdala in the temporal lobe, the ventrolateral part of the thalamus, the posterior limb of the internal capsule and the most rostral part of the midbrain.

The MCA supplies the lateral and superior surface of the cerebral hemisphere, except for a strip over the vertex (supplied by ACA), the occipital pole and inferomedial temporal lobe (supplied by PCA). The lateral lenticulostriate branches of the MCA supply most of the lentiform nucleus and the superior aspect of the internal capsule.

The ACA supplies the medial hemispheric surface except for the occipital lobe. The medial lenticulostriate branches of the ACA supply the caudate nuclei, the anteromedial aspect of the lentiform nucleus and the anterior limb of the internal capsule. The ACAs are joined by the anterior communicating artery.

## Posterior circulation

Each of the two vertebral arteries gives rise to an anterior and posterior spinal artery (which join with the corresponding vessel from the other side), and a posterior inferior cerebellar artery. The basilar artery gives rise to the superior and anterior inferior cerebellar arteries. These vessels supply the medulla oblongata, pons and midbrain, as do smaller branches of the vertebral and basilar arteries. The cerebellar vessels supply the corresponding parts of the cerebellum.

The terminal branches of the basilar artery are the two posterior cerebral arteries. On each side, the posterior cerebral artery (PCA) supplies the occipital poles and most of the undersurface of the temporal lobe except for its tip, which is supplied by the MCA. Branches of the PCA supply the midbrain and most of the thalamus.

With the exception of the most rostral part of the midbrain, the entire blood supply for the medulla oblongata, pons, midbrain and cerebellum comes from the posterior circulation.

## Watershed areas

Vascular watershed areas exist at the boundary of the main arterial territories (MCA, PCA and ACA). These areas are vulnerable to hypoperfusion during hypotensive episodes.

## PROBLEM 3.01

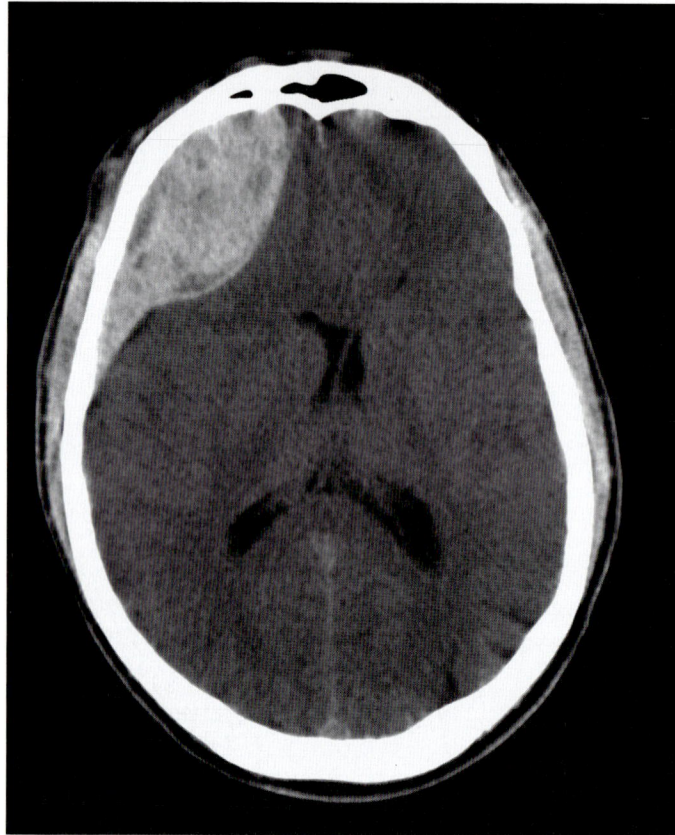

While intoxicated with alcohol, this 21-year-old man jumped off a roof. His GCS was 13 on presentation, but fell to 8 prior to intubation.

**Q**

1. What are the findings on the CT scan?
2. What intervention is required?

# A

1. There is a large hyperdense extra-axial collection in the right frontal region. It is convex towards the brain substance, an appearance typical of an extradural haematoma. The heterogeneous density within the lesion suggests acute and ongoing bleeding. There is significant midline shift, with subfalcine herniation.

No fractures are identified on the image in the book, though a small temporal fracture can be seen on the DVD images.

2. Urgent surgical evacuation of the extradural haematoma.

## LEARNING POINT

Identifying mass lesions that need urgent surgical evacuation is the main reason for performing CT head scans in severe head injuries.

# PROBLEM 3.02

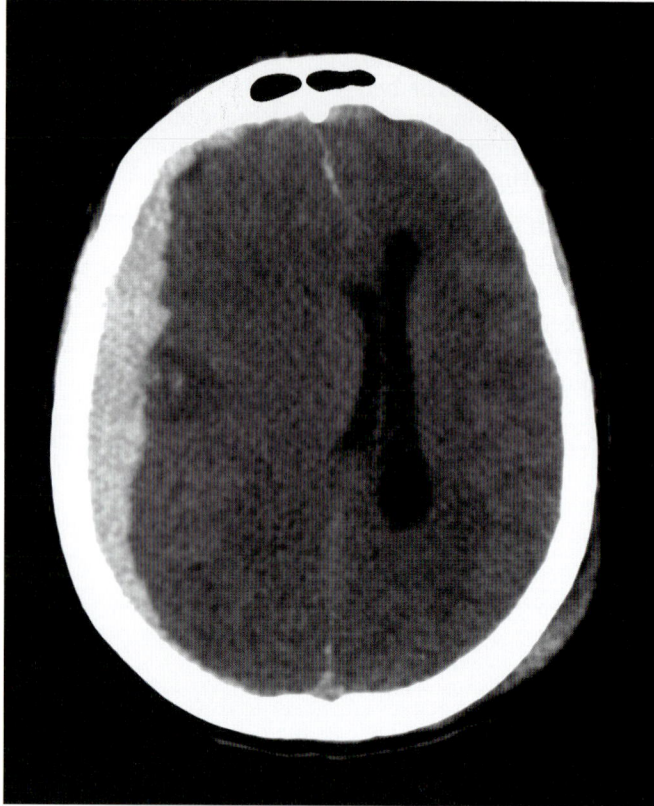

This 51-year-old woman fell down stairs and struck her head. Her GCS was 6 when the paramedics arrived.

**Q** Describe the findings on the CT scan.

# A

There is a large right-sided hyperdense extra-axial collection, concave towards the brain substance, an appearance typical of an acute subdural haematoma. There is significant mass effect. The ipsilateral ventricle is compressed and there is midline shift. There is a haemorrhagic cerebral contusion underlying the haematoma. The left-sided soft tissue swelling over the occipital region suggests a coup-contrecoup injury.

## LEARNING POINT

The age of an intracranial haemorrhage can be estimated by its appearance (Osborn, 2004). Unclotted blood is hypodense. Clotted blood is initially hyperdense, but gradually becomes less dense over several weeks as the blood components break down.

- A "hyperacute" haemorrhage (< 6 hours) has a significant hypodense component, due to unclotted blood. A fluid level may develop as the cellular and serous components separate.
- An acute haemorrhage (6 hours to 3 days) is typically homogeneously hyperdense. If there is ongoing active bleeding, it may be heterogenous, which is known as the "swirl sign" (see extradural in Problem 3.01).
- A subacute haemorrhage (3 days to 3 weeks) is isodense to the cerebral parenchyma and is the most difficult to see.
- A chronic haemorrhage that has not resorbed is hypodense to the brain, and may reach CSF density. When new hyperdensity is present within such a collection it suggests acute-on-chronic haemorrhage (see Problem 3.03).

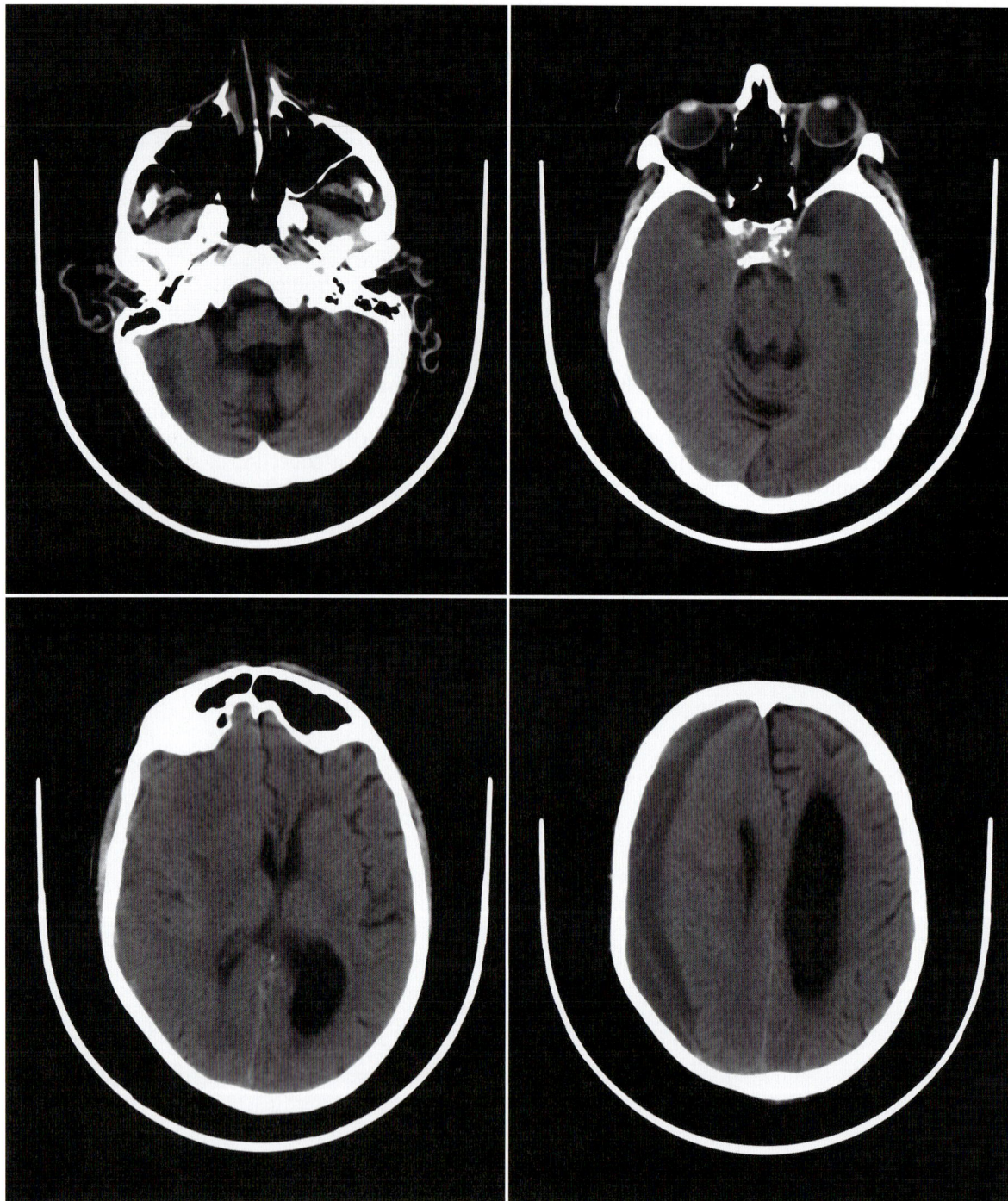

This 75-year-old man has a history of a high alcohol intake. He fell two days ago and struck his head. He is now confused and agitated.

**Q**
What explanation for the clinical picture is seen on the CT scans?

## A

There is a large right-sided hypodense extra-axial collection, concave towards the brain substance. This appearance is typical of a chronic subdural haematoma. There is significant mass effect, with effacement of the ipsilateral sulci, compression of the ipsilateral ventricle and midline shift.

There is a small hyperdense component within the collection, suggesting some acute-on-chronic component. The ventricular system is prominent, but there appears to be generalised cerebral atrophy. Furthermore, the temporal horns are not dilated and the basal cisterns are not effaced, which both argue against hydrocephalus.

## LEARNING POINT

Dilated ventricles are not always due to hydrocephalus.

# PROBLEM 3.04

3D CT angiogram

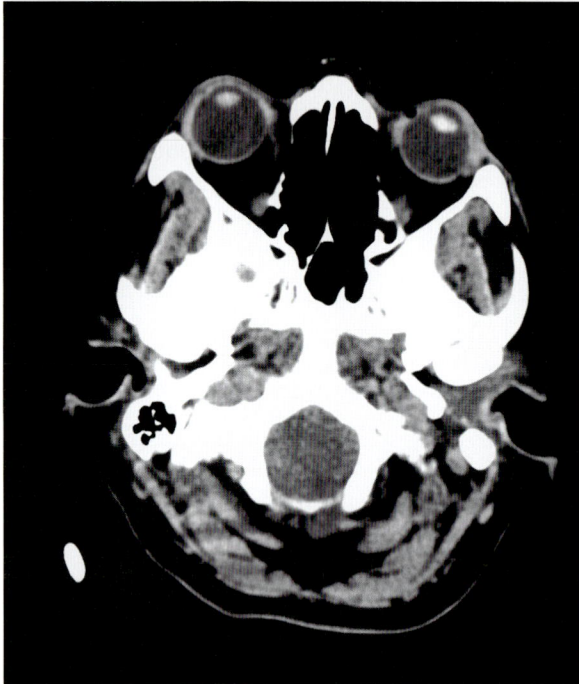

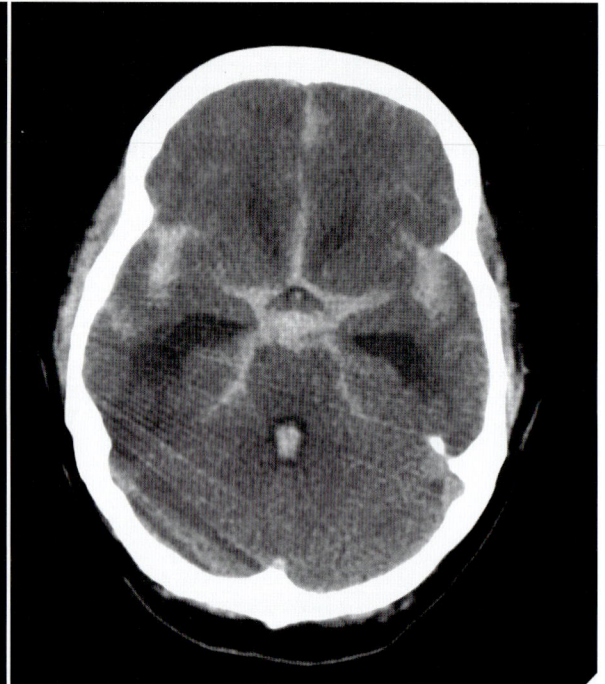

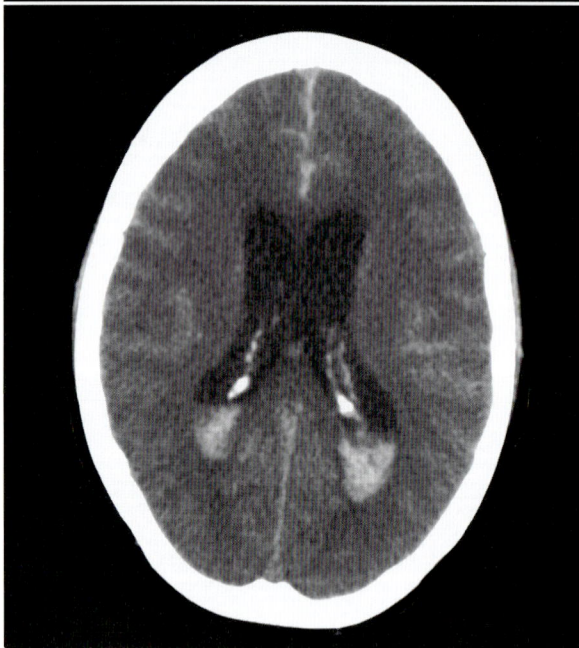

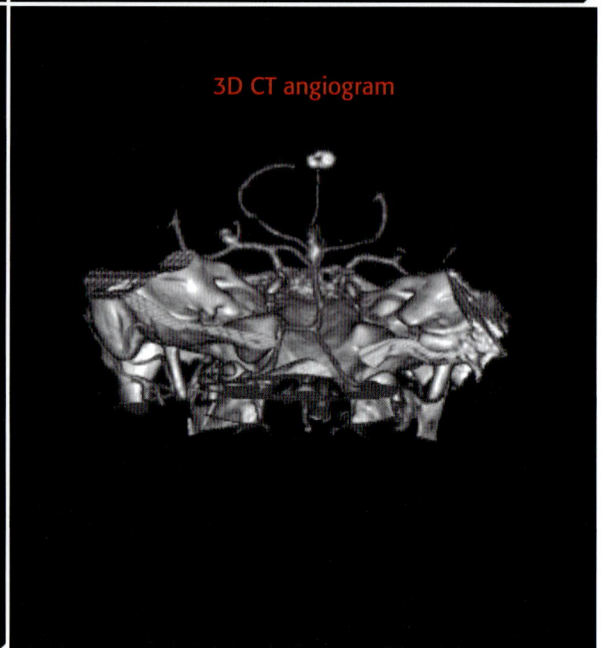

This 42-year-old woman was found unconscious at home by her daughter.

**Q**
1. What is the cause of the patient's condition?
2. What complications have occurred?

# A

1. The scans show extensive subarachnoid haemorrhage with an intraventricular component. The 3D reconstruction of the CT angiogram shows two aneurysms, one on the left middle cerebral artery near its trifurcation and the other at the tip of the basilar artery.

2. Hydrocephalus and cerebral oedema. There is reduced grey–white differentiation and the image at the level of the foramen magnum shows herniation of the cerebellar tonsils.

## LEARNING POINT

One of the early signs of hydrocephalus is that the temporal horns of the lateral ventricles dilate, becoming crescentic rather than having their normal slit-like appearance.

# PROBLEM 3.05

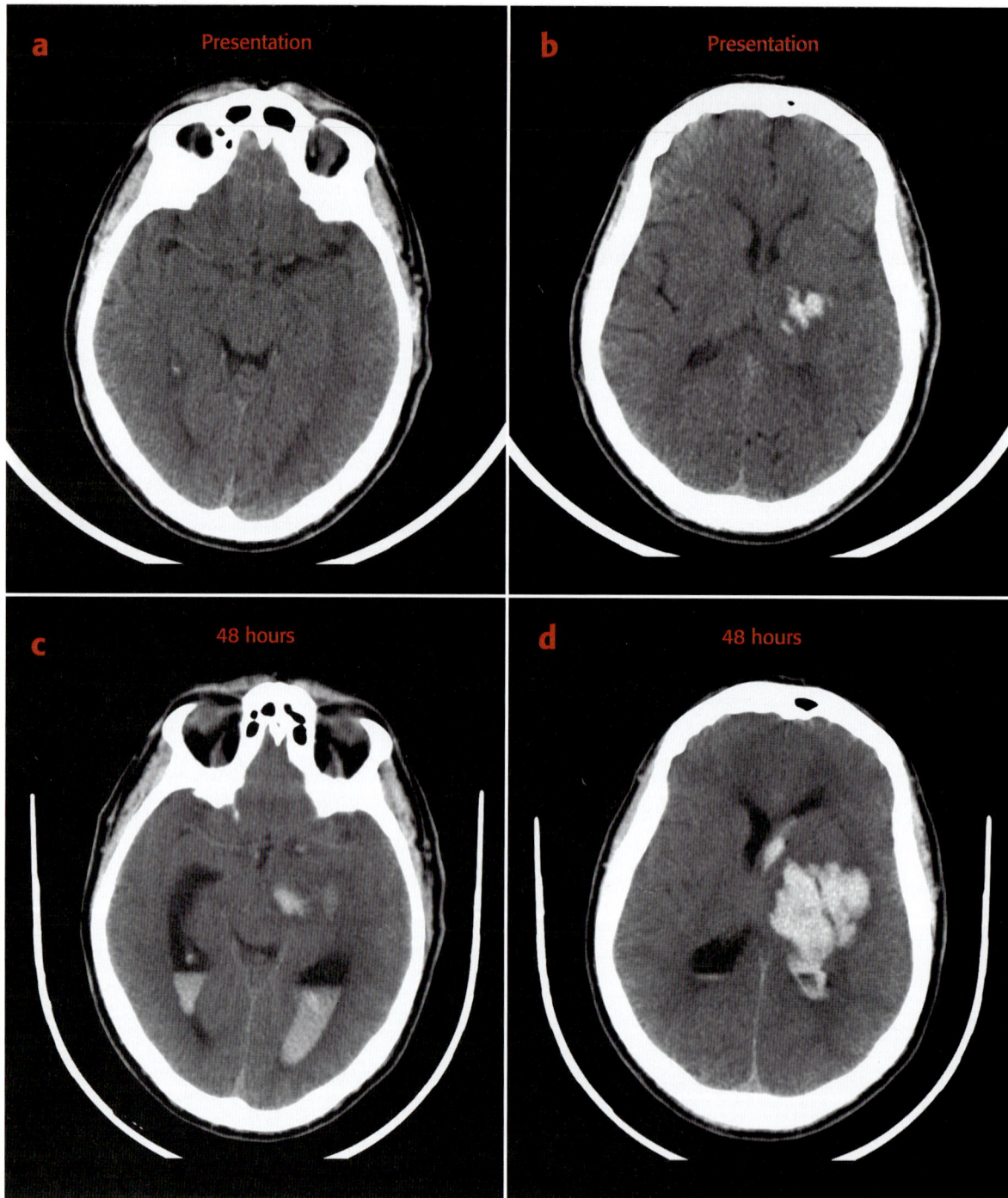

a  Presentation

b  Presentation

c  48 hours

d  48 hours

This 65-year-old woman presented with mild right hemiparesis and a GCS of 15 (images a and b). Forty-eight hours later, her GCS fell to 5 (images c and d).

**Q**

1. What caused the initial hemiparesis?
2. Why has the clinical deterioration occurred?

## A

1. There is hyperdensity in the left thalamus and posterior limb of the internal capsule, consistent with a small acute thalamic haemorrhage.

2. The size of the thalamic haemorrhage has increased and there is intraventricular extension. Transtentorial uncal herniation is seen, denoted by compression of the ipsilateral cerebral peduncle by the medial aspect of the temporal lobe. Significant hydrocephalus is also present.

## LEARNING POINT

Predisposing factors for thalamic bleeds include hypertension and anticoagulant therapy.

# PROBLEM 3.06

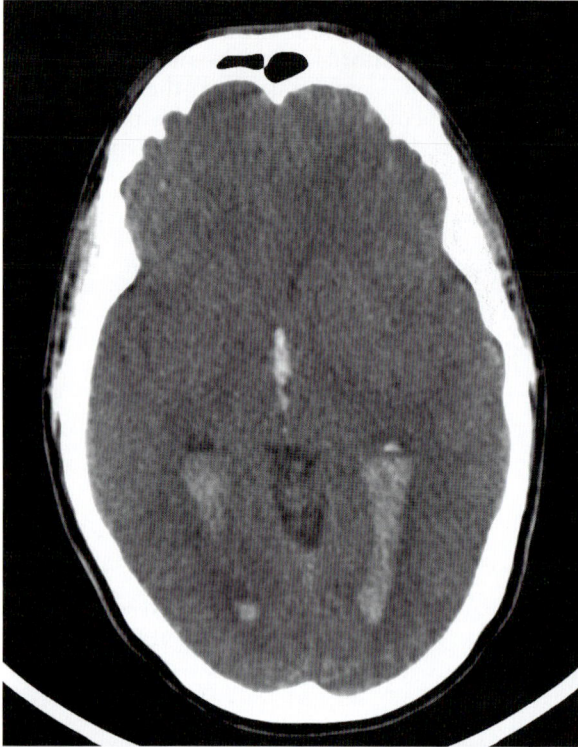

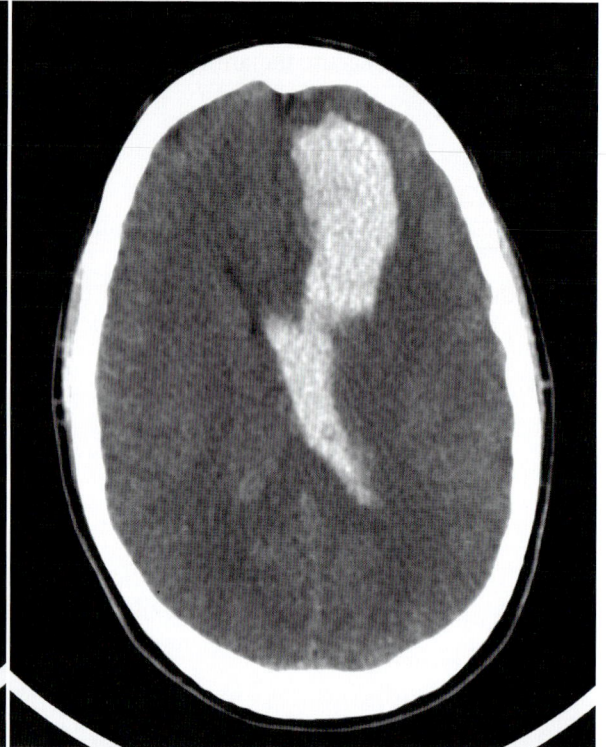

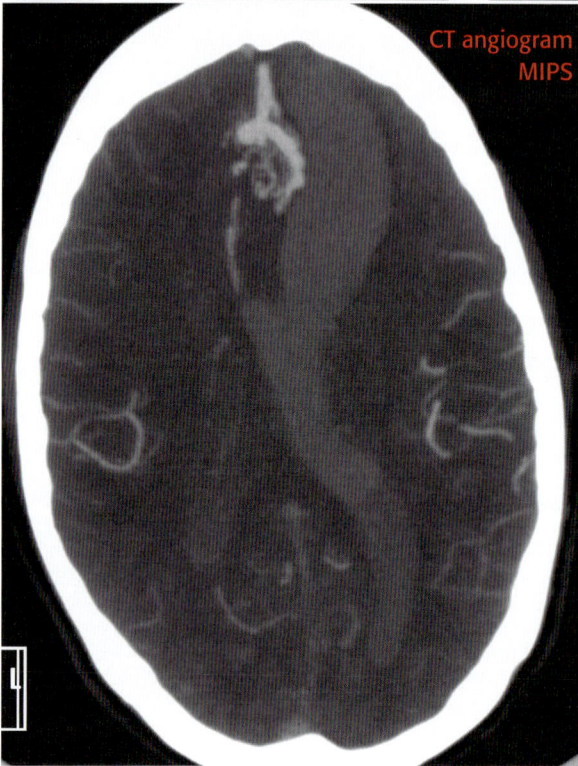

CT angiogram
MIPS

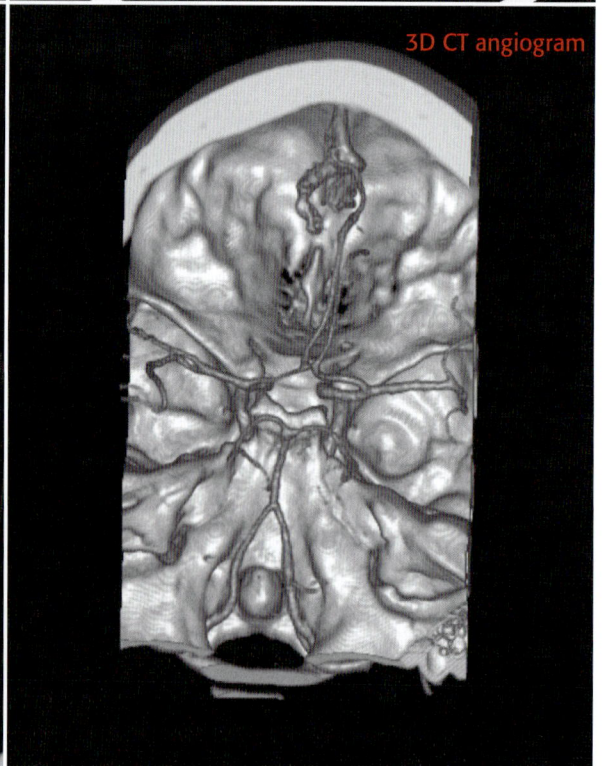

3D CT angiogram

After a sudden onset of headache at work, this 26-year-old man rapidly became unconscious.

## Q

What pathological process does the scan demonstrate?

## A

There is a large haematoma within the left frontal lobe, with significant mass effect producing mid-line shift. There is extension of the haemorrhage into the ventricular system. CT angiography shows an arteriovenous malformation, arising from the anterior cerebral vessels.

## LEARNING POINT

CT angiography should be considered when the initial CT study shows non-traumatic intracranial haemorrhage. While digital subtraction angiography (DSA) is still the "gold standard" against which other forms of angiography are compared, CT angiography using the modern generation of scanners performs almost as well as DSA and is relatively non-invasive.

## PROBLEM 3.07

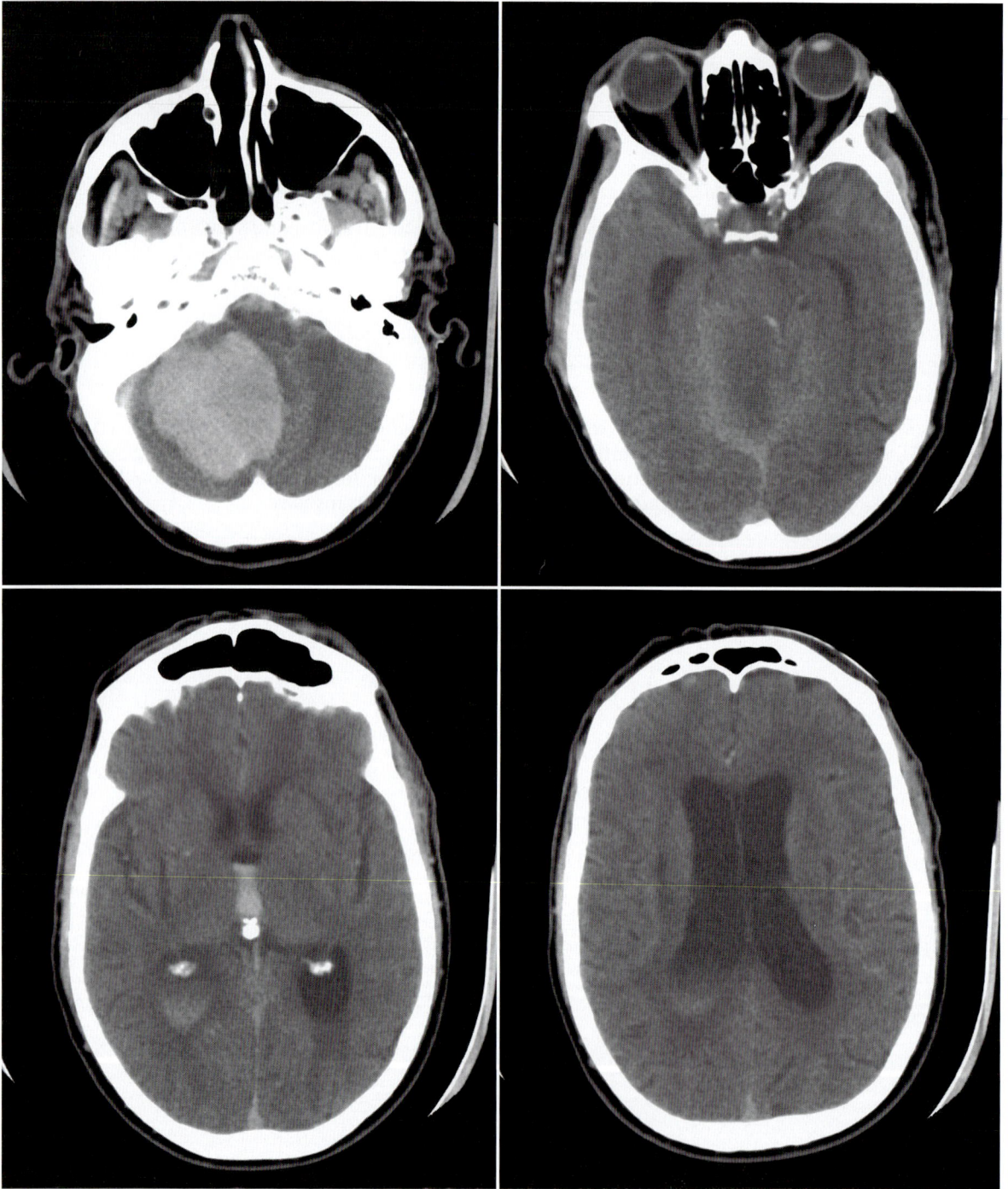

This 69-year-old man complained of a severe headache. The level of consciousness fell rapidly and his GCS was 6 by the time he arrived in the emergency department.

**Q** What is the cause of the clinical picture?

# A

There is a hyperdense area in the right cerebellar hemisphere, representing an acute haemorrhage. There is intraventricular extension, with blood seen in the dependent areas of the ventricular system, and moderate hydrocephalus.

A history of predisposing factors for cerebellar haemorrhage, such as hypertension and anticoagulant therapy, should be sought. Trauma is unlikely with this pattern of haemorrhage.

## LEARNING POINT

Posterior fossa haemorrhage may cause hydrocephalus by either directly compressing CSF outflow from the ventricles or by extending into the ventricular system, leading to obstruction of CSF outflow by blood. The hydrocephalus may need decompression with an external ventricular drain but, in the presence of posterior fossa hypertension, there is a risk of ventricular decompression producing transtentorial herniation of posterior fossa contents ("reverse coning").

## PROBLEM 3.08

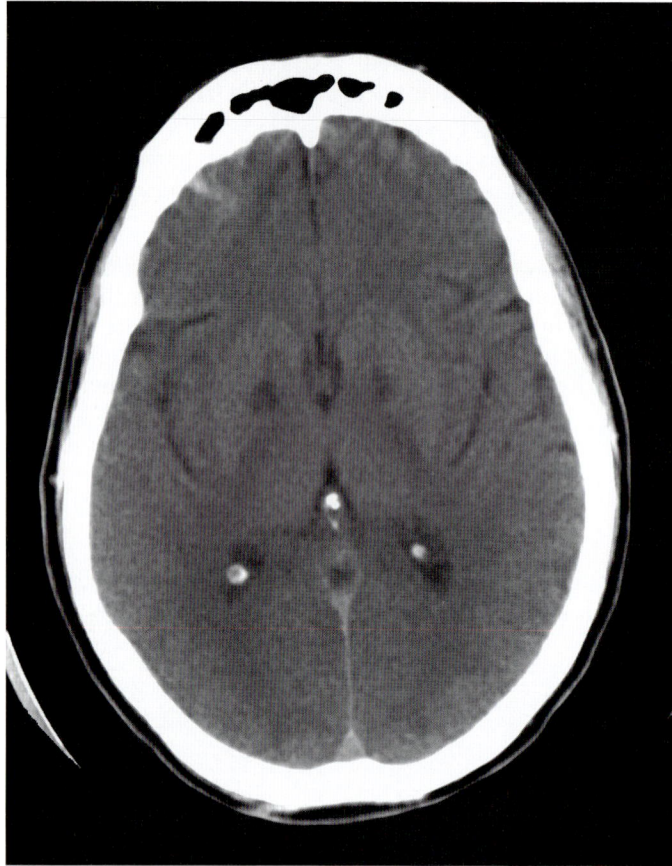

This 38-year-old man had an unexpectedly difficult airway to intubate during induction of anaesthesia for elective surgery. There was a prolonged period of severe hypoxia. Forty-eight hours later, he was agitated and confused when sedation was ceased.

Q
What significant abnormality is present on this CT scan?

## A

There are bilateral hypodense areas in the lentiform nuclei. This gives a characteristic "owl's eyes" appearance, typical of the basal ganglia infarction caused by hypoxia.

## LEARNING POINT

The basal ganglia are particularly sensitive to hypoxia. Severe hypoxia may cause basal ganglia infarction.

# PROBLEM 3.09

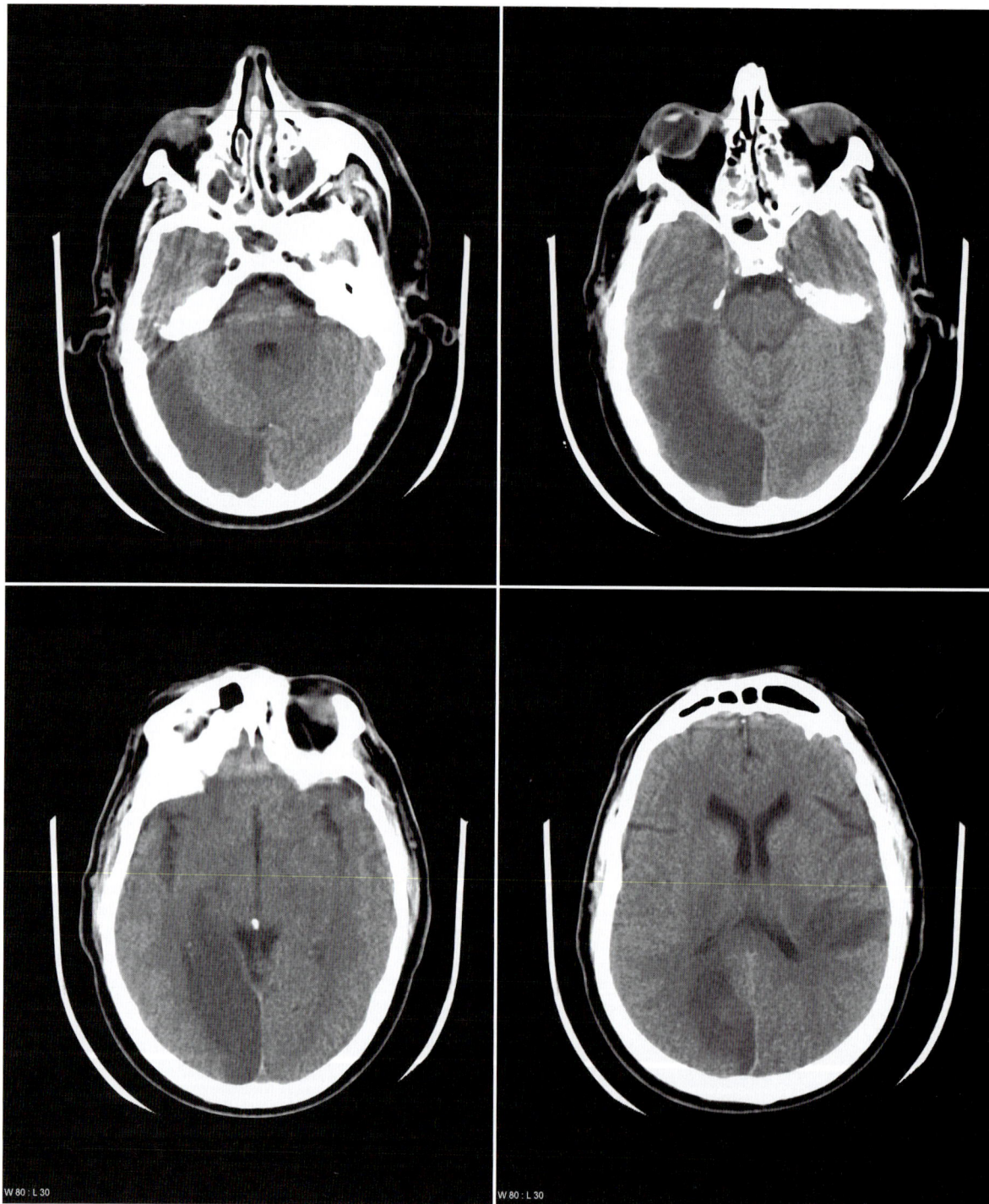

W 80 : L 30

W 80 : L 30

This 54-year-old man was slow to wake following aortic valve replacement. On examination, he appears to be moving all limbs symmetrically.

**Q** Which vascular territory is affected?

# A

There is hypodensity within the occipital lobe and the inferior and medial parts of the right temporal lobe. This is typical of a right posterior cerebral artery territory infarction. There is also a separate area of hypodensity within the left parietal lobe.

## LEARNING POINT

Infarction in the territory of the distal posterior cerebral artery often causes homonymous hemianopia without hemiparesis (Smith, 2005).

## PROBLEM 3.10

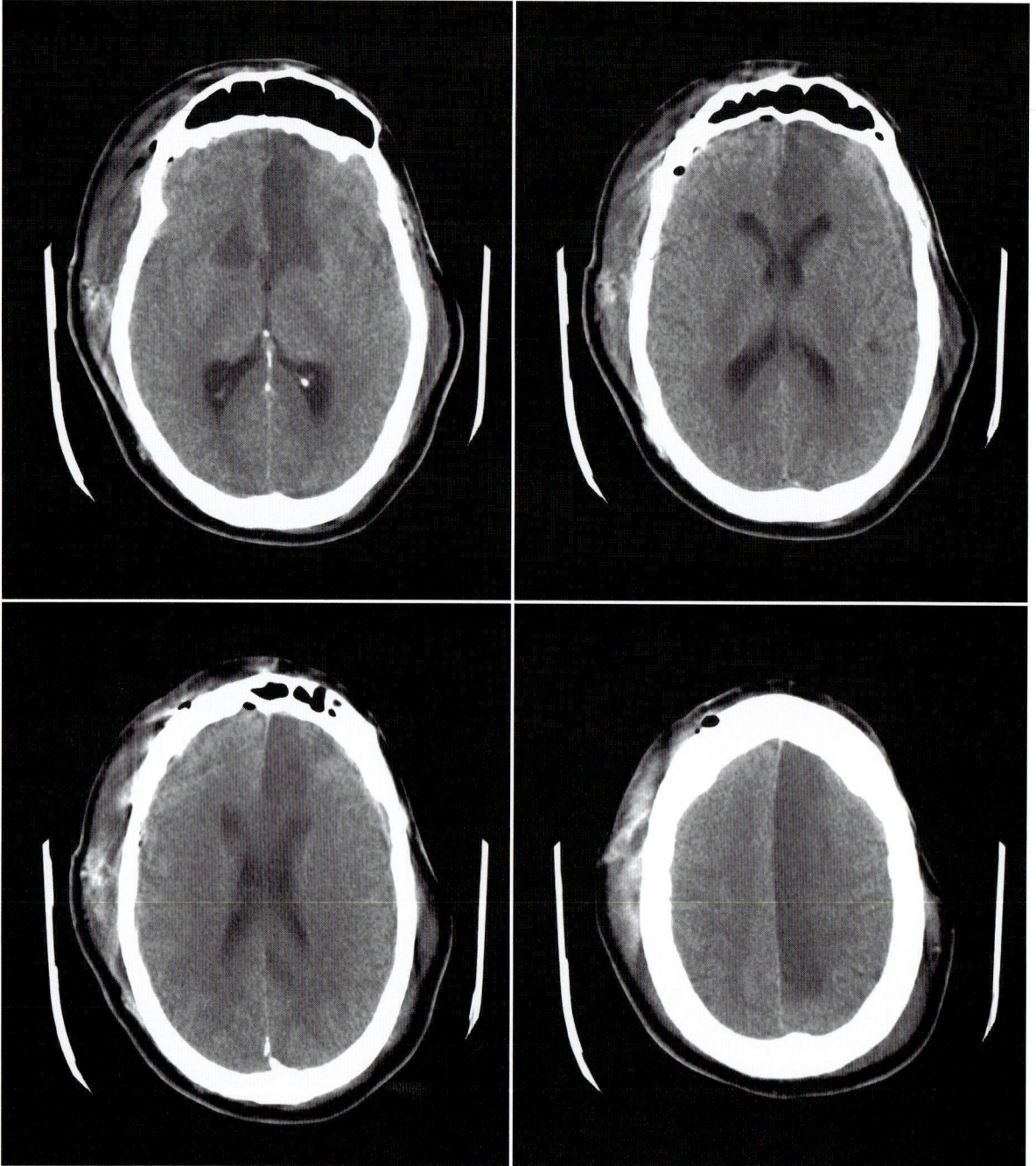

Five days ago, this 32-year-old woman had a grade I subarachnoid haemorrhage. The next day, an anterior communicating artery aneurysm was clipped. Weakness developed in her right leg 48 hours ago. Today, she has become progressively obtunded.

**Q** What is the likely cause of this clinical picture?

## A

There is hypodensity of the medial aspect of the left frontal and parietal lobes. This pattern is typical of anterior cerebral artery territory infarction. As the clinical features were not present in the immediate postoperative period, the problem is likely to be vasospasm rather than a misplaced clip. There is also a small area of hypodensity on the medial aspect of the right frontal lobe.

## LEARNING POINT

With an anterior cerebral artery territory infarct, leg weakness is often the predominant feature (Smith, 2005).

## PROBLEM 3.11

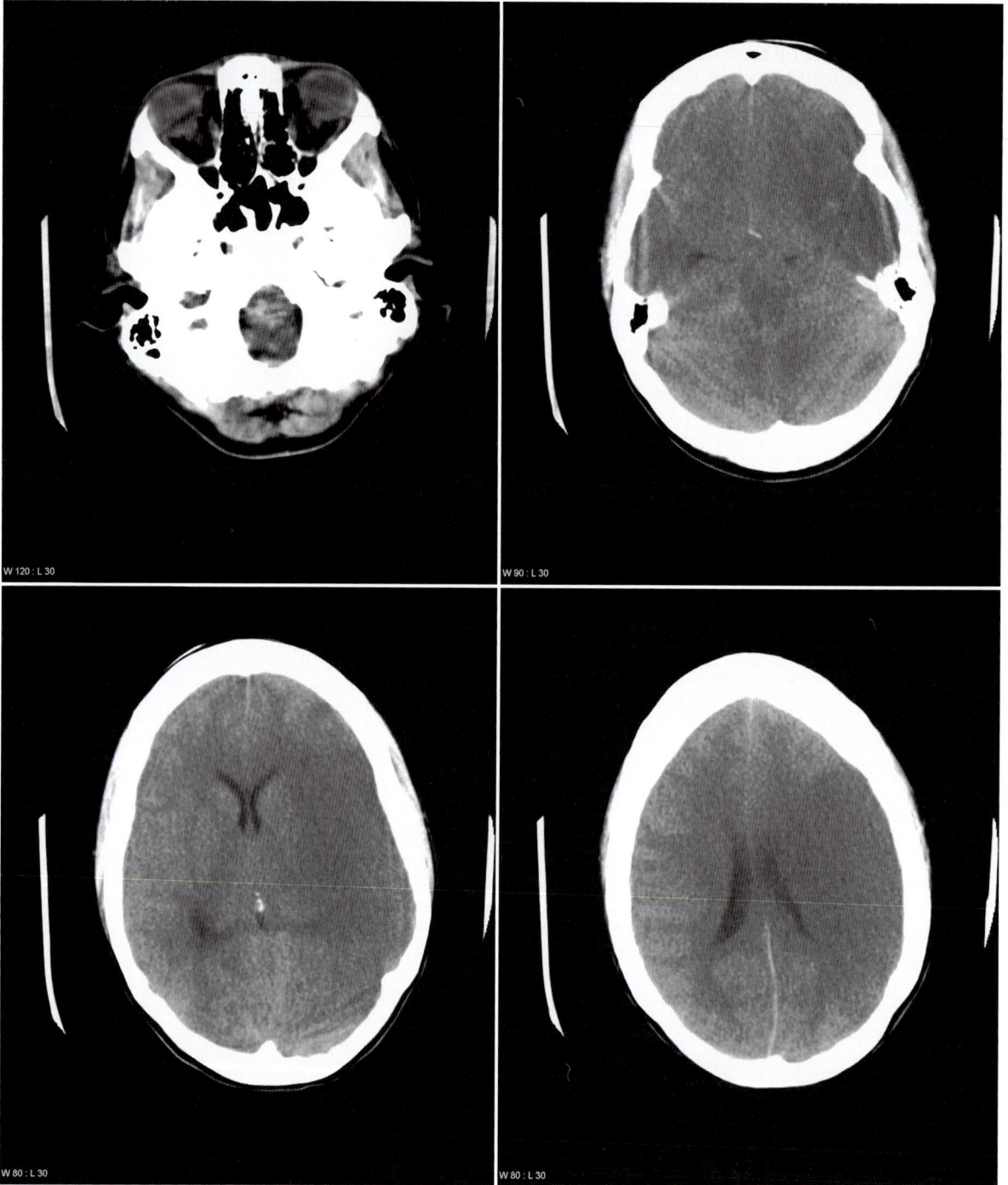

W 120 : L 30

W 90 : L 30

W 80 : L 30

W 80 : L 30

Forty-eight hours ago, this 58-year-old woman had a mitral valve repair. Off sedation, she has a GCS of 7 (E2, V1, M4) and is not moving her right arm or leg in response to pain.

**Q**

Are there any findings on this scan that could explain the clinical features?

## A

Over most of the left hemisphere, there is a subtle hypodensity with complete loss of grey–white differentiation. The occipital lobe, and the medial part of the frontal and parietal lobes are spared. There is evidence of mass effect and intracranial hypertension including: midline shift, obliteration of the basal cisterns and herniation of the cerebellar tonsils into the foramen magnum. These findings are consistent with a left middle cerebral artery territory infarct with significant mass effect.

## LEARNING POINT

CT features suggesting elevated intracranial pressure include:
- effacement of basal cisterns
- loss of grey–white differentiation
- loss of sulci
- midline shift
- herniation of cerebellar tonsils into the foramen magnum
- uncal herniation

The features of uncal herniation are:
- shift of the brainstem and distortion of adjacent cisterns
- dilation of contralateral temporal horn
- compression of the posterior cerebral artery as it crosses the tentorium, causing a posterior cerebral artery territory infarct (Osborn, 2004)

## PROBLEM 3.12

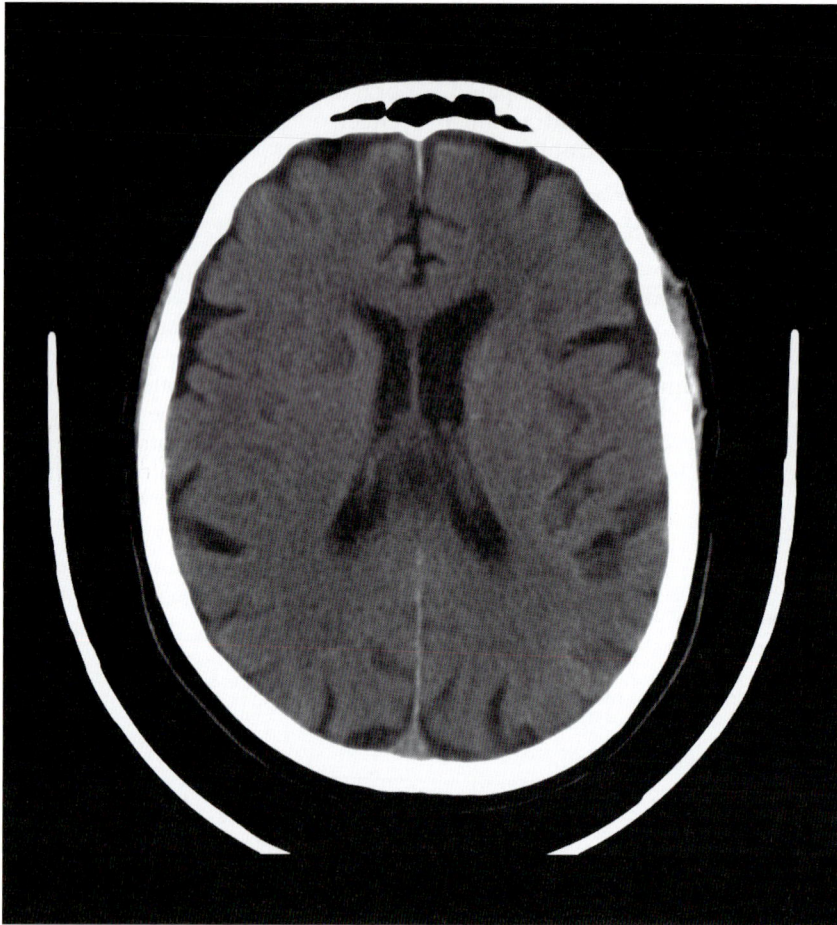

This 68-year-old man sustained chest and limb injuries when he fell from a ladder. He was slow to wake when sedation was withdrawn.

**Q** What is the likely cause of this clinical picture?

# A

There is generalised cerebral atrophy, consistent with advancing age. A small area of hypodensity is present in the region of the right corona radiata. On the DVD, it is seen to extend into the basal ganglia. This is a lacunar infarct. These findings do not explain the clinical picture. No cause for the altered level of consciousness is evident on this CT scan. Sedation often has prolonged effects in the elderly.

## LEARNING POINT

Lacunar infarcts are small, deep subcortical infarcts less than 1.5 cm in size. They usually occur in the basal ganglia, thalamus, internal capsule, corona radiata and brainstem. They are caused by occlusion of deep penetrating branches of major cerebral arteries and are particularly common in elderly patients with hypertension and diabetes, which are associated with severe atherosclerosis of small vessels and small vessel cerebral disease. Lacunar infarcts are often asymptomatic (Norrving, 2008).

## PROBLEM 3.13

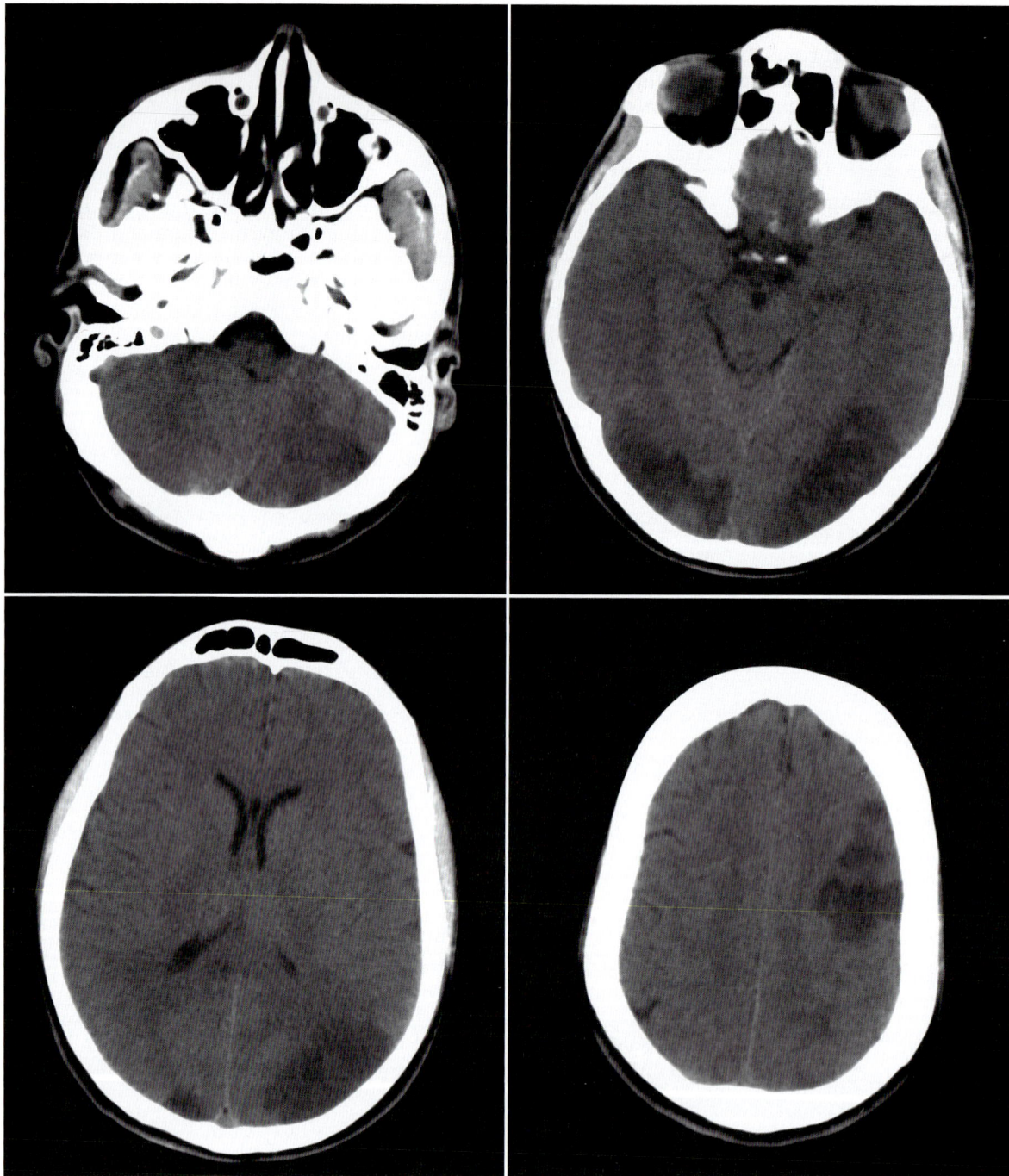

One week ago, this 38-year-old man was stabbed in the groin, sustaining a lacerated femoral artery that required emergency repair because of exsanguinating haemorrhage. He now has resolving acute renal failure. Sedation was ceased 48 hours ago, but he is still unresponsive. There are no localising signs.

**Q**
Are there any findings on this scan that could explain the clinical features?

**A**
There are multiple bilateral hypodense lesions involving both the grey and subcortical white matter. They are predominantly in watershed areas between the territories of the major vessels, but not exclusively so.

## LEARNING POINT

Prolonged severe hypotensive insults may result in watershed infarcts.

Watershed infarcts occur in areas with relatively poor blood supply, at the boundary between the territories of cerebral arteries. Two forms of watershed infarction may occur:

1. Cortical border zone infarctions between the territories supplied by the anterior, middle, and posterior cerebral arteries.

2. Internal border zone infarctions between the territory of the penetrating arteries arising from the superficial pial plexus and the territory of the deep penetrating arteries arising from the basal cerebral arteries. These infarcts lie in the corona radiata and the centrum semiovale adjacent to the lateral ventricles (Bladin, 1993).

## PROBLEM 3.14

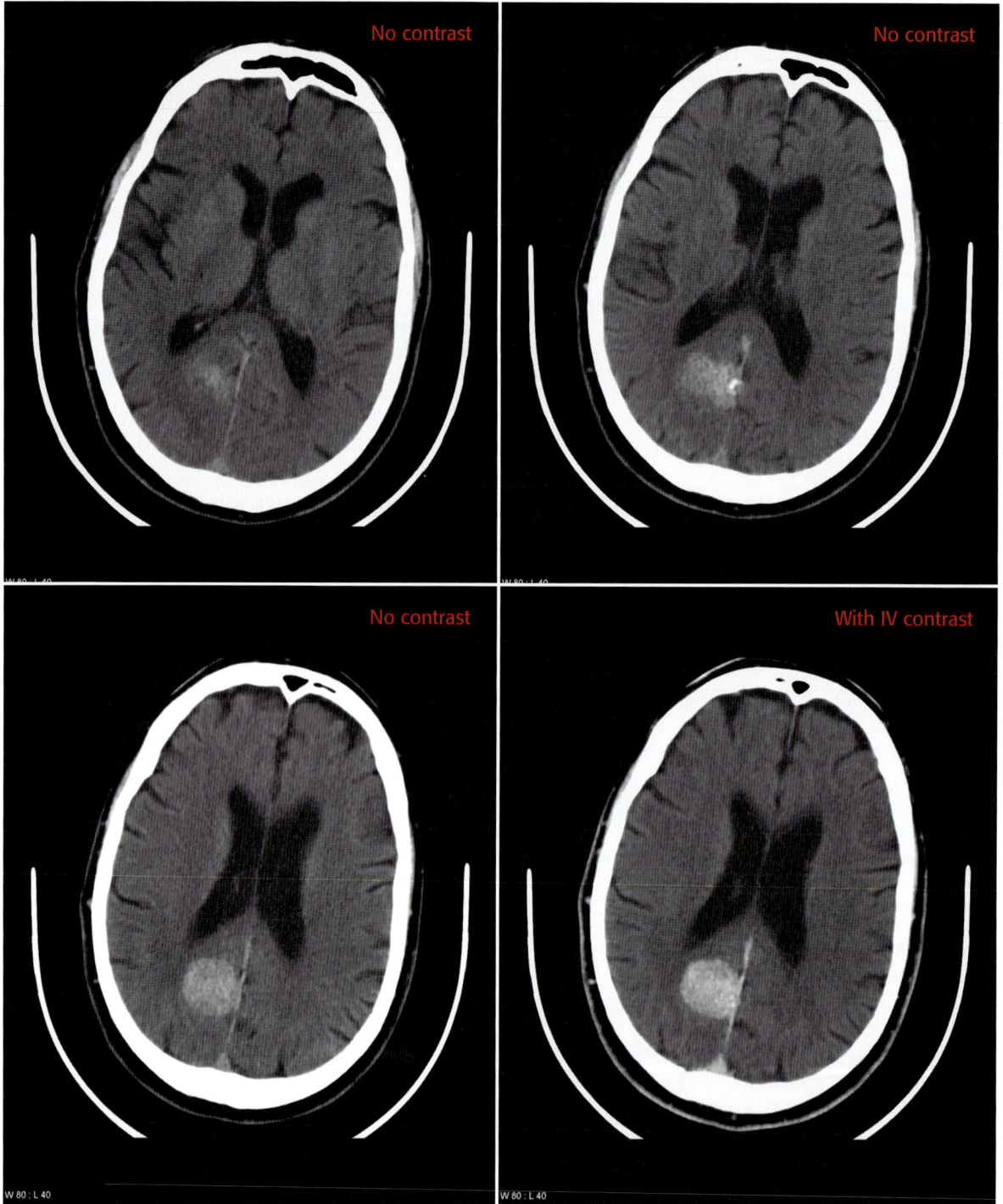

This 69-year-old man was admitted to ICU after a prolonged epileptic seizure. There was no previous history of seizures.

**Q**
Why does this patient have epilepsy?

# A

There is a well-circumscribed, hyperdense mass adjacent to the falx cerebri (dural based), with a small area of calcification. There is no significant mass effect and minimal surrounding oedema. There is homogeneous contrast enhancement of the mass. These findings are highly suggestive of a meningioma.

## LEARNING POINT

New onset epilepsy often has a structural intracranial cause. It requires investigation with CT and, if no diagnosis is apparent on CT, with MRI.

# PROBLEM 3.15

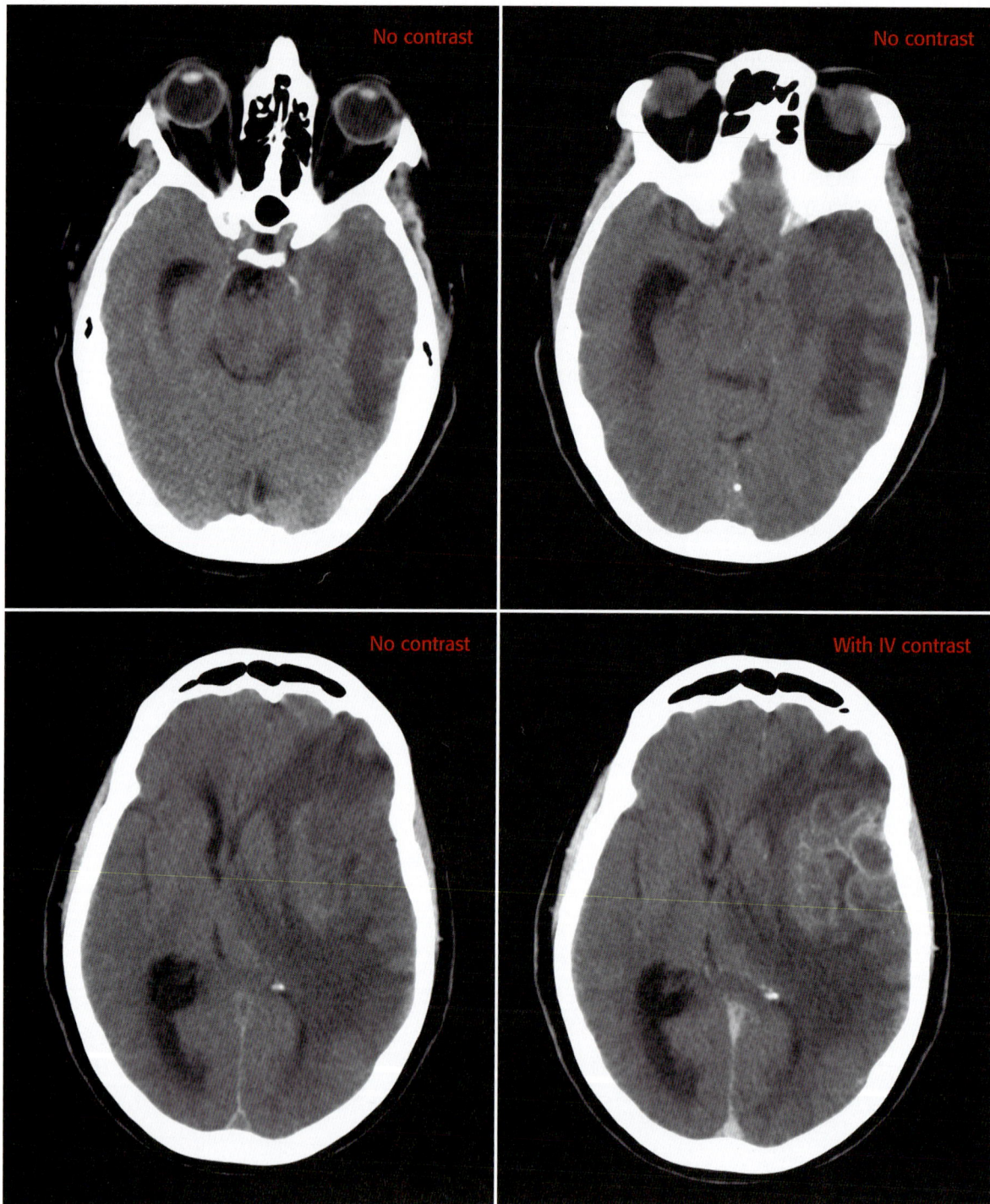

This 61-year-old woman was found at home unconscious. Her GCS was 7 and she was not moving her right arm or leg.

**Q**

What is the cause of this patient's clinical picture?

# A

There is a large, left-sided, mixed-density fronto-temporal lesion with variable enhancement and extensive surrounding vasogenic oedema. There is significant mass effect with midline shift. On the side of the lesion, there is sulcal effacement, effacement of the lateral ventricle, subfalcine herniation and transtentorial herniation of the uncinate process of the temporal lobe displacing the brainstem to the right. Contralaterally, there is obstructive dilatation of the lateral ventricle. The appearances of the lesion are most suggestive of a primary malignant brain tumour, such as a glioblastoma multiforme.

## LEARNING POINT

Patterns of brain herniation include (Ropper, 2005):

- uncal transtentorial herniation: the uncinate process of the temporal lobe herniates into the anterior part of the opening of the tentorium cerebelli.
- central tentorial herniation: there is symmetrical downward movement of the thalamic region through the opening of the tentorium cerebelli.
- subfalcine herniation: there is displacement of the cingulate gyrus under the falx and across the midline.
- foraminal herniation: there is downward herniation of the cerebellar tonsils into the foramen magnum.

There are two types of cerebral oedema (Osborn, 2004):

1. cytotoxic: intracellular oedema caused by cell swelling with an intact blood–brain barrier. Cytotoxic oedema affects predominantly grey matter, with subsequent loss in the grey–white matter differentiation. It generally accompanies stroke and hypoxia and gives a pattern of "restricted diffusion" on MRI sequences (see Chapter 6: Imaging modalities, p 375).
2. vasogenic: extracellular oedema caused by loss of integrity of the blood–brain barrier. Vasogenic oedema predominantly affects white matter and spreads along white matter tracts, accentuating the grey–white matter differentiation. It generally accompanies inflammatory disease and brain tumours. It does not give a pattern of "restricted diffusion" on MRI sequences.

## PROBLEM 3.16

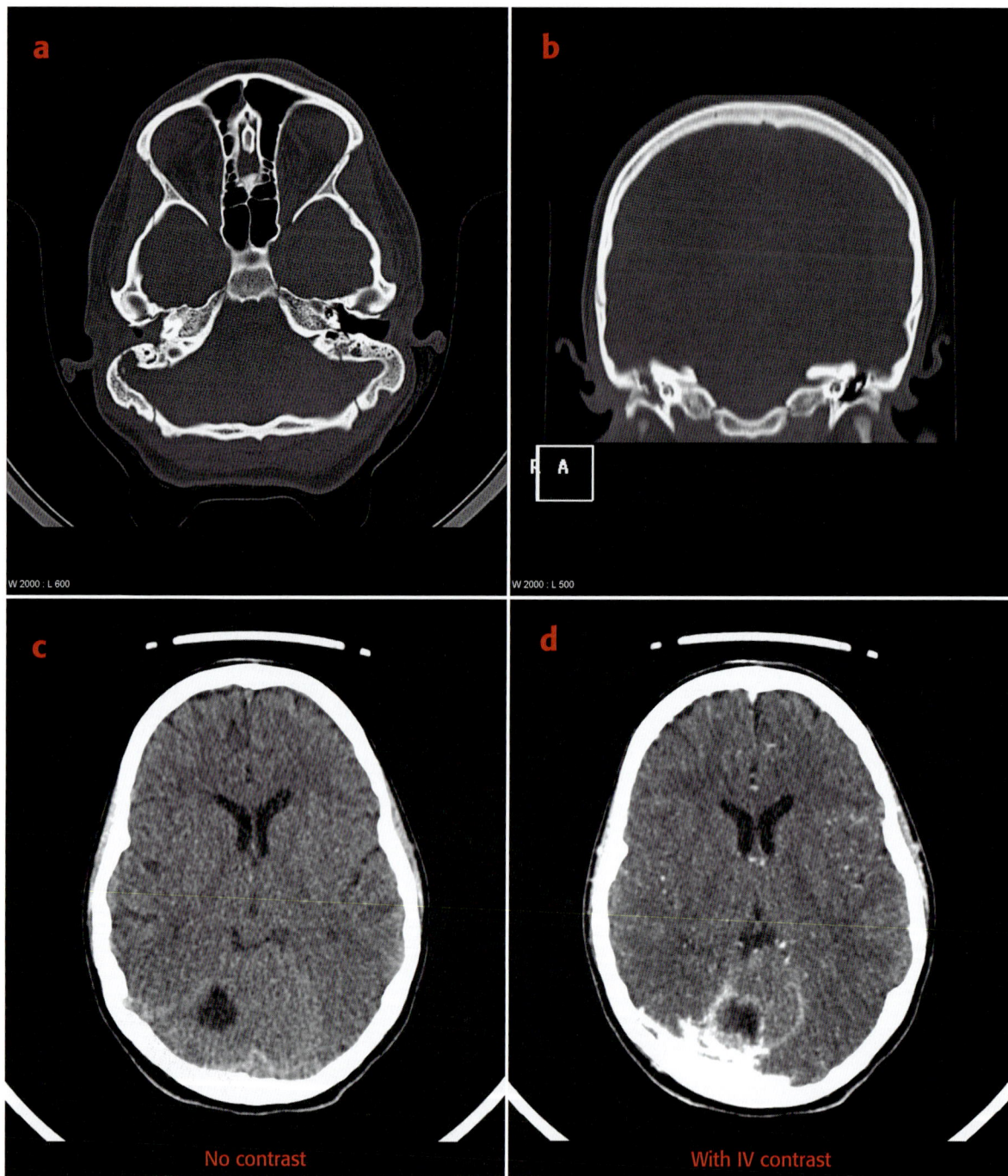

a

b

W 2000 : L 600

W 2000 : L 500

c

No contrast

d

With IV contrast

This 17-year-old woman was brought to the emergency department by her mother. On examination, she was febrile and confused.

Q
1. What is the likely cause of this illness?
2. Outline the important aspects of management.

# A

1. Otitis media and mastoiditis resulting in subdural empyema. Image a shows the right external auditory canal and middle ear filled with fluid. The right mastoid bone is eroded, suggesting the presence of mastoiditis. Image b shows a fluid-filled middle ear and erosion of the tegmen tympani (bony plate dividing middle ear from cranial cavity), which is pathognomonic of cholesteatoma.

   Image c shows a hypodense lesion adjacent to the tentorium cerebelli, while image d shows rim enhancement of the lesion with contrast.

2. Management should include antibiotics, myringotomy and debridement of the affected area of the mastoid, with drainage of the subdural empyema.

## LEARNING POINT

Examination of the ears is an important part of assessing the patient with an altered level of consciousness, especially if there is clinical suspicion of sepsis.

# PROBLEM 3.17

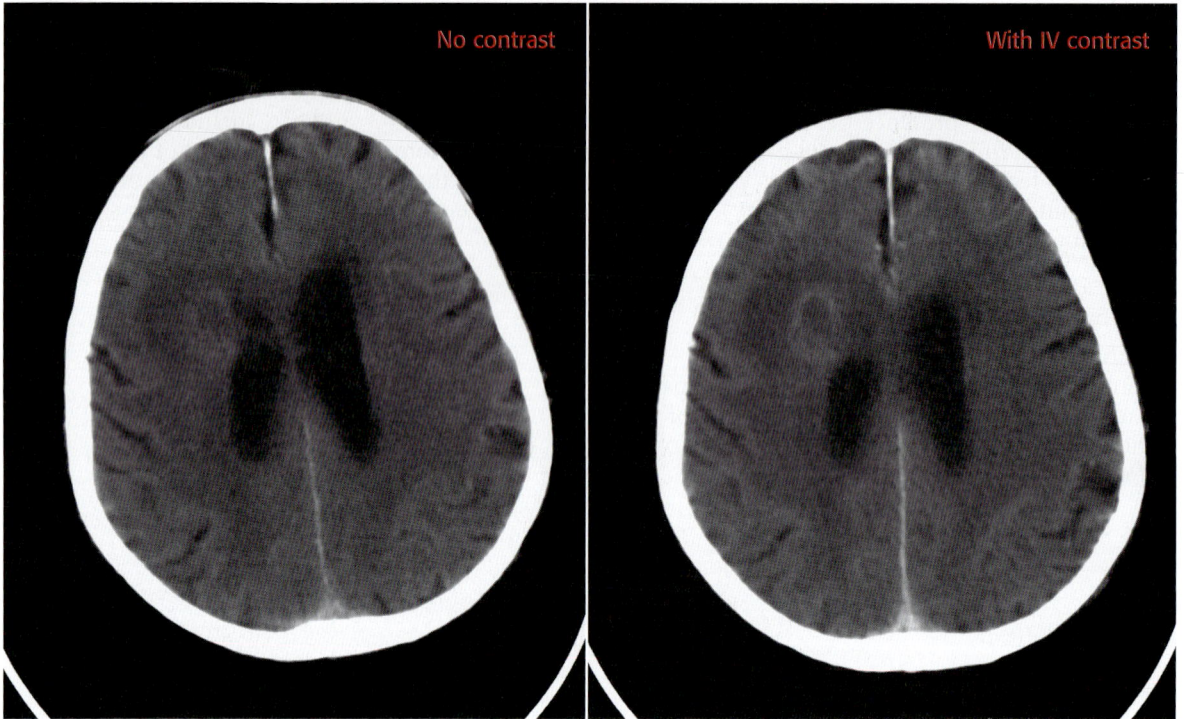

No contrast

With IV contrast

This 76-year-old man presented with fever, neutrophil leukocytosis and an altered level of consciousness. There were no focal neurological signs.

**Q** What does the scan demonstrate?

## A

There is a ring-shaped hyperdense lesion in the right periventricular white matter. The lesion rim enhances with contrast. This is consistent with a cerebral abscess.

## LEARNING POINT

Common causes for a rim-enhancing lesion are cerebral abscess, tumours of the brain parenchyma, such as glioma, and infections (e.g. toxoplasmosis).

## PROBLEM 3.18

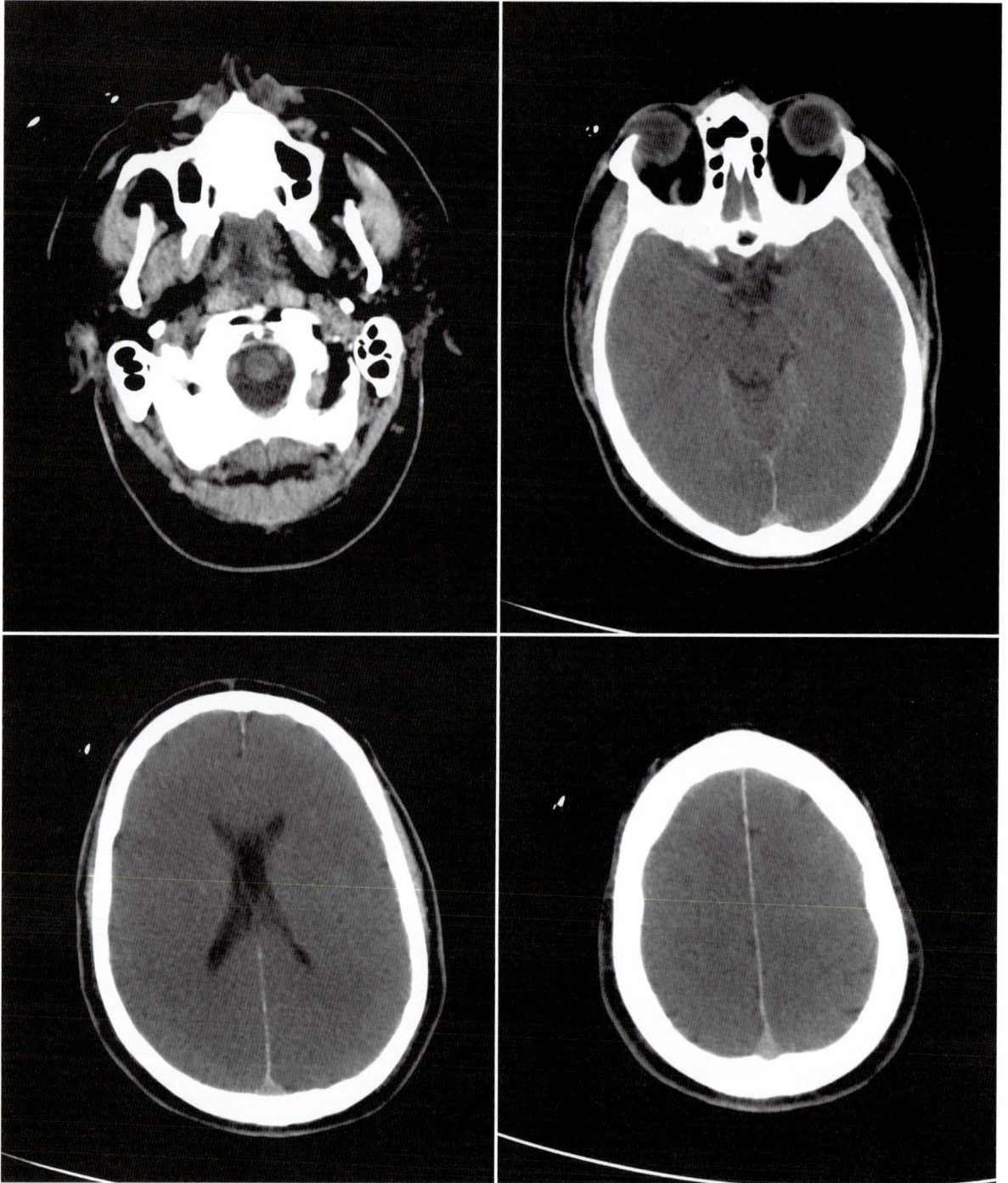

This 53-year-old man sustained severe chest trauma in a motor vehicle crash. There was prolonged entrapment at the scene. The GCS is 3 despite minimal sedation.

**Q** What does the scan demonstrate?

## A

There is generalised loss of grey–white differentiation, consistent with cerebral oedema. The basal cisterns are not effaced and there is no tonsillar herniation. An incidental finding of a cavum septum pellucidum is present. This is a congenital variant where the septum pellucidum is a cystic structure containing CSF; it is seen best in the DVD images.

## LEARNING POINT

Significant hypoxic cerebral damage can be present with an initially normal scan. The commonest abnormality on an acute CT scan is diffuse cerebral oedema.

## PROBLEM 3.19

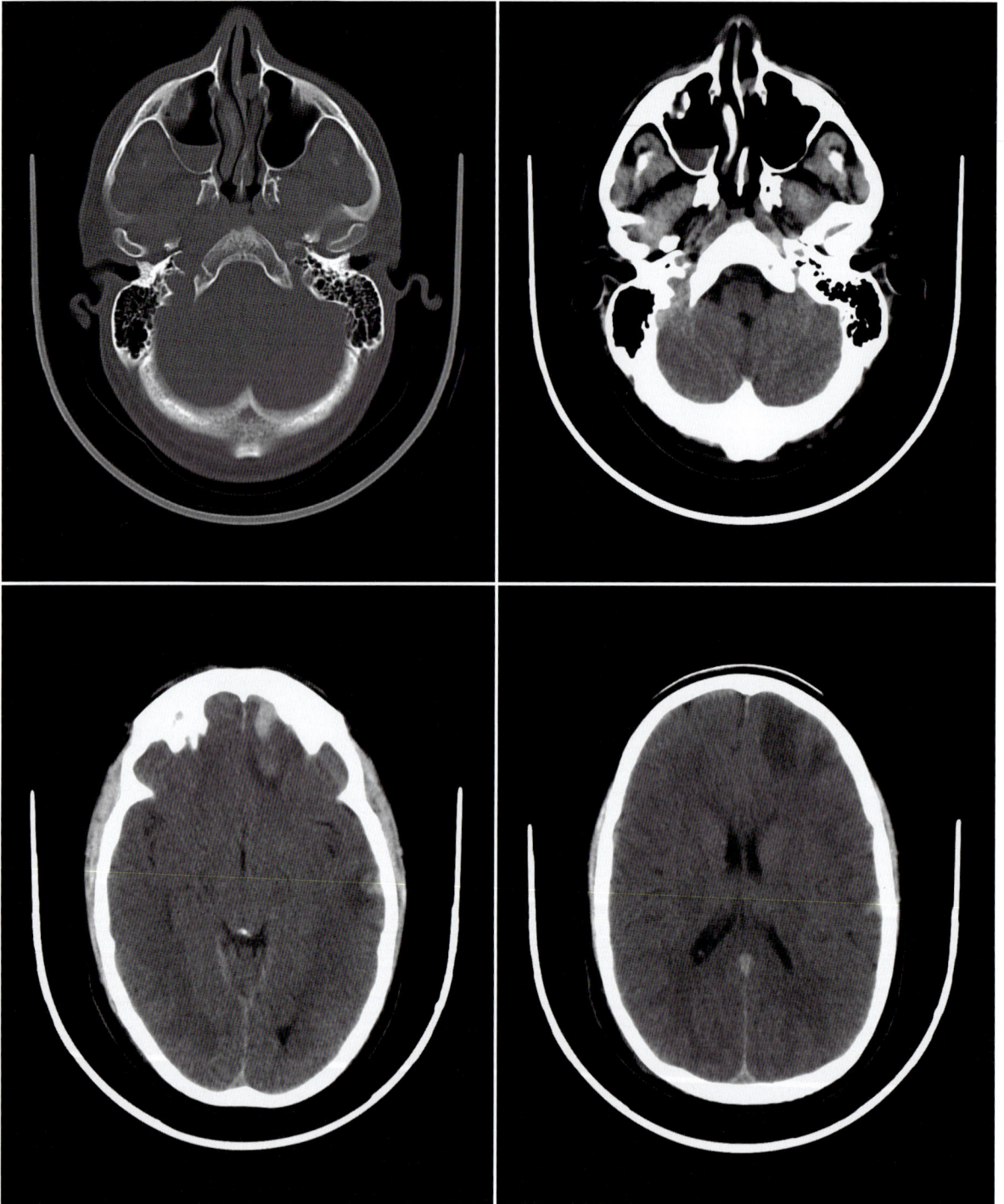

This 25-year-old man was punched in the face during an altercation at a nightclub. He was intubated because of agitation and confusion.

**Q** What intracranial pathology is shown on the scan?

# A

There are mixed-density lesions in the left frontal and temporal lobe, consistent with cerebral contusions. There is no significant mass effect. There is a fluid level in the right maxillary sinus, but no fracture is seen. In the context of trauma, a fluid level in a sinus may indicate an occult fracture. A small area of calcification is seen anterior to the quadrigeminal cistern, adjacent to the midbrain. This is consistent with pineal gland calcification.

## LEARNING POINT

Frontal and temporal lobes are common sites of traumatic contusions.

## PROBLEM 3.20

W 2500 : L 500

W 2500 : L 500

W 80 : L 40

W 80 : L 40

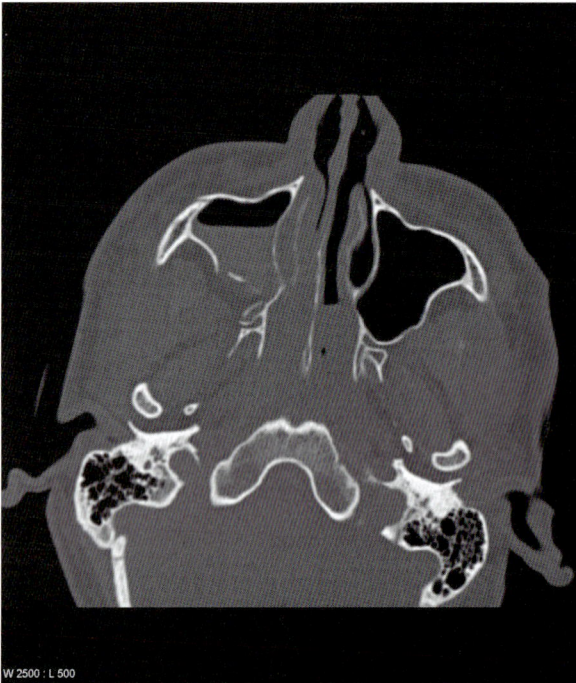

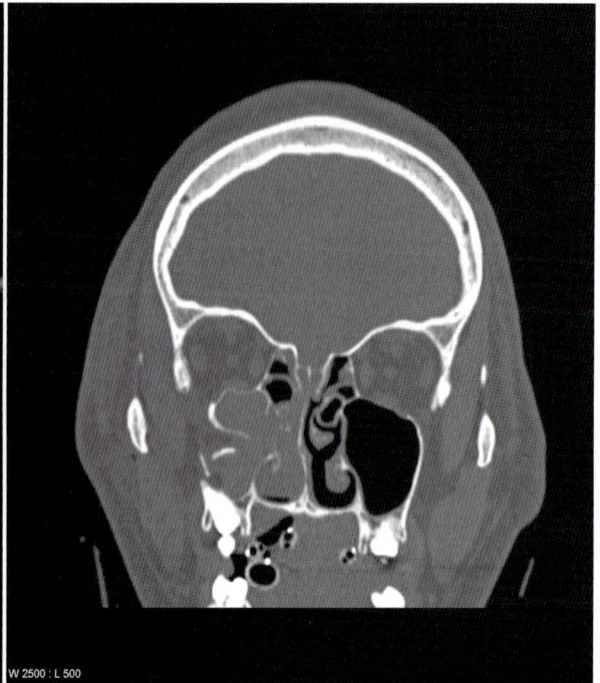

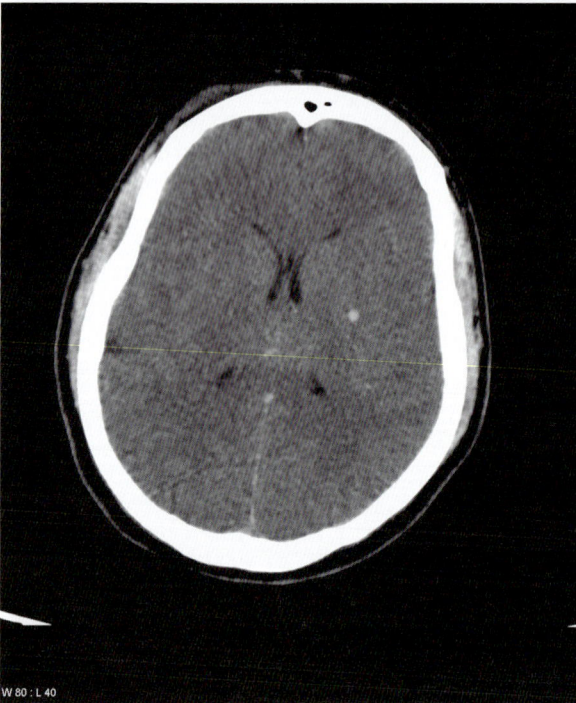

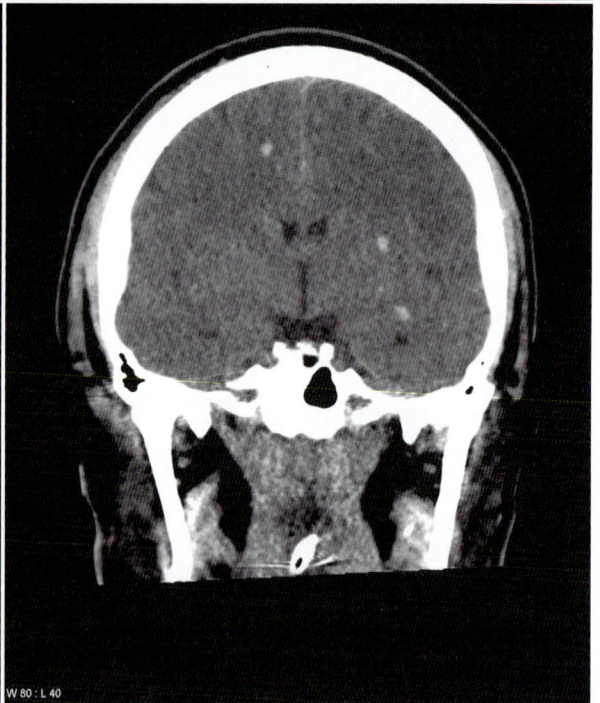

This 23-year-old man crashed his motorbike at high speed. He had a GCS of 5 at the scene.

**Q** What injuries are identified on the scan?

# A

There are multiple, small hyperdense lesions, predominantly within the white matter and the grey–white junction. These are petechial haemorrhages, consistent with diffuse axonal injury.

There is a fracture of the lateral wall of the right maxillary sinus, with an associated fluid level in the sinus (haemosinus).

## Learning POINT

Diffuse axonal injury is suggested by multiple petechial haemorrhages on the CT scan, classically at the grey–white interface, along the corpus callosum and within the white matter. MRI will give better information about the extent and nature of the injury, but is unlikely to change management in the acute phase (Osborn, 2004). MRI scanning is not without risk in the critically ill patient. This risk must be balanced against the likelihood of the information from the MRI providing real clinical benefit.

## PROBLEM 3.21

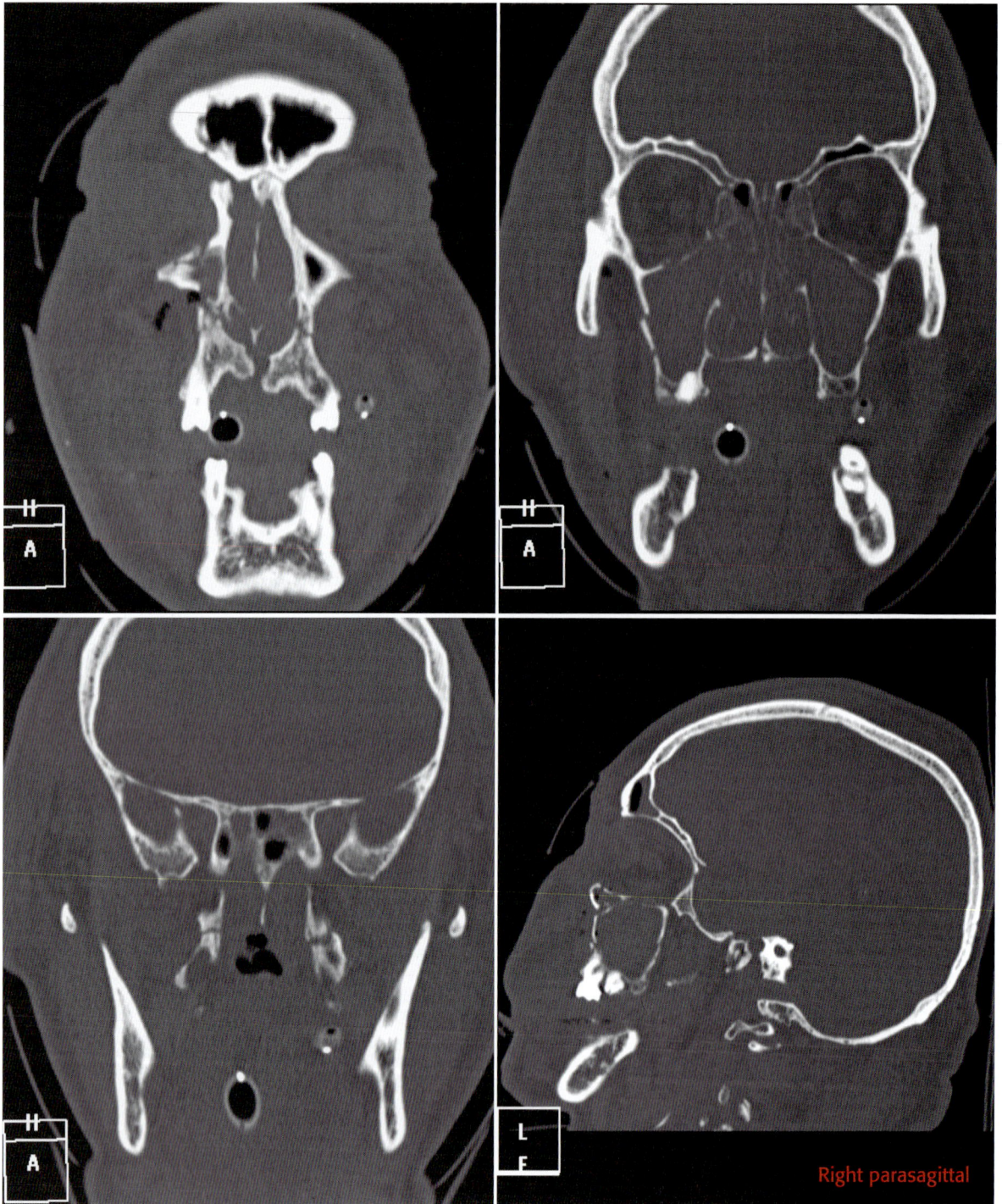

Right parasagittal

This 65-year-old man was the unrestrained driver in a high-speed motor vehicle crash.

**Q**
Describe the facial fractures.

## A

There are extensive facial fractures. The fractures pass through the pterygoid process bilaterally, extending horizontally through the walls of the maxillary sinuses and into the lateral margins of the nasal aperture bilaterally. On the right side the inferior orbital rim is fractured and this extends into the anteromedial orbital wall. The frontal process of the maxilla is fractured on the right and the right side of the frontonasal junction is disrupted. There is also a sagittal fracture of the hard palate. These findings are in keeping with a LeFort I fracture bilaterally and a LeFort II fracture on the right. On the images in the book, the right globe of the eye does not look entirely normal. The axial brain images on the DVD confirm that the globe is ruptured.

## LEARNING POINT

A LeFort fracture has two components (Jeffrey, 2007). Firstly, there must be disruption of the pterygomaxillary junction with fractures of the pterygoid processes and/or pterygoid plates. Secondly, there must be discontinuity between the skull and portions of the face (maxilla), which is usually manifest clinically by mobility of the face.

Other maxillary fractures that may be confused with LeFort fractures include zygomaticomaxillary complex fractures, nasoethmoid fractures and midface smash fractures. These fracture patterns do not involve the pterygoid processes or plates, unless there is a coexisting LeFort fracture, but this combination is common. Isolated pterygoid plate avulsion may occur with severe mandibular trauma.

LeFort fractures may be (Jeffrey, 2007):
- Type I: the fracture is horizontally oriented, separating the palate and maxillary alveolus from the remainder of the face and skull. The anterolateral wall of the nasal fossa, the medial and lateral walls of the maxillary sinus, and the nasal septum are fractured. The characteristic feature separating this type from the other LeFort types is a fracture of the lateral margin of the nasal aperture.
- Type II: the fracture separates the midface from the skull and is the commonest of the three types. The inferomedial orbital rim, the anteromedial orbital wall and the frontonasal junction are fractured. The characteristic feature of type II is a fracture of the inferior orbital rim.
- Type III: the fracture separates the entire face from the skull and is the least common type. The frontonasal junction, the medial and lateral orbital walls and the zygomatic arches are fractured.

Combinations of more than one type of LeFort fracture are common.

# PROBLEM 3.22

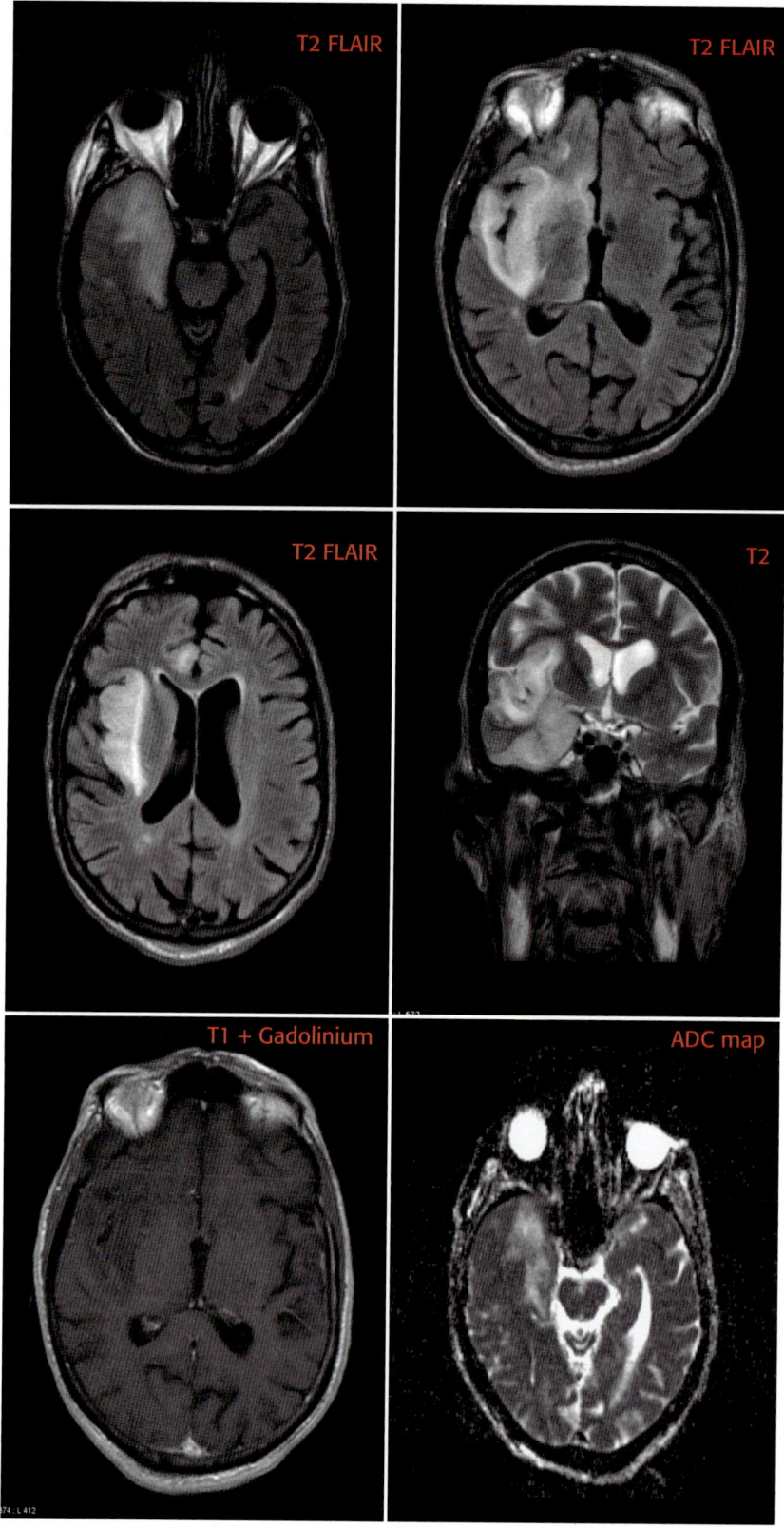

This 75-year-old man was admitted to the ICU with low grade fever, an altered level of consciousness and repeated seizures.

## Q
What diagnosis does the scan suggest?

## A
The T2-weighted images show increased signal (whiter areas) within the right temporal lobe, extending into the insula and frontal lobe inferiorly. There is reduced signal in these areas in the T1-weighted images. The lesion does not enhance with contrast. These findings are strongly suggestive of herpes encephalitis.

The apparent diffusion coefficient (ADC) map shows increased signal in the affected area. It is more typical that herpes encephalitis shows reduced signal (restricted diffusion), particularly in the early stages. However, the pattern is variable and the finding of increased ADC signal does not rule out the diagnosis in the presence of other typical features.

## LEARNING POINT
MRI is the imaging technique of choice for herpes encephalitis. Typically with herpes encephalitis, there is a hyperintense T2 signal in the temporal lobes, inferior frontal lobes and insula. It has a predilection for the medial temporal lobes and the basal ganglia are usually spared. The T1 signal is hypointense, consistent with oedema. Mild patchy gyral or cisternal contrast enchancement may occur. Diffusion weighted imaging may be more sensitive for early herpes than T2-weighted images (Dahnert, 2007).

See Chapter 6: Imaging modalities, p 375 for further explanation of terms used.

## PROBLEM 3.23

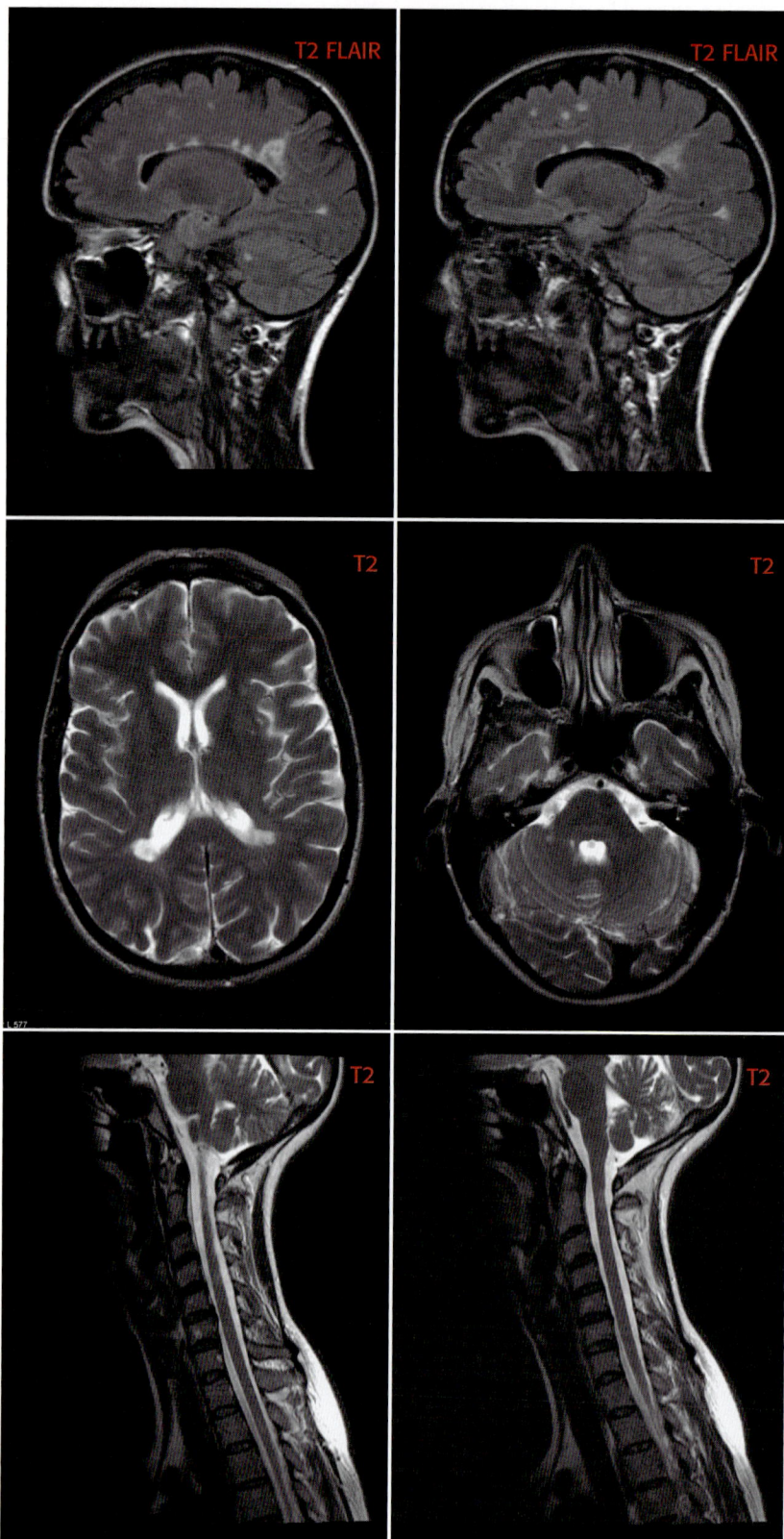

This 46-year-old woman presented with quadriparesis and respiratory failure. One year ago, she developed severe weakness in her right arm that resolved over a period of two months.

## Q

What pathological process is demonstrated in these images?

## A

There are multiple areas of increased intensity on the T2-weighted and the T2-FLAIR images in the cerebral white matter and the spinal cord. In this clinical context, these findings are strongly suggestive of multiple sclerosis. For this patient, dissemination in time is demonstrated by the two attacks and dissemination in space is demonstrated by the MRI.

## LEARNING POINT

To diagnose multiple sclerosis, there must be at least one clinically apparent neurological disturbance consistent with the multiple sclerosis and evidence that the disease process is disseminated in both space and time. This evidence may be clinical or based on MRI findings (Polman, 2005).

The lesions in multiple sclerosis are characteristically adjacent to the ventricles and oriented perpendicular to the ventricles. They involve regions such as the corpus callosum and the cerebellar peduncles. They show well in T2-weighted images. When gadolinium enhancement is present, this suggests active inflammation (Dahnert, 2007).

See Chapter 6: Imaging modalities, p 375 for further explanation of terms used.

## PROBLEM 3.24

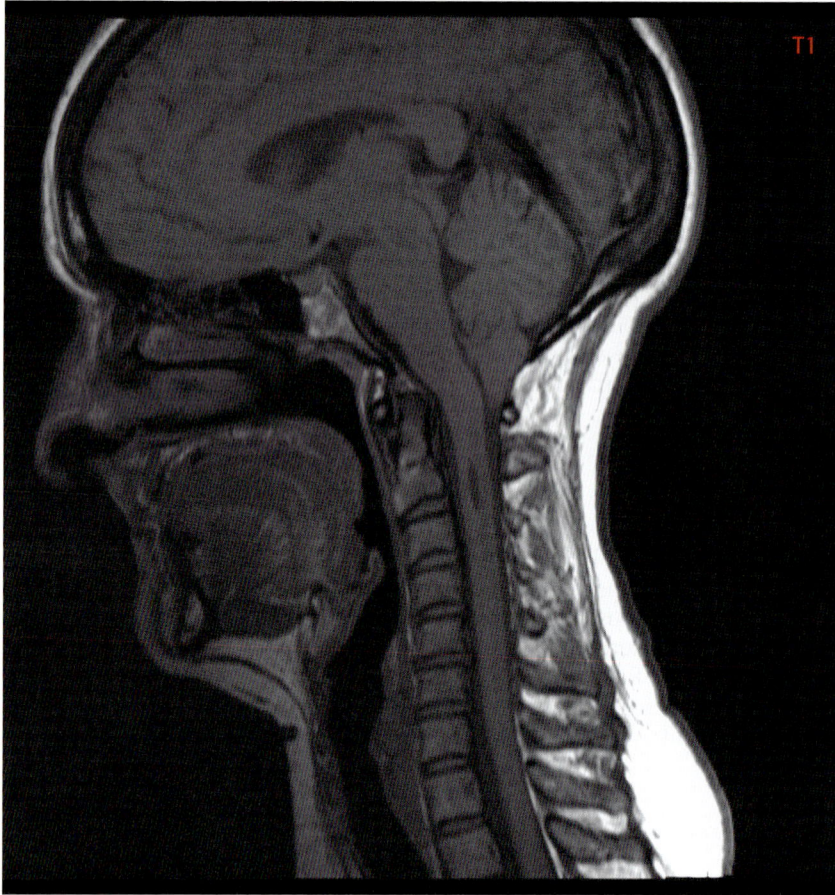

This 48-year-old woman suffered from episodes of syncope for two weeks. During a syncopal episode in the emergency department, she became apnoeic and required manual ventilation by facemask.

**Q**

What disease process is suggested by the image?

## A

The cerebellar tonsils extend well below the level of the foramen magnum and have an elongated pointed shape. The fourth ventricle is correspondingly elongated. At the C2 level, there is an oblong hypointense lesion within the spinal cord; consistent with hydromyelia (dilatation with CSF of the central canal of the cord). These features are in keeping with a Chiari 1 malformation.

## LEARNING POINT

With a Chiari 1 malformation, the following findings may be observed on MRI:
- displacement of the cerebellar tonsils below the level of the foramen magnum
- pointed and/or peg-like tonsils
- narrow posterior cranial fossa
- elongation of the fourth ventricle, which remains in the normal position
- hindbrain abnormalities
- obstructive hydrocephalus
- associated abnormalities such as syringomyelia or hydromyelia and skeletal abnormalities (Dahnert, 2007)

The most reliable diagnostic criterion is herniation of the cerebellar tonsils by at least 5 mm below the foramen magnum, in the absence of an intracranial mass lesion (Dahnert, 2007).

The level of the foramen magnum is measured on the sagittal T1 image. It is defined as a line between the front (basion) and the back (opisthion) of the foramen magnum. The signal of cortical bone, not marrow, must be used to define these landmarks.

## PROBLEM 3.25

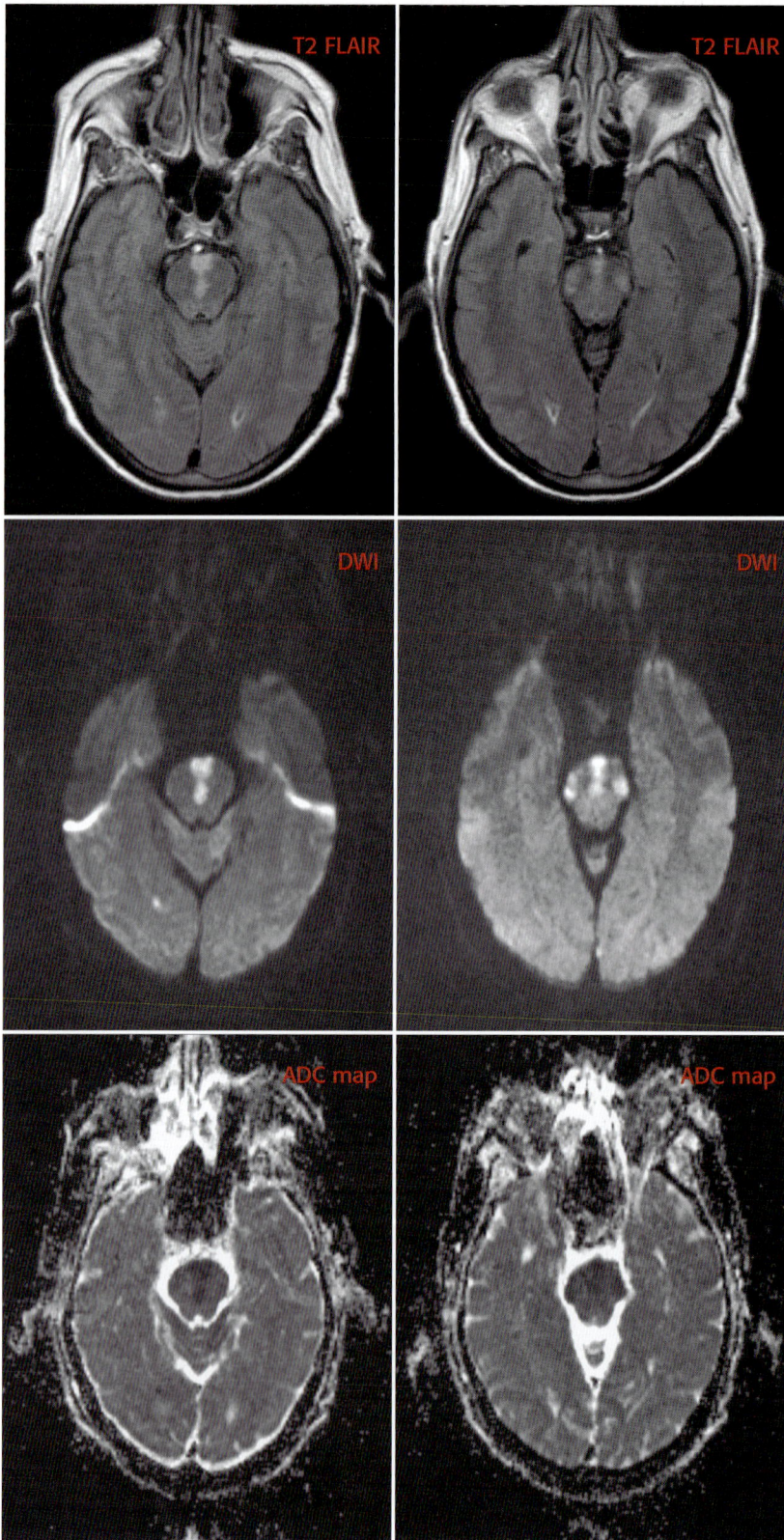

This 59-year-old woman had a rapid onset of quadriparesis. A CT scan of her head and cervical spine was normal. A provisional diagnosis of Guillaine-Barré syndrome has been made.

**Q**

Why has this patient become quadriparetic?

**A**

On the T2-FLAIR image, there are multiple areas of increased intensity within the pons and midbrain. On the diffusion weighted image, these same areas are of increased intensity while, on the apparent diffusion coefficient map, they appear hypointense. This is a pattern of reduced diffusion, suggesting cytotoxic oedema from acute ischaemia in these areas. On the DVD images, there are other similar areas consistent with acute posterior circulation ischaemia.

The other clue to the pathology is the absence of a flow void in the basilar artery, which appears hyperintense on the FLAIR sequence. This is strongly suggestive of basilar artery thrombosis, either as a primary event or secondary to dissection or embolism. This could be confirmed with MR angiography.

See Chapter 6: Imaging modalities, p 375 for further explanation of terms used.

**L**EARNING POINT

CT has a low sensitivity for brainstem ischaemic events because of the high incidence of bone-related artefact in the posterior fossa and inability to elicit ancillary signs such as cerebral swelling, sulcal effacement and loss of grey–white differentiation. MRI has a high sensitivity and specificity for detecting this disease process.

# PROBLEM 3.26

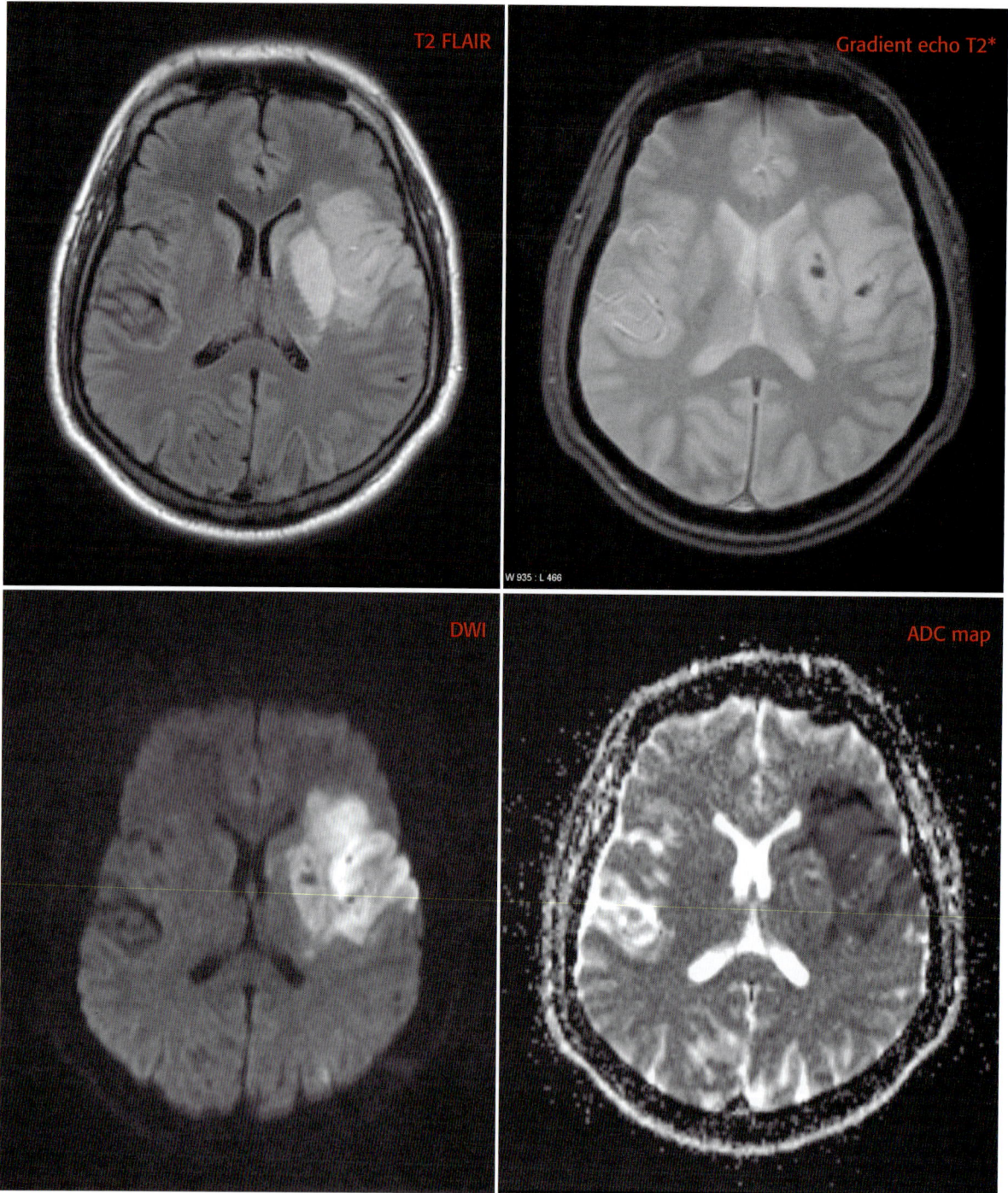

This 42-year-old man developed an acute right hemiplegia. He required mechanical ventilation after a massive aspiration episode resulted in hypoxaemic respiratory failure.

**Q**

What pathological process is suggested by these images?

## A

There is abnormal T2 signal in the left basal ganglia and adjacent cortex on the left. On the corresponding areas of the diffusion weighted image (DWI), there is increased signal and, in the apparent diffusion coefficient (ADC) map, there is reduced signal. This suggests acute ischaemia in the left middle cerebral artery territory. On the DWI image, there are some foci of reduced signal, which suggest some petechial haemorrhage within the infarct. This is best seen on the gradient echo sequence.

## LEARNING POINT

With cerebral ischaemia or acute infarction, there is a pattern suggestive of cytotoxic oedema. That is, intensity is high on the DWI and reduced on the ADC map before any changes are visible on T2-weighted images. The T2-signal subsequently becomes hyperintense. At around 7–10 days, the ADC map becomes bright, allowing the age of the infarct to be estimated (Rajeshkannan, 2006).

See Chapter 6: Imaging modalities, p 375 for further explanation of terms used.

# PROBLEM 3.27

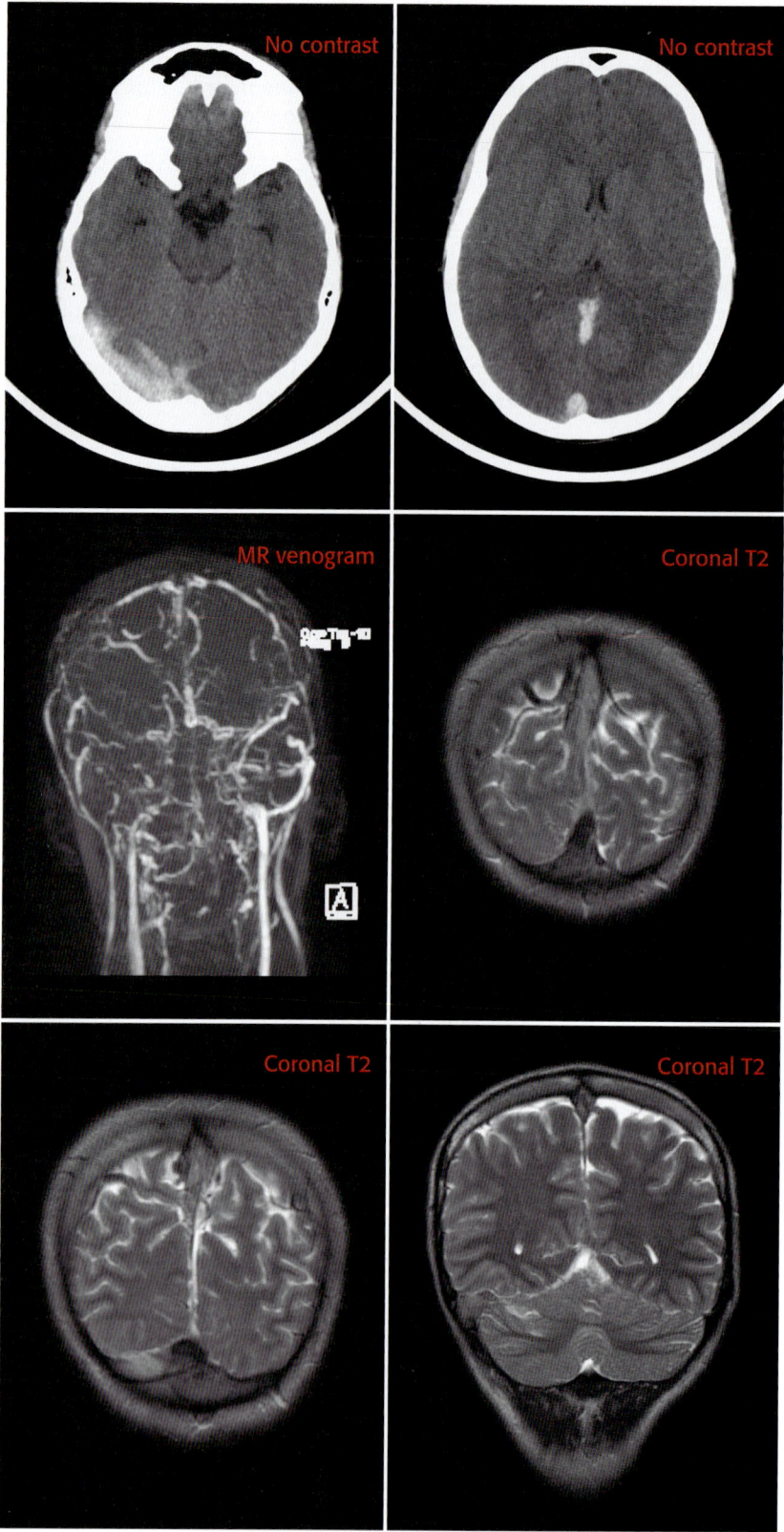

This 20-year-old woman presented with severe headache and subsequent seizures.

## Q

What pathological process is demonstrated by these images?

## A

The CT images are hyperdense in the positions of the right transverse sinus, superior sagittal sinus and straight sinus. This suggests thrombosis of these vessels.

The coronal T2 images show normal flow voids in cortical vessels. However, there is abnormal signal and absence of flow voids in the positions of the superior sagittal sinus, the right transverse sinus and the right sigmoid sinus. The MR venogram shows flow defects in the superior sagittal sinus, right and left transverse sinuses, and right sigmoid sinus. The left sigmoid sinus is relatively normal. Despite this extensive cerebral venous sinus thrombosis, there is no evidence of infarction.

## LEARNING POINT

A hyperdense appearance of an artery or vein on non-contrast CT suggests vascular thrombosis. Filling defects may be demonstrated on contrast enhanced CT. On both T1- and T2-weighted MRI images, the features suggesting arterial or venous thrombosis are the absence of normal flow voids and the presence of abnormal signal within the affected vessels.

MRI is the imaging modality of choice for cerebral venous thrombosis. MR venography demonstrates flow defects in the affected veins, while the other imaging sequences assess for the presence of venous infarction. Venous infarction is characteristically haemorrhagic and does not conform to the territories of the arterial supply.

## PROBLEM 3.28

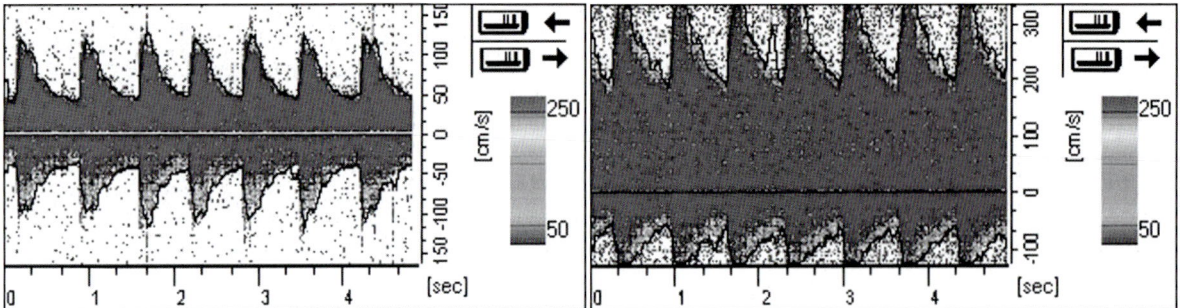

**Three days after admission**
Site:  L middle cerebral artery
Depth:  60 mm; Scale: 8500 Hz; Gain: 60%

|  | +ve | -ve |
|---|---|---|
| Peak velocity (cm/sec) | 139 | 125 |
| Mean velocity (cm/sec) | 75 | 65 |
| Pulsatility index | 1.25 | 1.37 |

Mean velocity at extracranial L ICA was 42 cms$^{-1}$

**Five days after admission**
Site:  L middle cerebral artery
Depth:  50 mm; Scale: 12000 Hz; Gain: 70%

|  | +ve | -ve |
|---|---|---|
| Peak velocity (cm/sec) | 334 | 134 |
| Mean velocity (cm/sec) | 259 | 98 |
| Pulsatility index | 0.57 | 0.81 |

Mean velocity at extracranial L ICA was 48 cms$^{-1}$

After having a grade 1 aneurysmal subarachnoid haemorrhage, this 24-year-old woman developed a right hemiparesis on day seven after admission.

The transcranial Doppler studies shown use a window in the temporal region to study the left middle cerebral artery. The sample volume for the pulse-wave Doppler study is placed at the junction of the middle cerebral artery (MCA) and anterior cerebral artery (ACA). Hence, forward flow in the MCA is above the baseline and forward flow in the ACA is below the baseline.

## Q

What pathological process is demonstrated by these transcranial Doppler studies?

## A

The transcranial Doppler (TCD) study three days after admission is normal. There is systolic and diastolic flow signal above the baseline (towards the transducer) from the left MCA. There is similar flow pattern below the baseline (away from the transducer). With a sample depth of 60 mm during a MCA study (temporal window), this indicates that the sample volume is at the bifurcation of the MCA and ACA, respectively.

The TCD study five days after admission shows a marked increase in the mean flow velocity in the MCA (above the baseline). The Lindegaard ratio is moderately elevated at 5.4. The pulsatility index is normal. These findings suggest vasospasm in the MCA. The flow velocity remains normal in both the ACA (below the baseline) and the extracranial internal carotid.

## LEARNING POINT

The Lindegaard ratio (LR) is a parameter derived from TCD recordings.

**Lindegaard ratio =**

$$\frac{\text{mean velocity in MCA}}{\text{mean velocity in ipsilateral extracranial carotid artery}}$$

High flow velocities in the MCA (mean velocity in MCA > 120 cms$^{-1}$) may be due to hyperaemia or vasospasm. The LR is used to distinguish these conditions. In the setting of a high flow velocity, a LR < 3 suggests the problem is hyperaemia, while a LR > 3 suggests the problem is vasospasm (White, 2006).

Mild vasospasm is suggested by a LR of 3–6. Severe vasospasm is suggested by a mean velocity in the MCA > 200 cms$^{-1}$ or a LR > 6. An increase in systolic velocity > 50 cms$^{-1}$ over 24 hours predicts the onset of delayed ischaemic deficit (White, 2006).

## PROBLEM 3.29

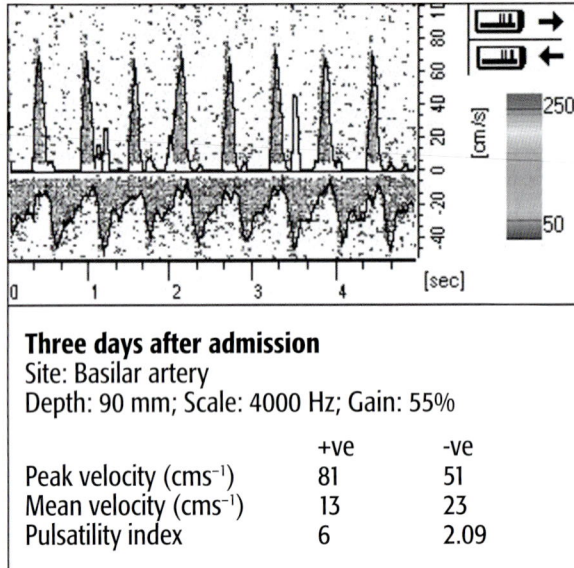

**Three days after admission**
Site: Basilar artery
Depth: 90 mm; Scale: 4000 Hz; Gain: 55%

|  | +ve | -ve |
|---|---|---|
| Peak velocity (cms$^{-1}$) | 81 | 51 |
| Mean velocity (cms$^{-1}$) | 13 | 23 |
| Pulsatility index | 6 | 2.09 |

This 19-year-old motorcyclist was admitted with a severe head injury. On day three following admission, his pupils have become fixed and dilated.

The image shown is from a transcranial Doppler study, using a window through the foramen magnum to study the basilar artery. Forward flow in the basilar artery is above the baseline.

**Q**
What does this transcranial Doppler study demonstrate?

## A

There is a "reverberant flow" pattern, in which there is forward flow during systole and backward flow during diastole. This indicates that the cerebral blood flow during systole is not retained during diastole and there is no sustainable cerebral perfusion (Moppett, 2004).

## LEARNING POINT

Transcranial Doppler (TCD) is a useful ancillary investigation in the setting of suspected brain death. When the clinical criteria for brain death cannot be used, TCD may assist with the timing of definitive studies such as four-vessel angiography.

The pulsatility index (PI) is a parameter derived from TCD recordings. The PI is an index of the vascular resistance of the more distal cerebral circulation. It is normal in vasospasm, but rises with elevation in the intracranial pressure. Values over 1.5 are abnormal.

**Pulsatility index** =

$$\frac{(\text{Peak systolic velocity} - \text{end diastolic velocity})}{\text{mean velocity}}$$

## REFERENCES

Berman SA, Hayman LA, Hinck VC. Correlation of CT cerebral vascular territories with function. I: Anterior cerebral artery. Am J Roentgenol 1980; 135(2): 253–7

Berman SA, Hayman LA, Hinck VC. Correlation of CT cerebral vascular territories with function. 3: Middle cerebral artery. Am J Roentgenol 1984; 142(5): 1035–40

Bladin CF, Chambers BR. Clinical features, pathogenesis, and computed tomographic characteristics of internal watershed infarction. Stroke 1993; 24: 1925–32

Carpenter MB. Chapter 13. Blood supply of the central nervous system. In: Carpenter MB, ed. Core text in neuroanatomy. 4th edn. Baltimore: Williams and Wilkins; 1991

Dahnert W, ed. Radiology review manual. 6th edn. Philadelphia: Lippincott Williams and Wilkins; 2007

Harnsberger HR, Osborn AG, Ross JS, et al (eds). Diagnostic and surgical imaging anatomy. Brain, head and neck, spine. Int edn. Salt Lake City: AMIRSYS; 2006

Hayman LA, Berman SA, Hinck VC. Correlation of CT cerebral vascular territories with function. II: Posterior cerebral artery. Am J Roentgenol 1981; 137(1): 13–19

Jeffrey RB, Manaster BJ, Gurney JW, et al (eds). Diagnostic imaging. Emergency. 1st edn. Salt Lake City: AMIRSYS; 2007

Moppett IK, Mahajan RP. Transcranial Doppler ultrasonography in anaesthesia and intensive care. Br J Anaesth 2004; 93(5): 710–24

Moeller TB, Reif E (eds). Pocket atlas of sectional anatomy: CT and MRI. 2nd edn. Stuttgart, Thieme; 2000

Nakano S, Yokogami K, Ohta H, et al. CT-defined large subcortical infarcts: Correlation of location with site of cerebrovascular occlusive disease. Am J Neuroradiol 1995; 16(8): 1581–5

Norrving B. Lacunar infarcts: no black holes in the brain are benign. Pract Neurol 2008; 8(4): 222–8

Osborn AG, Hedlund GL, Blaser SI, et al (eds). Diagnostic imaging brain. 1st edn. Salt Lake City: AMIRSYS; 2004

Polman CH, Reingold SC, Edan G, et al. Diagnostic criteria for multiple sclerosis: 2005 revisions to the "McDonald criteria". Ann Neurol 2005; 58(6): 840–6

Rajeshkannan R, Moorthy S, P. SK, et al. Clinical applications of diffusion weighted MR imaging: a review. Indian J Radiol Imaging 2006; 16(4): 705–10

Ropper AH. Chapter 257: Acute confusional states and coma. In: Kasper DL, Braunwald E, Fauciet AS, eds. Harrison's principles of internal medicine. 16th edn. New York: McGraw-Hill; 2005: 1624–31

Smith WS, Johnston SC, Easton JE. Chapter 349: Cerebrovascular diseases. In: Kasper DL, Braunwald E, Fauciet AS, eds. Harrison's principles of internal medicine. 16th edn. New York: McGraw-Hill; 2005: 2372–2393

White H, Venkatesh B. Applications of transcranial doppler in the ICU: a review. Intensive Care Med 2006; 32(7): 981–94

# CHAPTER 4

# NECK AND BACK

Computed tomography (CT) is the preferred imaging modality for assessment of suspected spinal injuries in critically ill trauma patients, with supplementary MRI used when spinal cord or ligamentous injury is suspected. This chapter will focus on these imaging modalities.

# APPLIED ANATOMY

## Craniocervical junction

The skull base, atlas (C1) and axis (C2) form the craniocervical junction that in conjunction with associated ligaments, acts as a single functional unit. Classification of injury is based on anatomical site. Injury patterns include occipitocervical dissociation, occipital condyle fracture, atlas fracture, atlantoaxial rotatory instability, atlantodens instability, odontoid fracture and traumatic spondylolisthesis of the axis (Torretti, 2007).

On sagittal CT images (Figure 4.1), check for the following normal features :
- space between anterior arch of C1 and the odontoid peg (atlantodental space) should be < 3 mm in an adult and < 5 mm in a child
- anterior cortex of the odontoid peg and posterior cortex of anterior arch of C1 are parallel
- anterior aspects of the laminae of C1–C3 form a straight line, the spinolaminar line
- bodies of C2 and C3 are in alignment, with a normal disc space

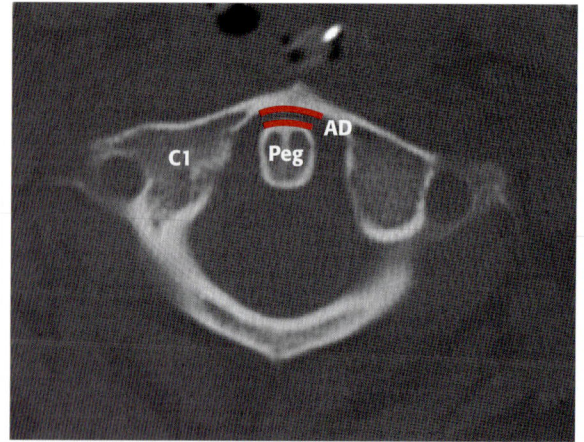

**FIGURE 4.2** Craniocervical junction: Axial image. AD = Atlantodental space.

- no subluxation or widening of the atlanto-occipital joints
- facet joints between C1/C2 and C2/C3 are aligned

On axial images (Figure 4.2), check for the following normal features:
- space between anterior arch of C1 and the odontoid peg should be < 3 mm
- C1 is symmetrically aligned around the odontoid peg
- no significant rotation of C0/1 or C1/2 (up to 15 degrees of C1/2 rotation may be normal)
- absence of soft tissue swelling

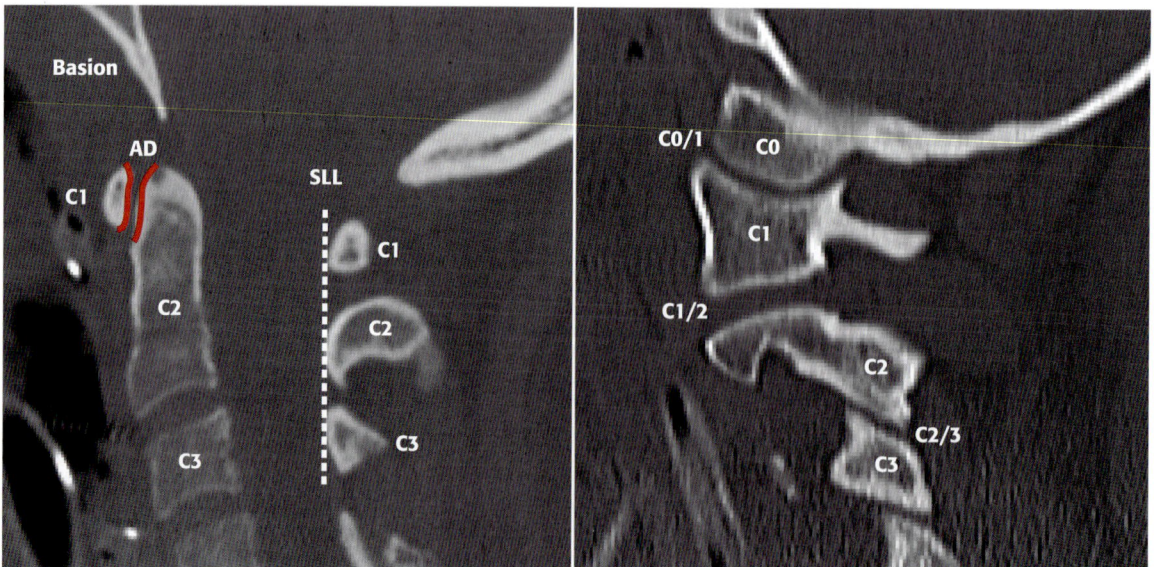

**FIGURE 4.1** Craniocervical junction: Sagittal and parasagittal images.
AD = Atlantodental space; SLL = Spinolaminar line; C0 = occipital condyle; C0/1 = Atlanto-occiptal joint; C1/2 = C1/2 facet joint; C2/3 = C2/3 facet joint.

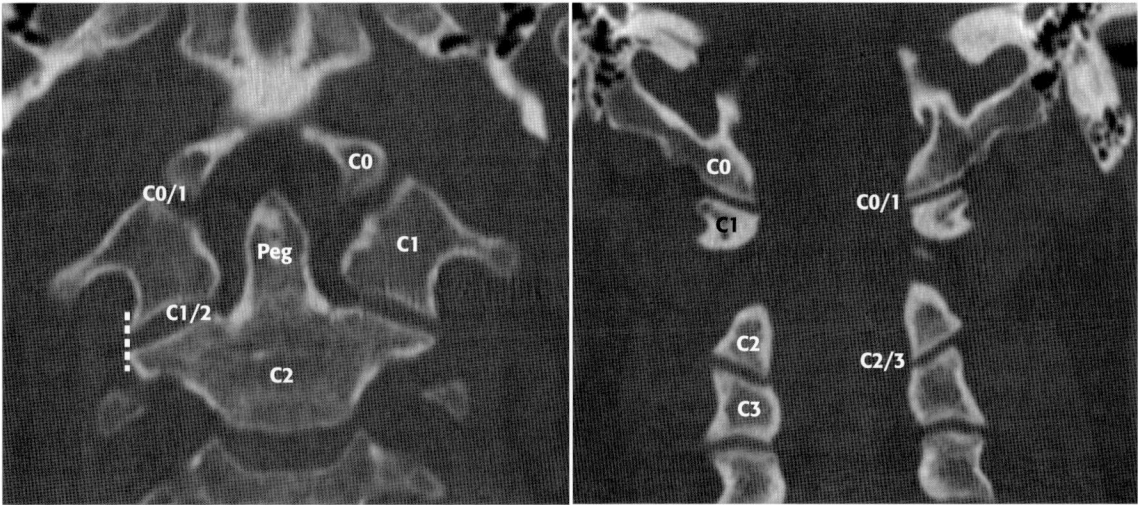

**FIGURE 4.3** Craniocervical junction: Coronal views.
C0 = Occipital condyle; C0/1 = Atlanto-occiptal joint; C1/2 = C1/2 facet joint; C2/3 = C2/3 facet joint; Peg = Odontoid peg; Dashed line indicates lateral borders of lateral masses of C1 and C2.

On coronal images (Figure 4.3), check for the following normal features:

- space between odontoid peg and lateral mass of C1 is the same on both sides
- there is no subluxation or widening of the atlanto-occipital joints
- the facet joints between C1/C2 and C2/C3 are aligned
- the edge of the lateral mass of C1 does not overhang C2 at the facet joint

The major ligaments of the craniocervical junction are (Torretti, 2007):

- the paired alar ligaments that extend from the odontoid peg to the medial aspect of the occipital condyles
- the posterior longitudinal ligament that runs posterior to the vertebral bodies and extends as the tectorial membrane to insert into the basion
- the anterior longitudinal ligament that runs anterior to the vertebral bodies and extends as the anterior atlanto-occipital membrane to insert into the basion
- the transverse atlantal ligament that extends between the lateral masses of C1, passing posterior to the odontoid peg

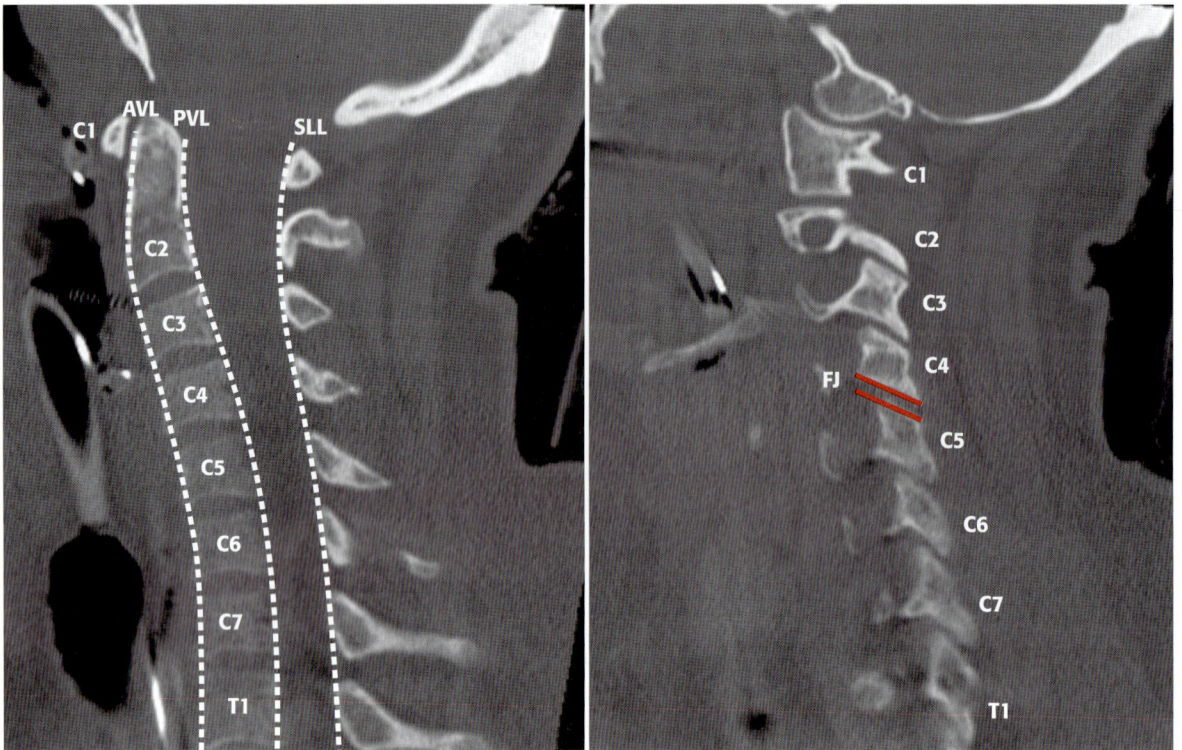

**FIGURE 4.4** Subaxial cervical spine: Sagittal and parasagittal images.
AVL = Anterior vertebral body line; PVL = Posterior vertebral body line; SLL = Spinolaminar line; FJ = Facet joint.

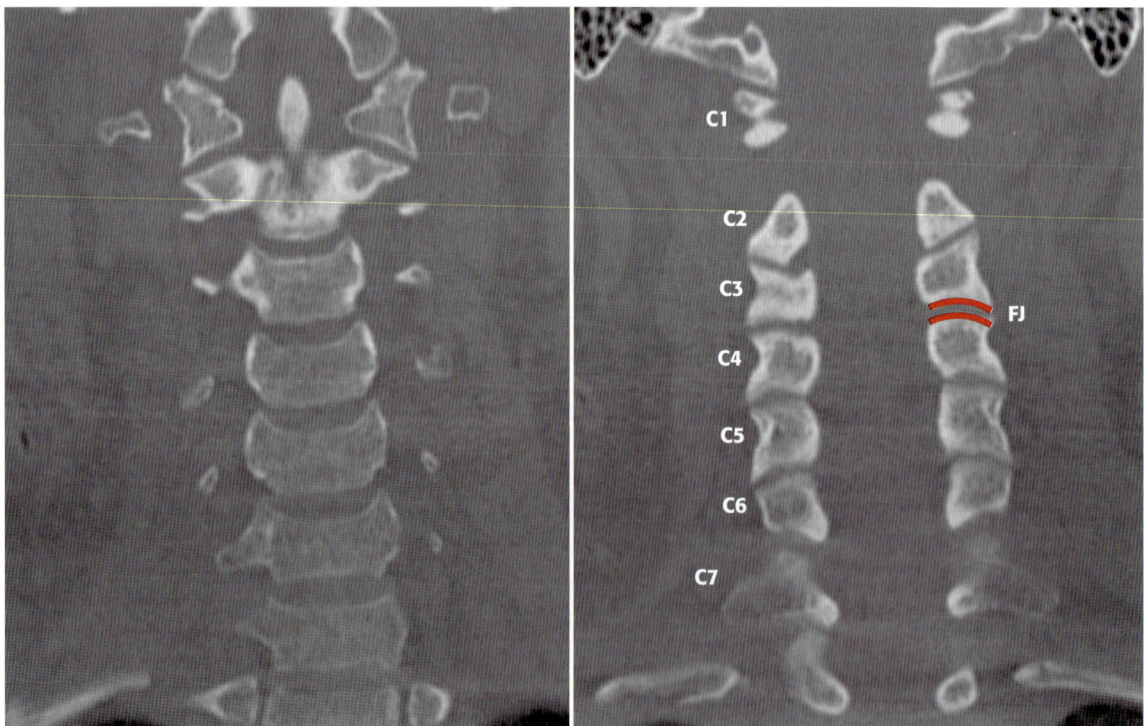

**FIGURE 4.5** Subaxial cervical spine: Coronal images. FJ = Facet joint.

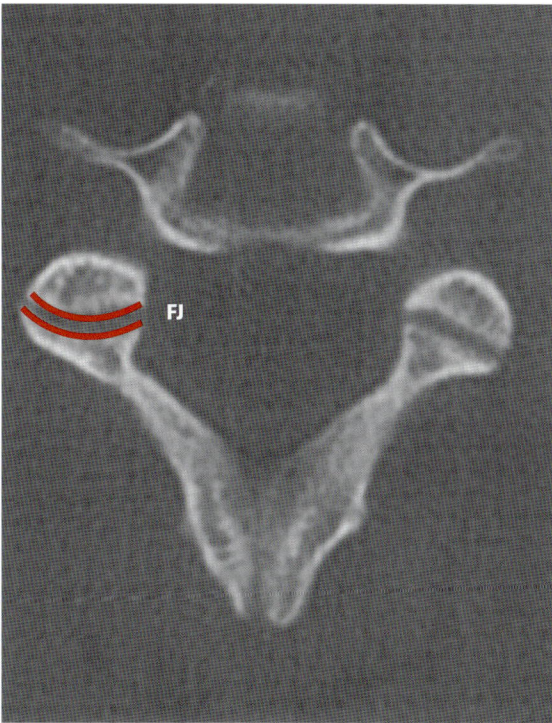

**FIGURE 4.6** Subaxial cervical spine: Axial images.
FJ = Facet joint.

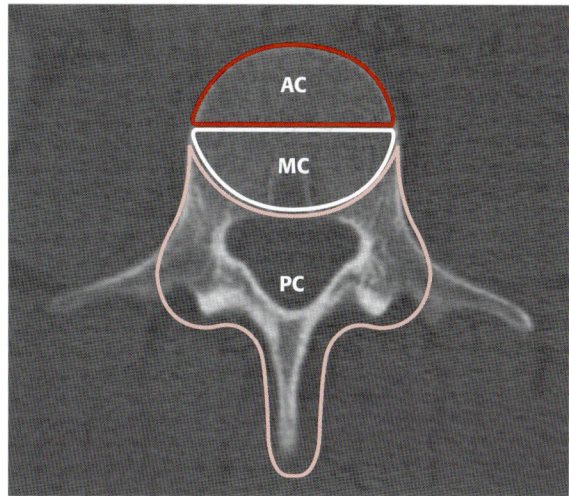

**FIGURE 4.7** Columns of thoracic spine.
AC = Anterior column; MC = Middle column; PC = Posterior column.

## Lower (subaxial) cervical spine

Classification of injury is based on the mechanism of injury. Common injury patterns include distractive flexion, compressive flexion, lateral flexion, vertical compression, distractive extension and compressive extension injuries (Allen, 1982; Torretti, 2007).

On sagittal reconstructions (Figure 4.4), check for the following normal features:

- anterior and posterior vertebral body lines and spinolaminar line are uninterrupted
- vertebral body height is the same anteriorly and posteriorly
- no prevertebral swelling
- no widening of distances between spinous processes
- facet joints aligned, appearing as stacked parallelograms
- disc spaces intact

On coronal images (Figure 4.5), check for the following normal features:

- height of each side of the vertebral body is the same
- disc spaces are intact
- facet joints are aligned

On axial images (Figure 4.6), check for the following normal features:

- no soft tissue swelling
- facet joints aligned
- no significant rotation

## Thoracolumbar spine (Figure 4.7)

Classification of injury to the thoracolumbar spine is based on the three column concept. Common injury patterns include compression fractures, burst fractures, flexion distraction (seat-belt type) injuries, and fracture dislocations (Denis, 1983). The anterior column is formed by the anterior longitudinal ligament, the anterior half of the vertebral body and the anterior annulus fibrosus. The middle column is formed by the posterior longitudinal ligament, the posterior half of the vertebral body and posterior annulus fibrosus. The posterior column is the posterior osseous arch, the supraspinous and interspinous ligaments, the ligamentum flavum, and the facet joint capsule.

The features sought on sagittal, coronal and axial images of the thoracolumbar spine are similar to those described for lower cervical spine injuries. The pattern of injuries differs between these two sites.

## PROBLEM 4.01

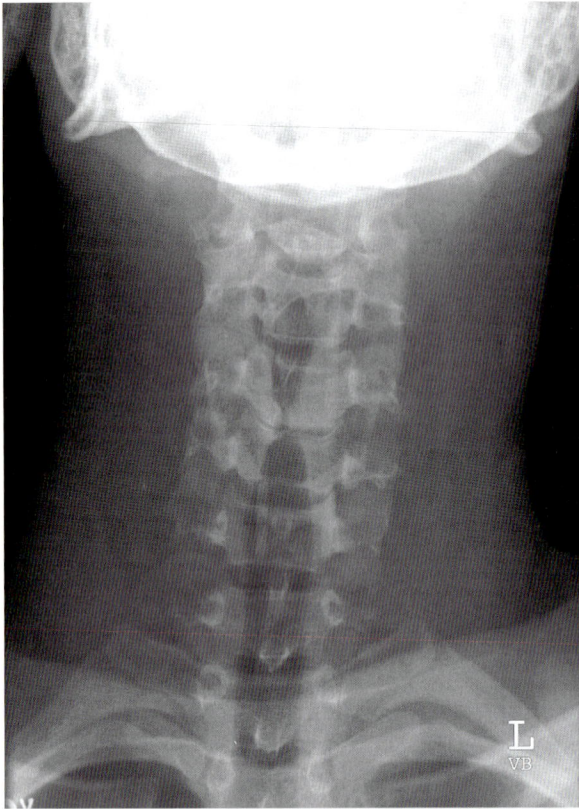
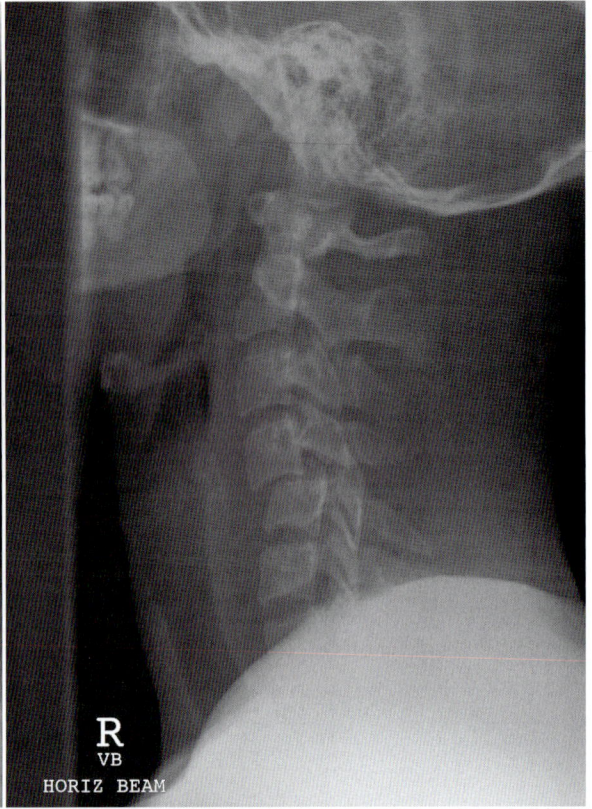
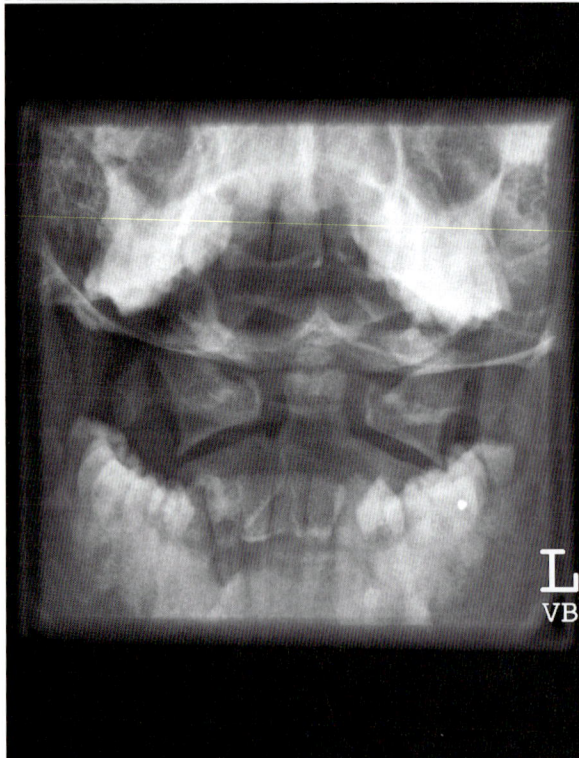
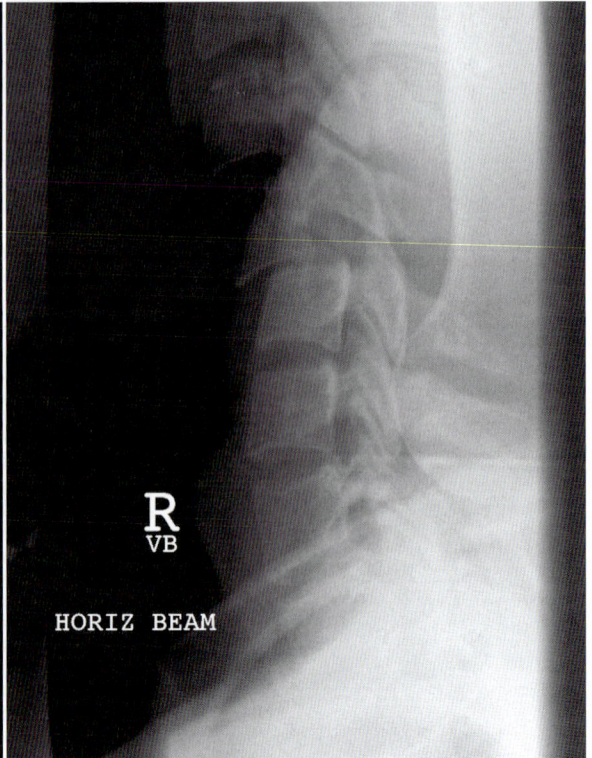

This 21-year-old man was knocked over by a wave while swimming in the surf four hours ago. He hit the back of his head on the sea floor. He has weakness and abnormal sensation in all limbs. The clinical signs suggest an incomplete spinal cord injury.

# Q

Describe the injury.

# A

On the AP view, the main abnormality is a narrowing of the C4/5 interspace. On the lateral view, there is disruption of the anterior and posterior vertebral body lines and the spinolaminar line at the C4/5 level. The inferior facets of C4 lie in front of the superior facets of C5. In addition, there is 50% shift of the body of C4 on C5 with angulation at this level. These features are typical of a bilateral facet joint dislocation. This is a severe form of a distractive flexion injury, often associated with spinal cord injury.

## LEARNING POINT

Recognition of a bilateral facet joint dislocation is important, as it is one of the few true surgical emergencies related to spinal injury. The dislocation may be reduced with traction or open reduction. If reduction cannot be achieved with traction, then immediate open reduction should be considered, particularly if the neurological signs are normal or incomplete (Thumbikat, 2007).

A unilateral facet joint dislocation is a less severe form of distractive flexion injury than a bilateral facet joint dislocation and can usually be distinguished from it on plain X-rays. On the AP image the spinous processes below the dislocation do not align with those above it and the interspinous gap is widened. The lateral image may show the facet joint dislocation but this is better seen on oblique views. At the level of the dislocation there is usually around 25% shift forward of the superior vertebral body on the inferior one. Traction is used to reduce unilateral facet joint dislocations but, even if this is unsuccessful, emergency surgery is seldom required (Thumbikat, 2007).

# PROBLEM 4.02

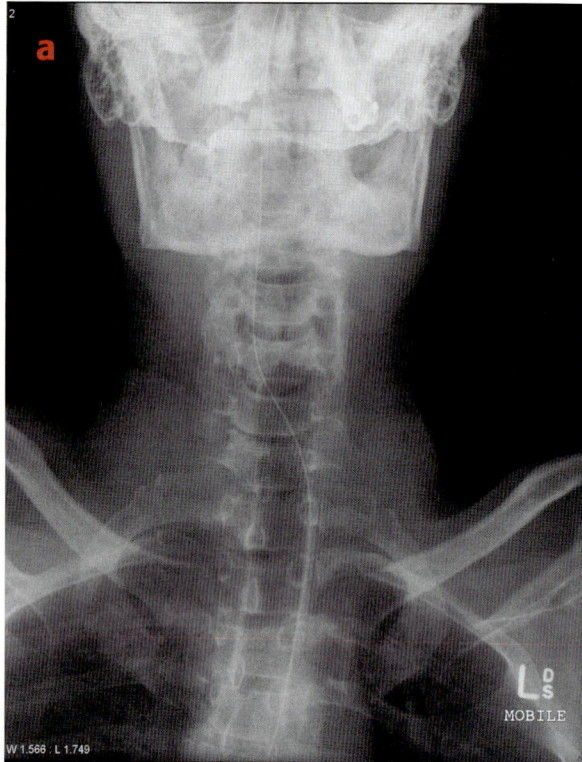

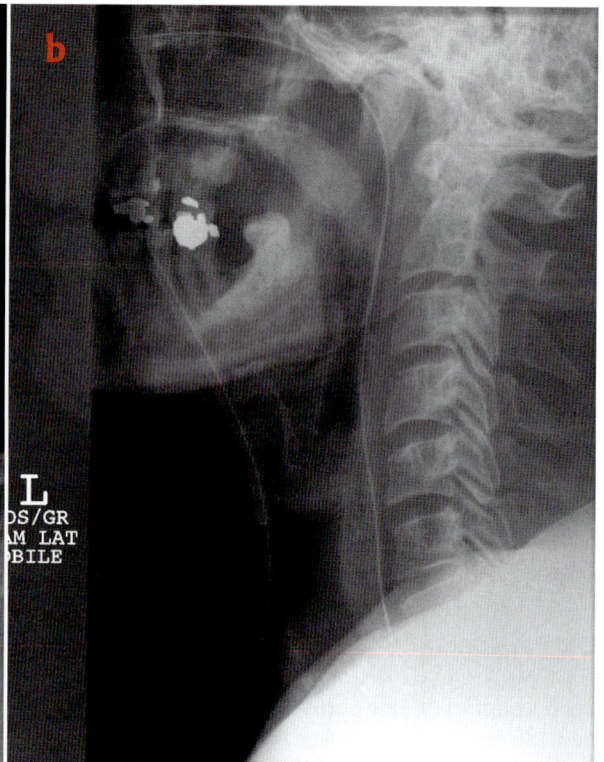

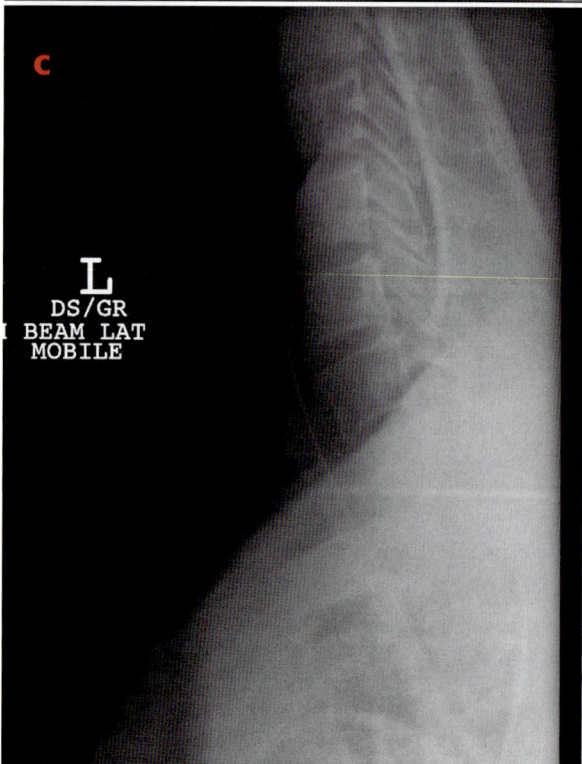

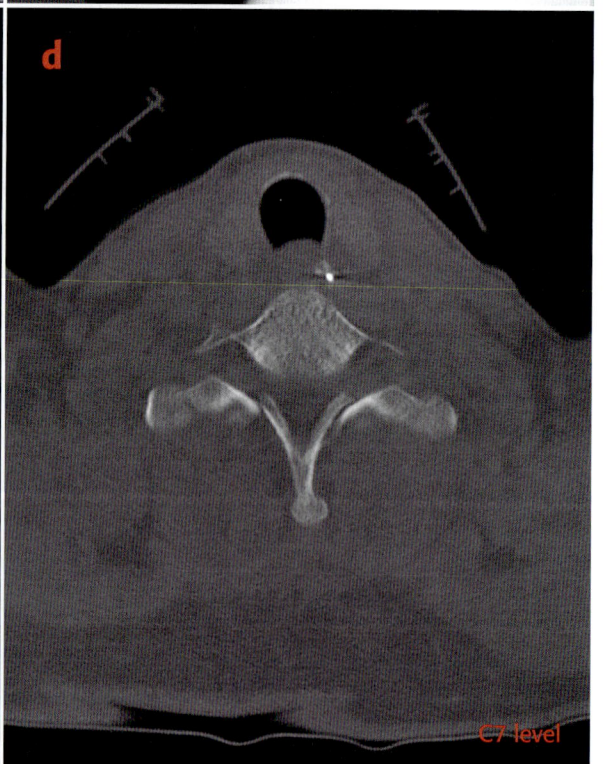

This 52-year-old man was an unrestrained passenger in a high-speed car crash today. He has multiple limb injuries and a major pelvic injury. He was intoxicated with alcohol and had a GCS of 12.

## Q

Describe the findings on the plain films and the CT scan.

## A

The plain films show no clear evidence of bone injury. At the antero-inferior border of the C5 and C6 vertebral bodies, there are small, well-corticated bone fragments that have the appearance of osteophytes. With the inclusion of a Swimmer view (image c), the alignment at the cervicothoracic junction is seen to be appropriate.

The CT scan presents a very different picture. The image in the book shows a bilaminar fracture at the C7 level, with anteropulsion of the fracture fragments into the vertebral canal. This indicates a compressive extension injury, which is potentially unstable. The images in the DVD show a similar injury at the C6 level.

## LEARNING POINT

The best approach to clearing the cervical spine in the patient with multiple trauma remains controversial. In this group of patients, plain X-rays miss a significant proportion of bony cervical spine injuries. In a study of patients with multiple trauma, a single cross table lateral view missed 37% of significant bony cervical spine injuries, a three-view series (AP, lateral, peg view) missed 10%, while cervical spine CT missed none (Platzer, 2006).

Ligamentous injuries are not well imaged with CT scan. When multiple trauma patients are imaged with CT scan, 6% have discoligamentous injuries that are not detected (Platzer, 2006).

The consequences of a missed cervical spine injury are potentially devastating. There is a relatively high incidence of missed fractures when plain radiography alone is used to image the cervical spine in patients with multiple trauma. CT is the imaging modality of choice in this group of patients, with supplementary MRI when spinal cord or ligamentous injury is suspected.

# PROBLEM 4.03

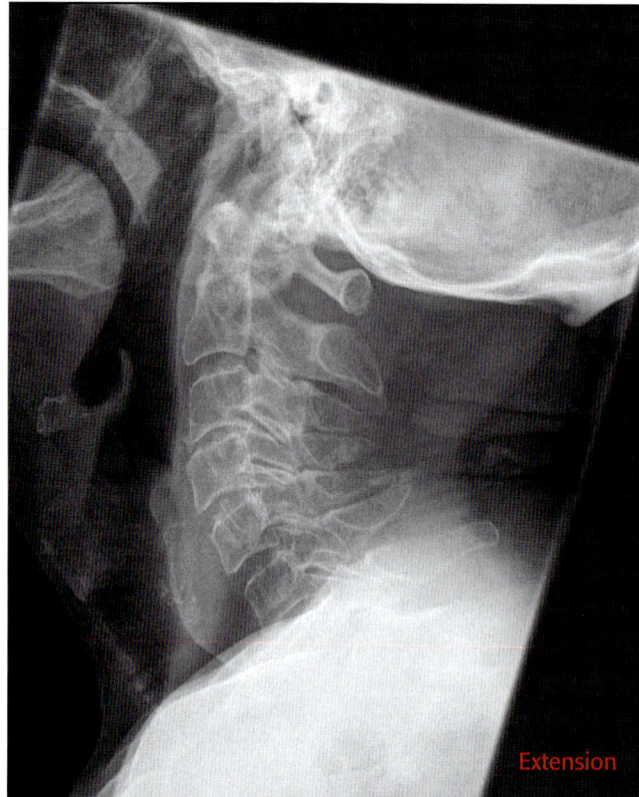

Extension

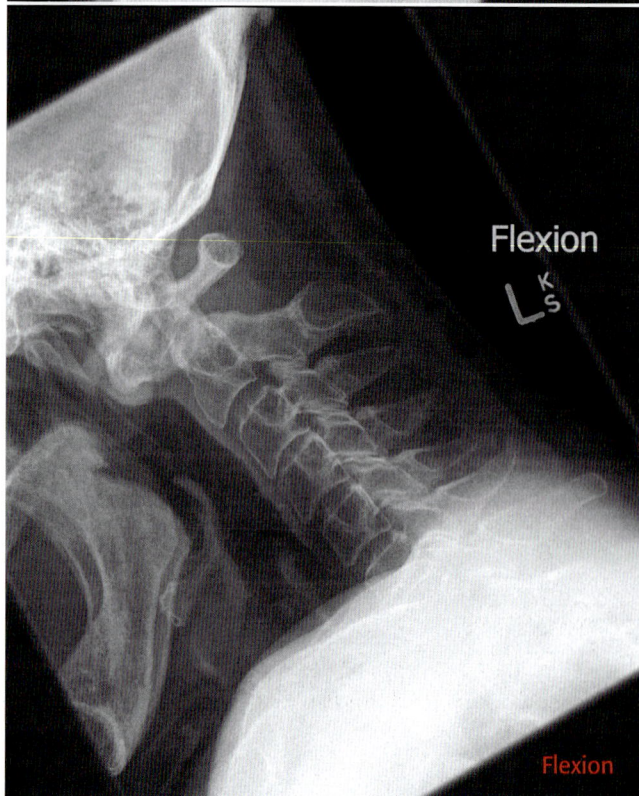

Flexion

Flexion

This 66-year-old man underwent elective coronary artery bypass grafting earlier today. He was extubated four hours after the procedure, but now requires reintubation because of atelectasis and sputum retention. These images were taken preoperatively because of a history of rheumatoid arthritis.

# Q

1. Describe the findings on these images.
2. What particular risk does reintubation pose for this patient?

# A

1. The major finding on these images is marked atlantoaxial subluxation that occurs when the neck is flexed. There is loss of the cortical outline of the upper part of the odontoid peg. This amount of subluxation is indirect evidence of rupture of the transverse atlantal ligament. There is osteoporosis of the spine.

These features are typical of severe rheumatoid arthritis. One feature of rheumatoid arthritis in the neck that is not seen on these images is fusion of the posterior elements of the spine.

2. There is a risk of cervical spinal cord injury with intubation.

# LEARNING POINT

Rheumatoid arthritis can have an important impact on airway management (Matti, 1998).
- Cervical spine involvement may produce subluxation at the atlanto-occipital joint or at subaxial joints. If this is present, manipulation of the position of the head during airway management may produce spinal cord compression or vertebrobasilar ischaemia.
- The range of motion of the neck may be limited by fibrosis and ankylosis.
- Temporomandibular joint involvement may lead to poor mouth opening.
- Cricoarytenoid joint arthritis may narrow the laryngeal inlet.

## PROBLEM 4.04

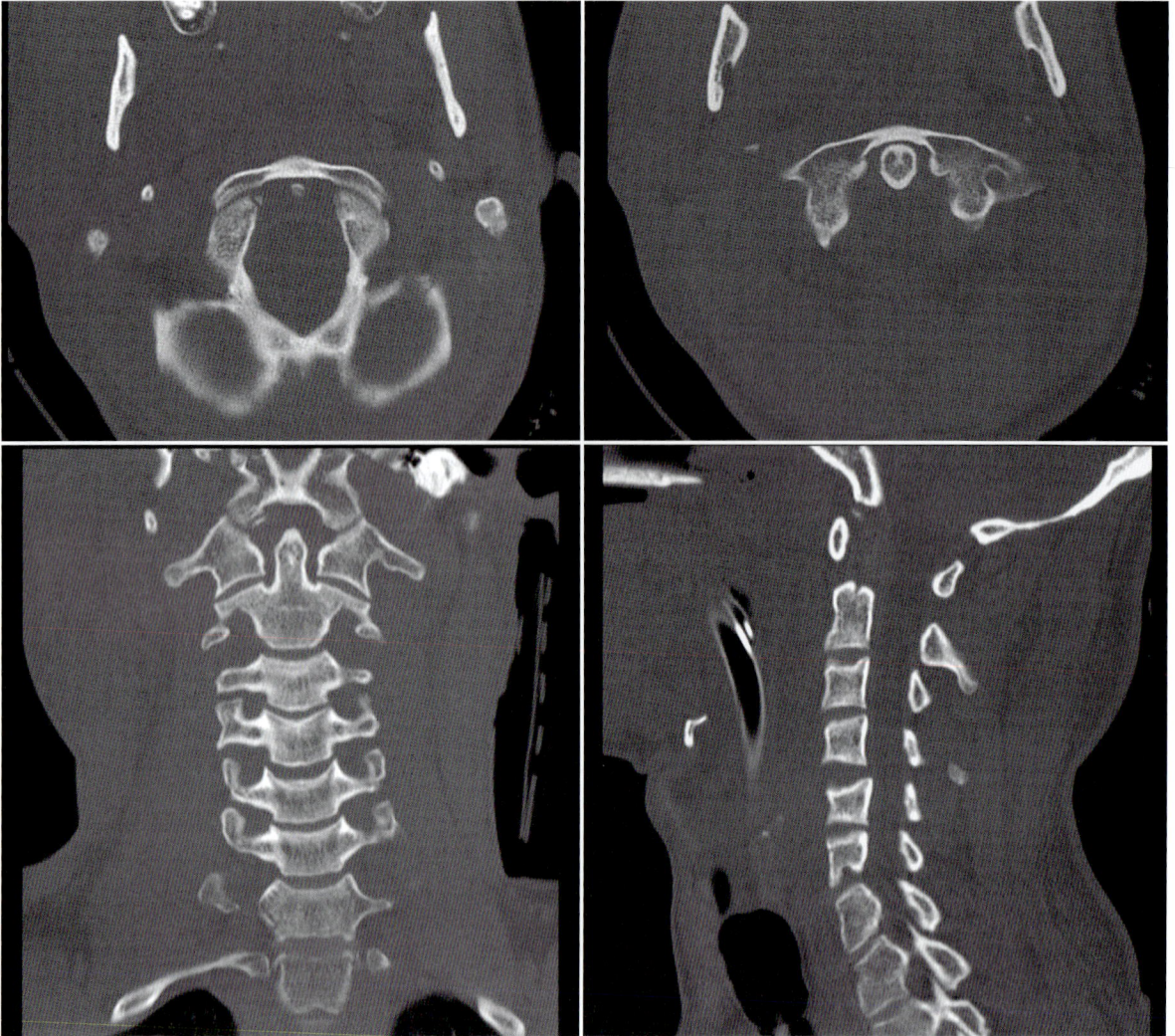

This 19-year-old woman fell off a horse while show jumping. She was confused and combative on arrival at hospital.

**Q** Describe the injury.

# A

There is a right occipital condyle fracture. The position of the fracture suggests that it may be an avulsion fracture at the insertion of the alar ligament. In the images provided, C1 is not displaced in relation to the occipital condyle.

The coronal views on the DVD show a fracture dislocation of the right mandibular ramus.

## LEARNING POINT

Common fracture patterns of the occipital condyle include crush fractures, fractures that are extensions of basal skull fractures and avulsion fractures related to the alar ligament (Anderson, 1988).

## PROBLEM 4.05

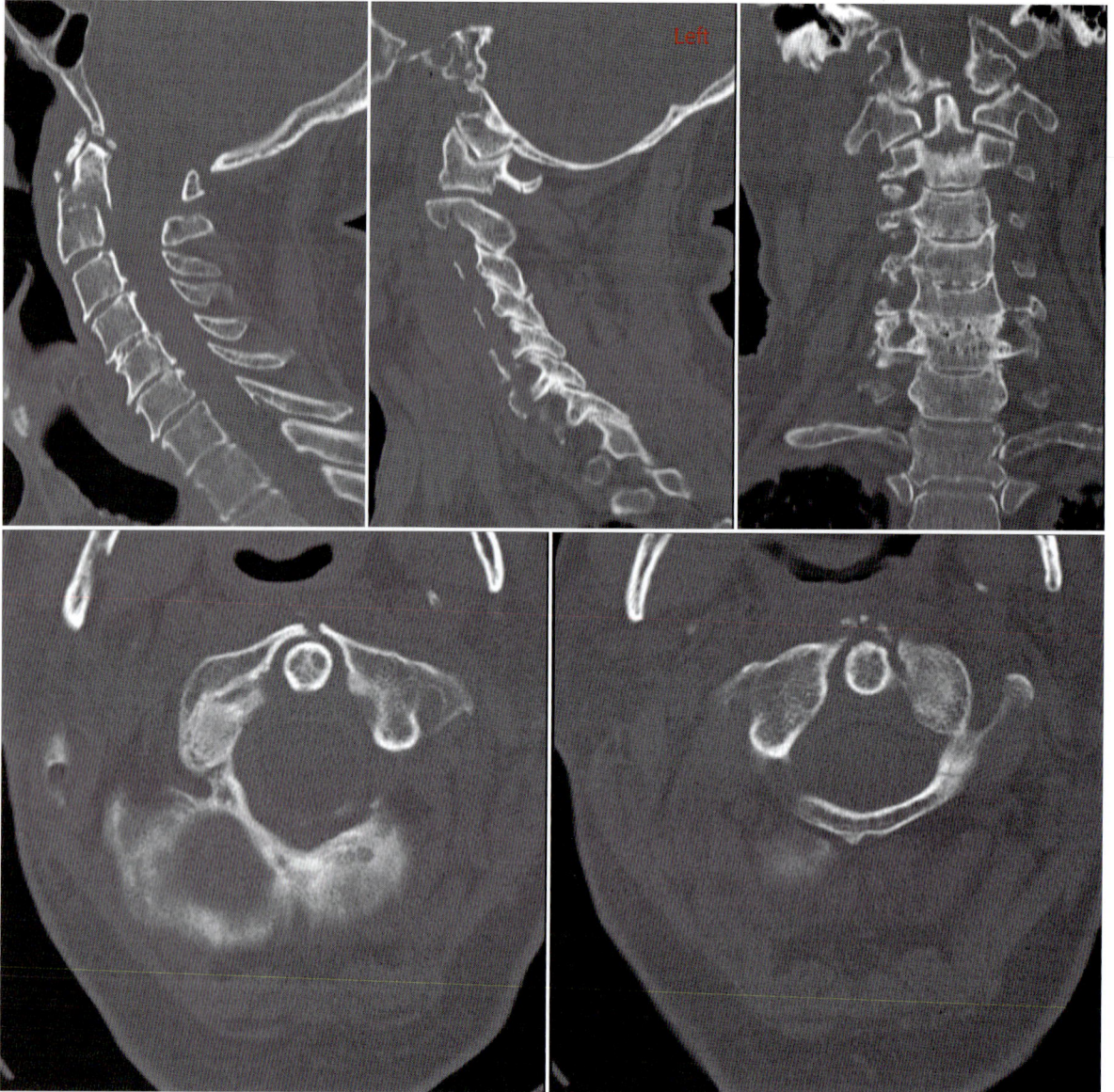

This 79-year-old front seat passenger was unconscious at the scene following a high-speed car crash.

**Q** Describe the injury.

## A

There are fractures of the anterior arch of C1 in the mid line and the posterior arch on the left side. In the coronal image, the right lateral mass of C1 overhangs C2, consistent with expansion of the C1 ring.

There is a fracture at the base of the odontoid peg extending into the body of C2 with posterior displacement of the peg (type 3 odontoid fracture). The spinolaminar line is disrupted at the C1/2 level. There is posterior displacement of C1 on C2 at both C1/2 facet joints.

There are extensive arthritic changes.

## LEARNING POINT

Odontoid fractures are classified as type 1 (tip of odontoid), type 2 (junction of dens and body) and type 3 (extending into the body of C2) (Anderson, 1974).

When the C1 ring is broken, it usually fractures in at least two places.

## PROBLEM 4.06

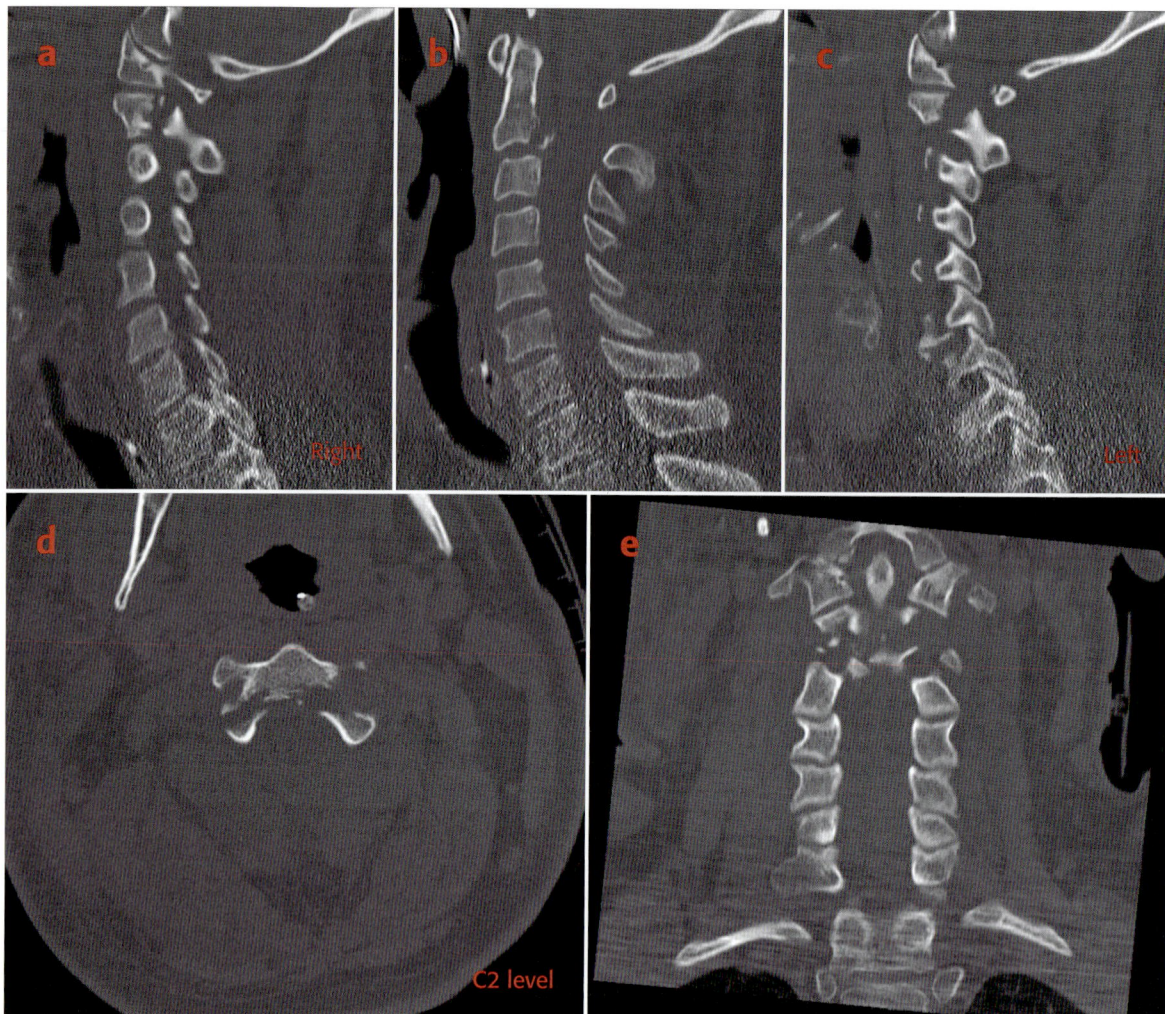

This 41-year-old man was a driver involved in a high-speed car crash in which two people died at the scene.

**Q**
Describe the injury pattern.

# A

There is a traumatic spondylolisthesis of C2 (Hangman's fracture) with a fracture through the pedicles bilaterally. The anterior aspects of the posterior arch of C1, C2 and C3 do not align correctly (disruption of the spinolaminar line). The astute interpreter will also note that there are fractures of the posterior arch of C1 (images a and c) and an avulsion fracture of the right occipital condyle (image e), though these fractures are relatively subtle on these sections (best seen on the full set of images on the DVD, which also show fractures of the lateral masses of C1). A well corticated detached osteophyte is seen at the anterosuperior corner of C6.

## LEARNING POINT

Injuries of the craniocervical junction often involve more than one anatomical site.

# PROBLEM 4.07

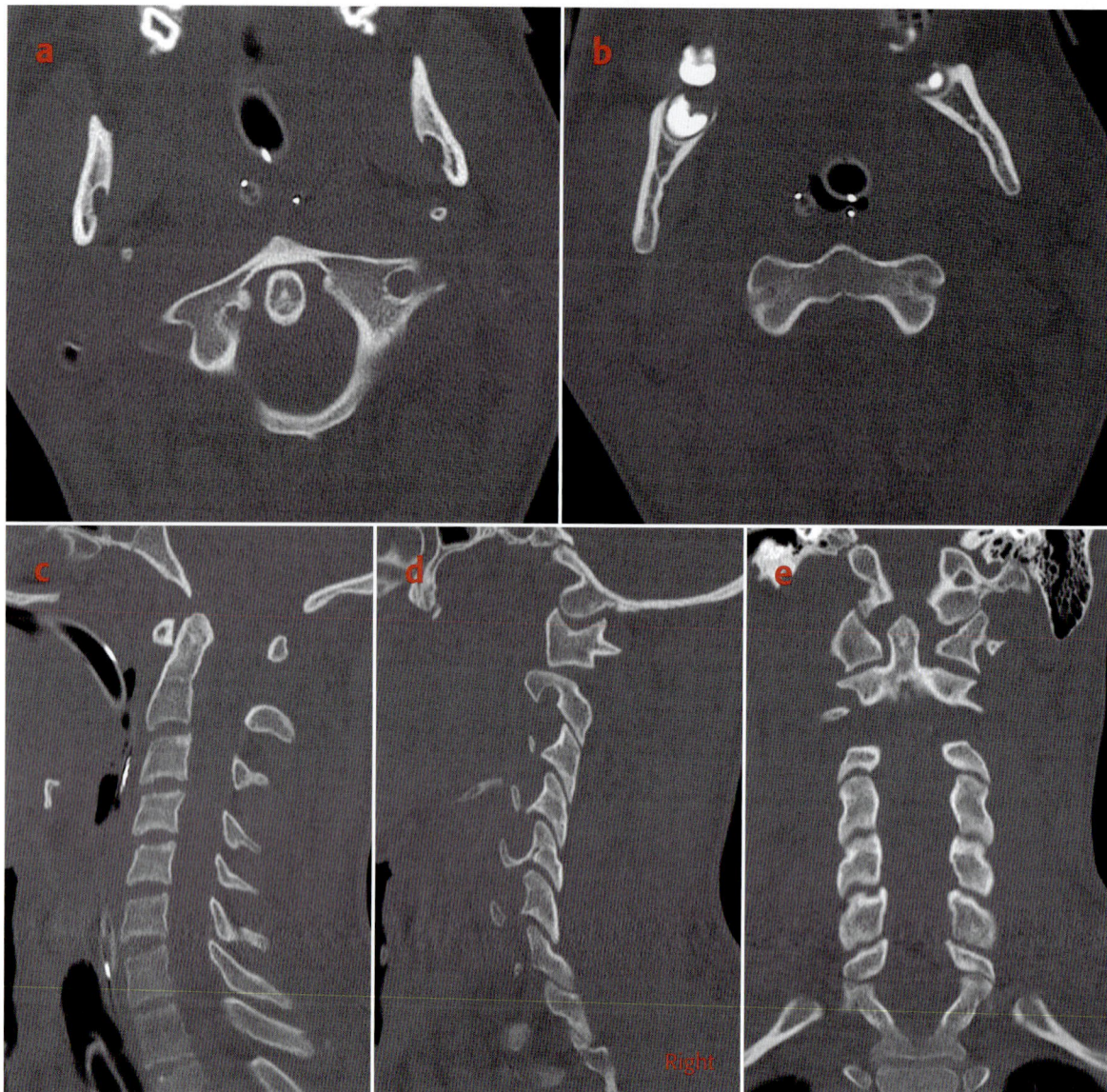

This 17-year-old man sustained multiple traumatic injuries in a single vehicle roll-over crash.

**Q** Can the spinal collar be removed?

# A

There is rotatory subluxation of C1 on C2 (up to 15–20 degrees of rotation of C1 on C2 is normal). The posterior cortex of the anterior arch of C1 and the anterior cortex of C2 are not parallel on the midline sagittal image (image c). In the right parasagittal view (image d), the facet of C2 is displaced forwards on C1, and the intervening facet joint is widened posteriorly. In the coronal view, the lateral masses of C1 are asymmetrically aligned around the peg. The left atlantoaxial joint is widened and the right lateral mass of C1 is not congruent with that of C2. This combination of findings is highly suspicious of a ligamentous injury, and spinal precautions, including the cervical collar, should remain in place until the injuries are further delineated. The coronal images on the DVD show a tiny avulsion fracture of the right occipital condyle.

There is a fracture of the T1 spinous process, which is separate to the craniocervical junction injury.

## LEARNING POINT

Significant injuries to the craniocervical junction can occur without bony injury. A high index of suspicion is required. MRI is more sensitive than CT for detecting unstable ligamentous injuries.

## PROBLEM 4.08

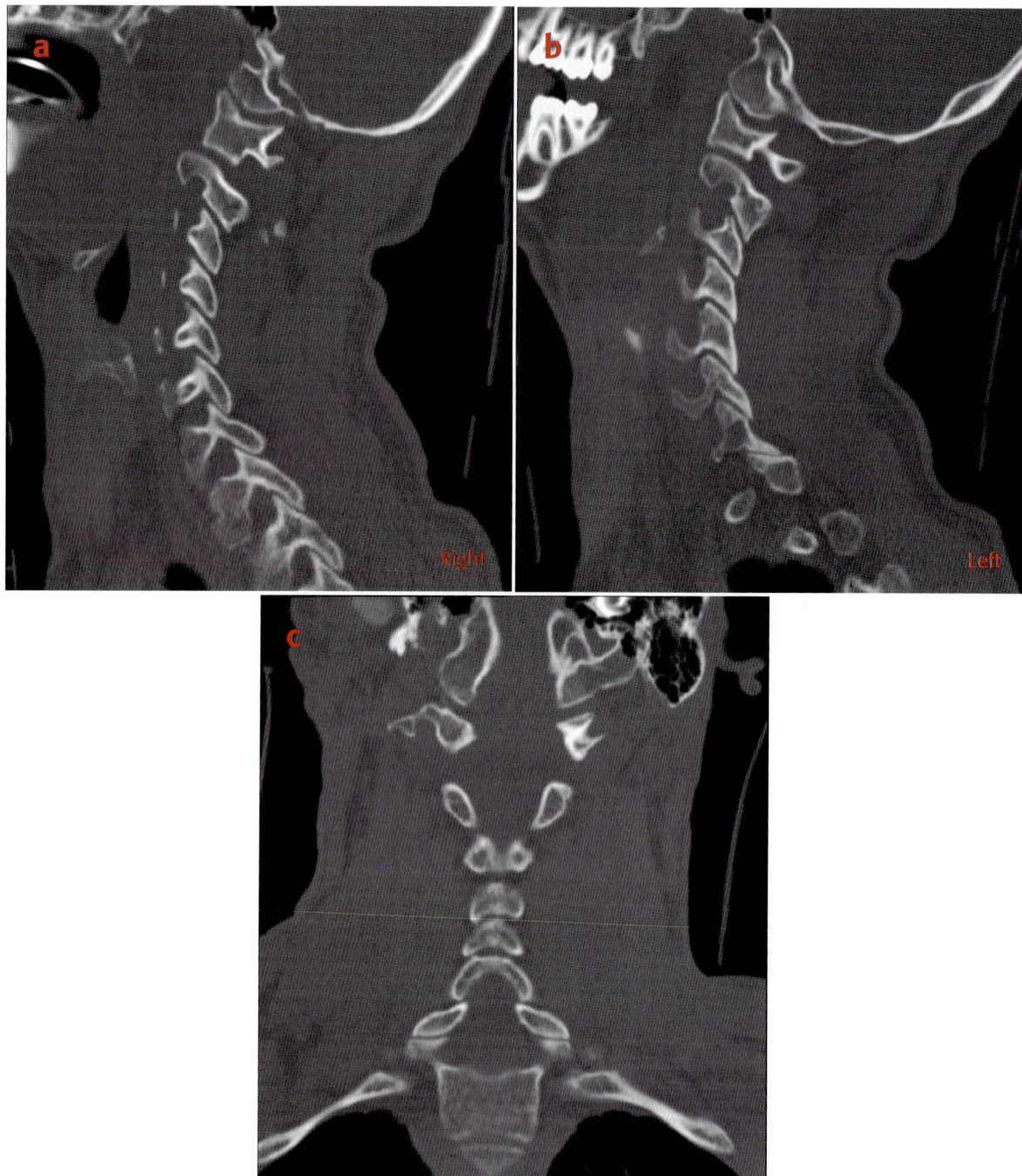

This 25-year-old man hit the median barrier on a motorway and was found eight metres away from his motorbike.

**Q**

Describe the injury pattern.

## A

The most significant abnormality is widening (vertical distraction) of the posterior aspect of the atlanto-occipital joints bilaterally, which indicates type 2 occipitocervical dissociation.

There is an avulsion fracture of the right occipital condyle (seen on DVD images only). Rotatory subluxation of C1 on C2 is noted on the right parasagittal reformatted images (image a), where the lateral mass of C2 is not aligned with that of C1. This rotatory subluxation of C1 on C2 is best appreciated in the axial images on the DVD.

## LEARNING POINT

Occipitocervical dissociation (also known as atlanto-occipital subluxation) is easily missed on plain radiography, and is potentially fatal. It may be type 1 (anterior subluxation), type 2 (vertical distraction of atlanto-occipital joint > 2 mm), or type 3 (posterior dislocation) (Torretti, 2007). It is frequently associated with significant injury of the craniocervical junction or brain stem.

## PROBLEM 4.09

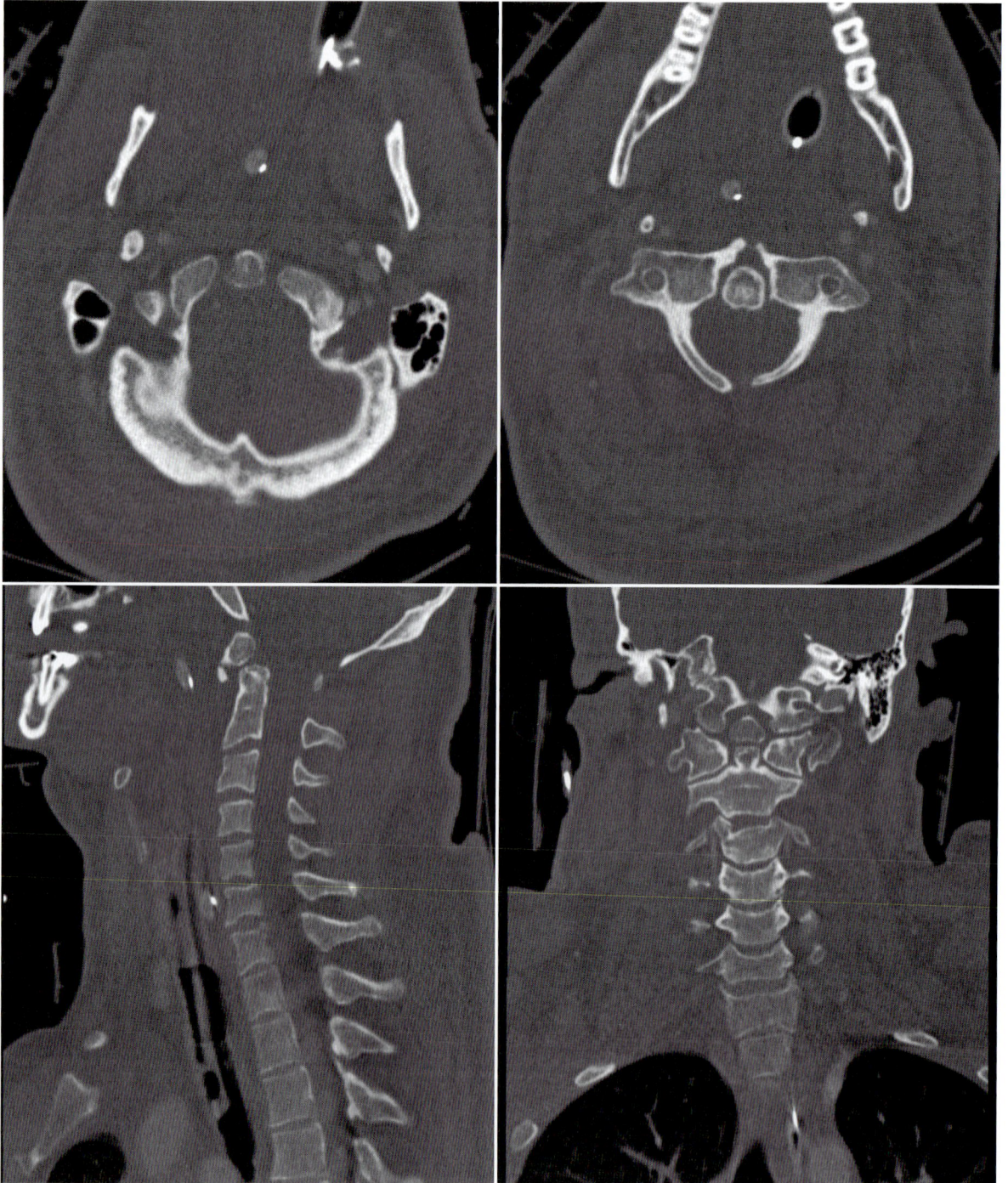

This 29-year-old man was injured in a high-speed car crash. Concerns have been raised that there may be a fractured odontoid peg and a Jefferson fracture of C1.

**Q** What do you think of the images?

## A

No fractures are present. Three congenital anomalies of the craniocervical junction are present on the scan. Firstly, there is a deficiency of the posterior arch of C1. This is not a fracture, as the bony ends are well corticated and rounded. In addition, the lateral mass of C1 does not overhang that of C2, which suggests that the C1 ring is not expanded. Secondly, there is an os odontoideum, a condition where the dens is separated from the body of C2 (Truumees, 2008). The edges of this ossicle are well corticated and the position that it has separated from C2 would be unusual for a fracture. Thirdly, there is a congenital defect of the anterior arch of C1.

## LEARNING POINT

Knowledge of common congenital anomalies may avoid misdiagnosis and incorrect management.

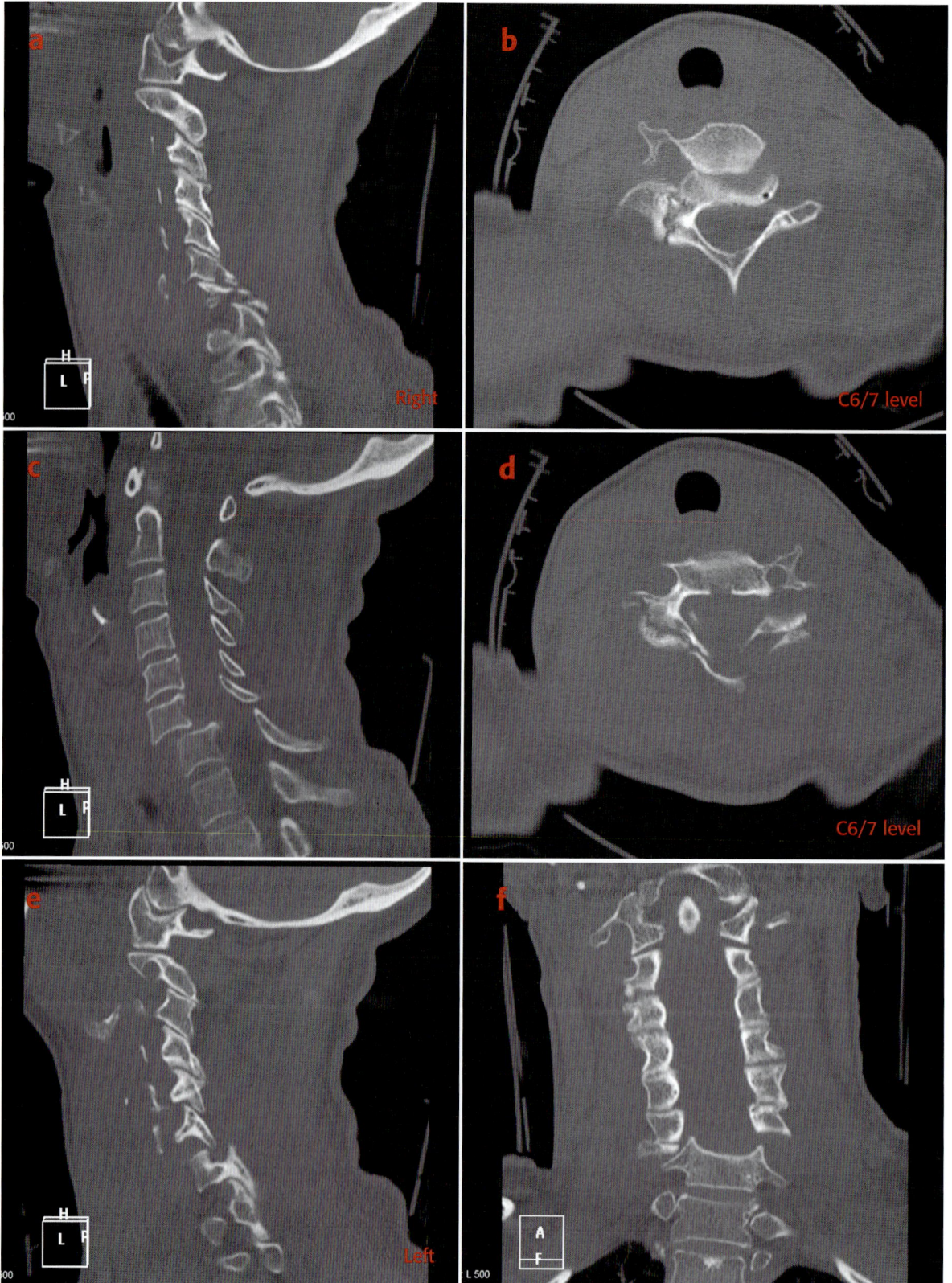

# PROBLEM 4.10

Right

C6/7 level

C6/7 level

Left

Following a high-speed car crash, this 52-year old woman was tetraplegic with a C7 neurological level.

**Q**

Describe the injury.

---

**A**

This is a distractive flexion injury at the C6/7 level. There is a greater than 50% shift of C6 forward on C7 (image c), with a facet joint dislocation on the left (images e and f) and fractures of the articular processes of C6 and C7 on the right (images a, b, d).

In image b, one vertebral body appears anterior to the other, indicating significant subluxation. Similarly, in image d, two posterior arches are visible. There is an uncovered facet, also termed "bare facet" or "naked facet", on the left in image b, indicating a facet dislocation (McConnel, 1995).

**L**EARNING POINT

Distractive flexion injuries range from facet sub-luxation, through unilateral facet fracture or dislocation to bilateral facet joint fracture or dislocation (Allen, 1982).

# PROBLEM 4.11

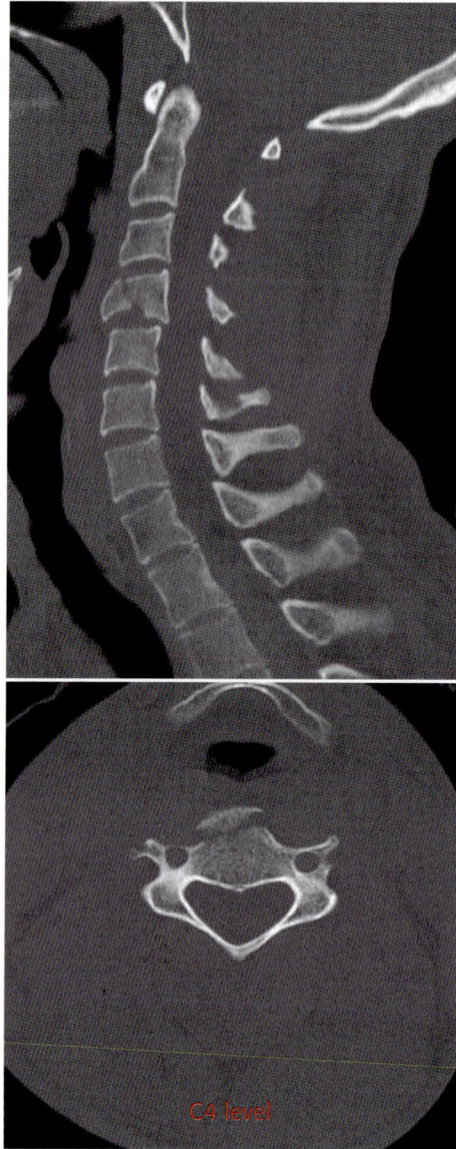

C4 level

This 34-year-old man was cutting down a tree, which fell on the back of his head while he was trying to avoid it.

**Q**

Describe the injury.

## A

There is loss of anterior height and a "beak-like" appearance of the anterior aspect of the C4 vertebral body. There is a vertical fracture of C4 vertebral body and mild displacement of the inferoposterior aspect of C4 relative to C5. The vertebral arch is intact. This is consistent with a grade 4 compressive flexion injury.

## LEARNING POINT

With stage 1 compressive flexion injury, there is blunting of the anterior–superior vertebral margin. With stage 2, there is a beak-like appearance to the anterior vertebral body with loss of anterior vertebral height and an oblique contour. With stage 3, there is a fracture extending from the anterior surface of the vertebral body into the disc space. With stage 4, there is posterior displacement of the inferoposterior aspect of the vertebral body < 3 mm. When this displacement relative to the vertebra below is > 3 mm, it becomes stage 5. Occasionally, a fracture of the laminae due to distraction may occur, though this is not typical. Retropulsion of fragments does not occur (Allen, 1982).

# PROBLEM 4.12

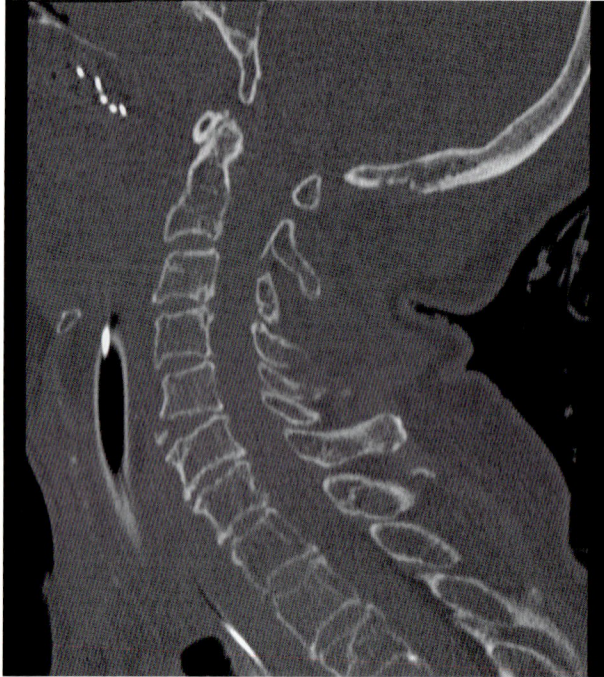

This 73-year-old woman was hit by a truck while crossing the road. She has been unconscious since the time of injury.

**Q**
Describe the injury.

# A

There is a stage 1 distractive extension injury at the C5/6 level. There is widening of the disc space anteriorly with an avulsed inferior corner fragment from C5 vertebral body. There is no loss of height of the posterior vertebral bodies or displacement of the cephalad vertebrae into the spinal canal. On the DVD, a number of additional injuries may be seen, including fractures of the occipital and hyoid bones, and a fracture of the fourth rib.

## LEARNING POINT

Distractive extension injuries are classified as stage 1, in which there is abnormal widening of the disc space (representing disruption of the anterior longitudinal ligament and disc) or stage 2, in which the posterior ligaments are disrupted and the cephalad vertebrae are displaced into the spinal canal (Allen, 1982). Patients with ankylosing spondylitis and diffuse idiopathic skeletal hyperostosis are at risk of these injuries with minimal trauma (Torretti, 2007).

## PROBLEM 4.13

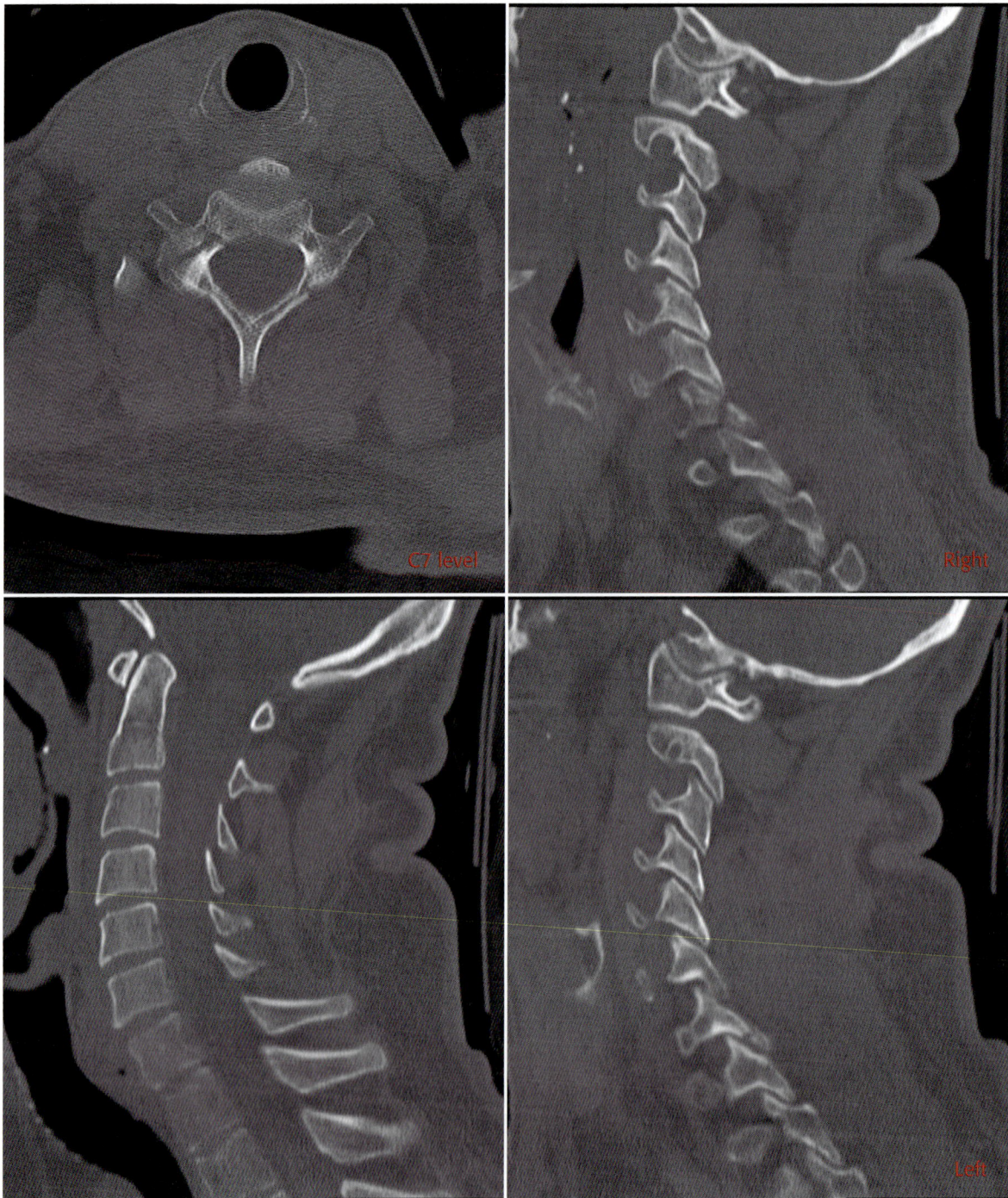

This 42-year-old man crashed his motorcycle when riding home from a party while intoxicated with alcohol.

**Q** Describe the injury pattern.

## A

There are bilateral fractures of the C7 vertebral arch. On the left the fracture involves the articular process and extends into the lamina. On the right, the fracture involves the articular process and extends into both the lamina and pedicle. This pattern is consistent with a compressive extension injury.

## LEARNING POINT

With compressive extension injury, there is damage to the vertebral arch but the body of the affected vertebra remains intact. The vertebral arch fractures may be unilateral or bilateral, involving the pedicle, articular process, the lamina or a combination of these. With more severe injuries, the affected vertebra may be displaced anteriorly relative to the subjacent vertebra and the antero-superior aspect of the subjacent vertebra may be sheared off (Allen, 1982).

# PROBLEM 4.14

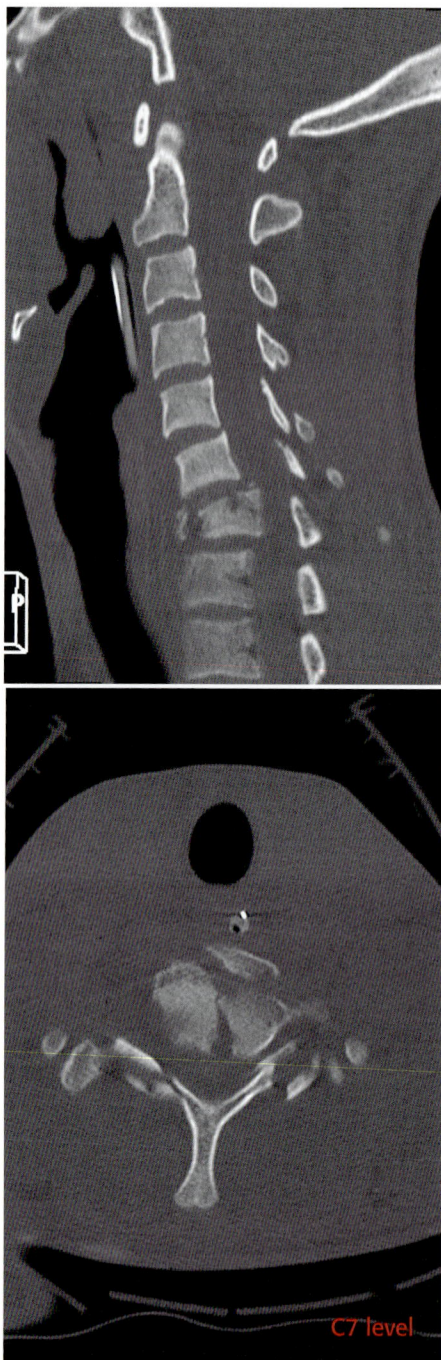

C7 level

This 20-year-old man was one of the drivers in a high-speed, multiple vehicle crash. He is now quadriplegic with a C7 neurological injury level.

**Q**
Describe the injury pattern.

## A

There is a comminuted fracture of the body of C7, with loss of height of the vertebral body and fractures of the elements of the posterior vertebral arch. There is significant retropulsion of bone fragments into the vertebral canal (which does not occur with compressive flexion injuries). There is kyphosis at the C7 level. In the images on the DVD (but not the book) fractures of the vertebral arch of C5 and C6 are seen. This pattern is consistent with a vertical compression injury.

On the axial images on the DVD, there is some asymmetry of C1 around the odontoid peg. In the absence of other findings suggesting an injury to the craniocervical junction, the significance of this finding is uncertain. MRI may be helpful to exclude ligamentous injury.

## LEARNING POINT

Vertical compression injuries are classified as stage 1, in which there is a central fracture of either the superior or inferior endplate with a "cupping" deformity of the endplate. In stage 2 injuries, both endplates are involved. In stage 3 lesions, the vertebral body is fragmented with fragments displaced in multiple directions. The vertebral arch may or may not be involved (Allen, 1982).

## PROBLEM 4.15

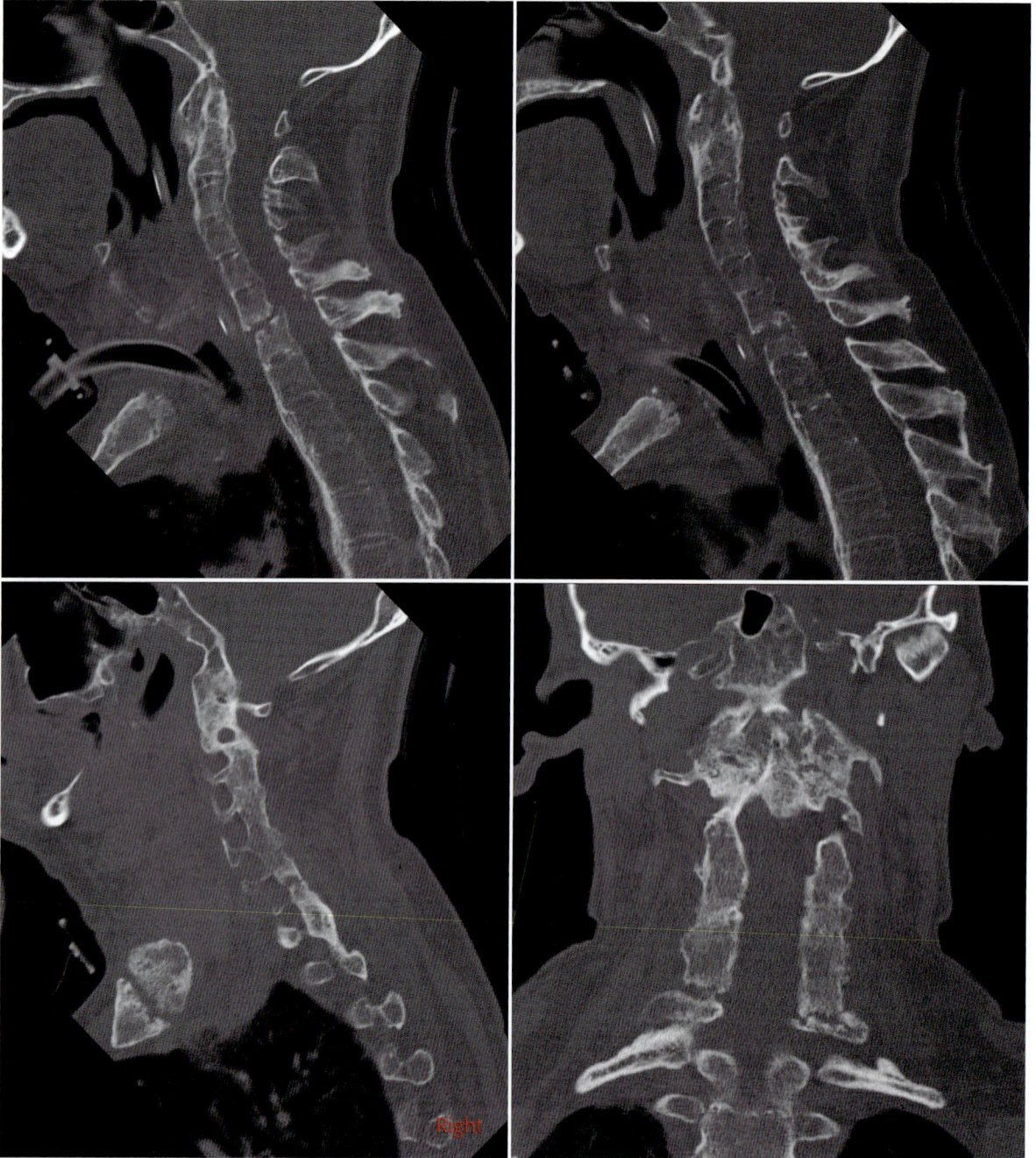

This 61-year-old man hurt his neck when he slipped and fell over earlier today. Now he is quadriparetic and required emergency tracheostomy because of respiratory distress.

Q

1. What condition does he have that predisposed him to a neck injury?
2. What injury has he sustained?
3. Why was a tracheostomy used to secure his airway?

## A

1. All the vertebral bodies are fused together, given the appearance of a piece of bamboo. This appearance is typical of ankylosing spondylitis, in which the facet joints also become fused. In addition, the annulus fibrosus, the anterior longitudinal ligament and the interspinous ligament calcify.

2. The fused vertebral column has fractured through the C6/7 disc. There is anterior displacement of C6 on C7 with some narrowing of the vertebral canal. The facet joints are also involved, hence the fracture involves all three columns.

3. Patients with severe ankylosing spondylitis are often extremely difficult to intubate by conventional means.

## LEARNING POINT

Patients with ankylosing spondylitis, or diffuse idiopathic skeletal hyperostosis (DISH), are at high risk of unstable cervical fractures, usually from extension injury (Torretti, 2007). Ankylosing spondylitis patients may develop unstable stress fractures with no history of significant trauma.

## PROBLEM 4.16

Right

C4 level

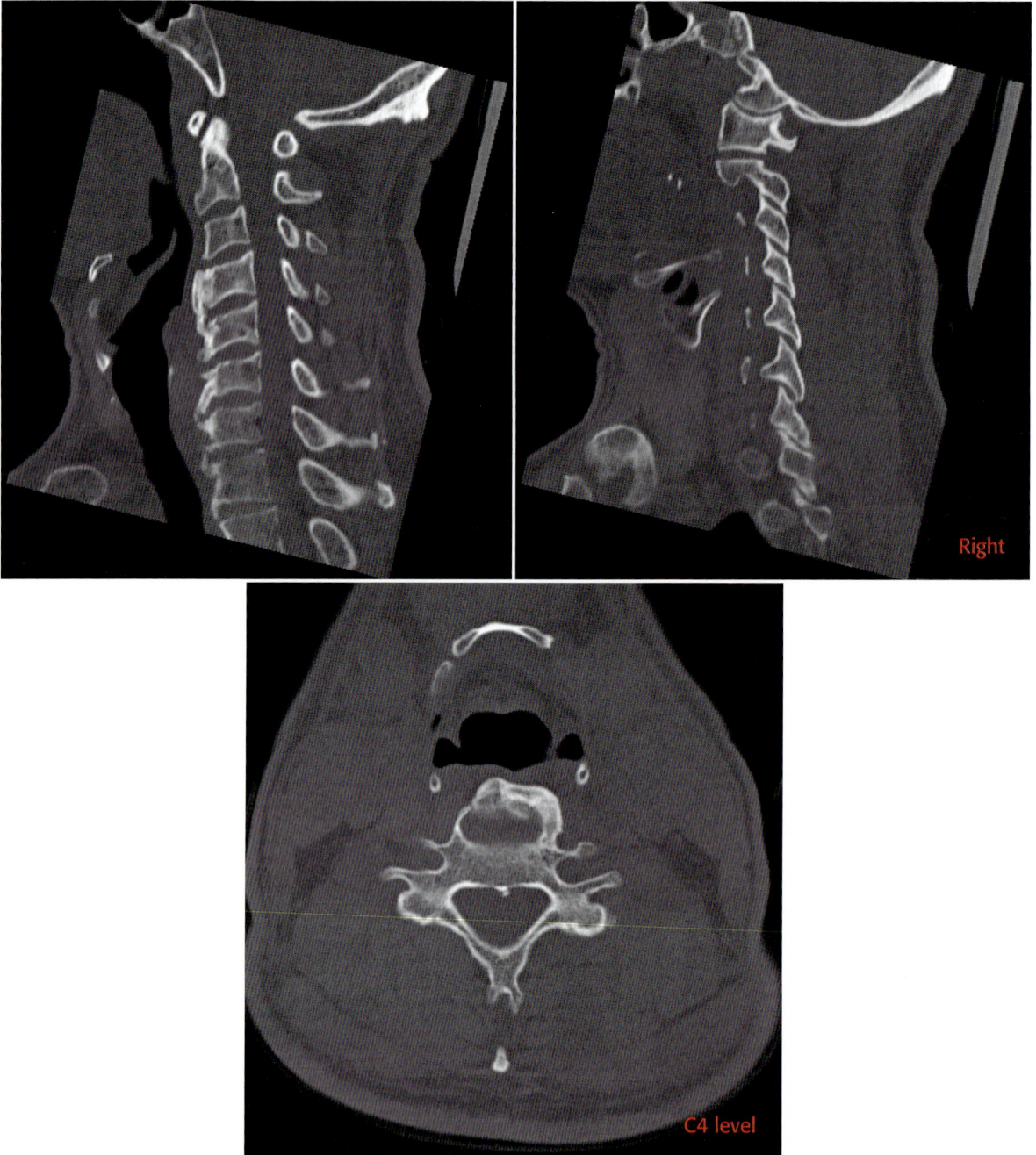

This 59-year-old man slipped over in the bathroom and hit his forehead. He initially complained of some neck pain, then became progressively confused and agitated. A CT scan of the head shows minor frontal contusions.

### Q

1. What condition is present?
2. What are the implications of this condition for your management in this clinical scenario?

# A

1. There is extensive ossification along the anterior aspect of five contiguous vertebral bodies, together with bridging osteophyte formation. The disc spaces are preserved and there is no ankylosis of the facet joints. Minimal ossification of the posterior longitudinal ligament is also noted on the axial image and is better seen on the DVD images. These features are suggestive of diffuse idiopathic skeletal hyperostosis (DISH).

2. Patients with DISH who have neck pain after minor trauma require MRI, even if no fractures are identified on CT or plain radiography (Torretti, 2007).

## LEARNING POINT

DISH predisposes to vertebral fractures due to the rigidity of the spine. Cord injury may occur with relatively minor trauma, due to narrowing of the spinal canal.

# PROBLEM 4.17

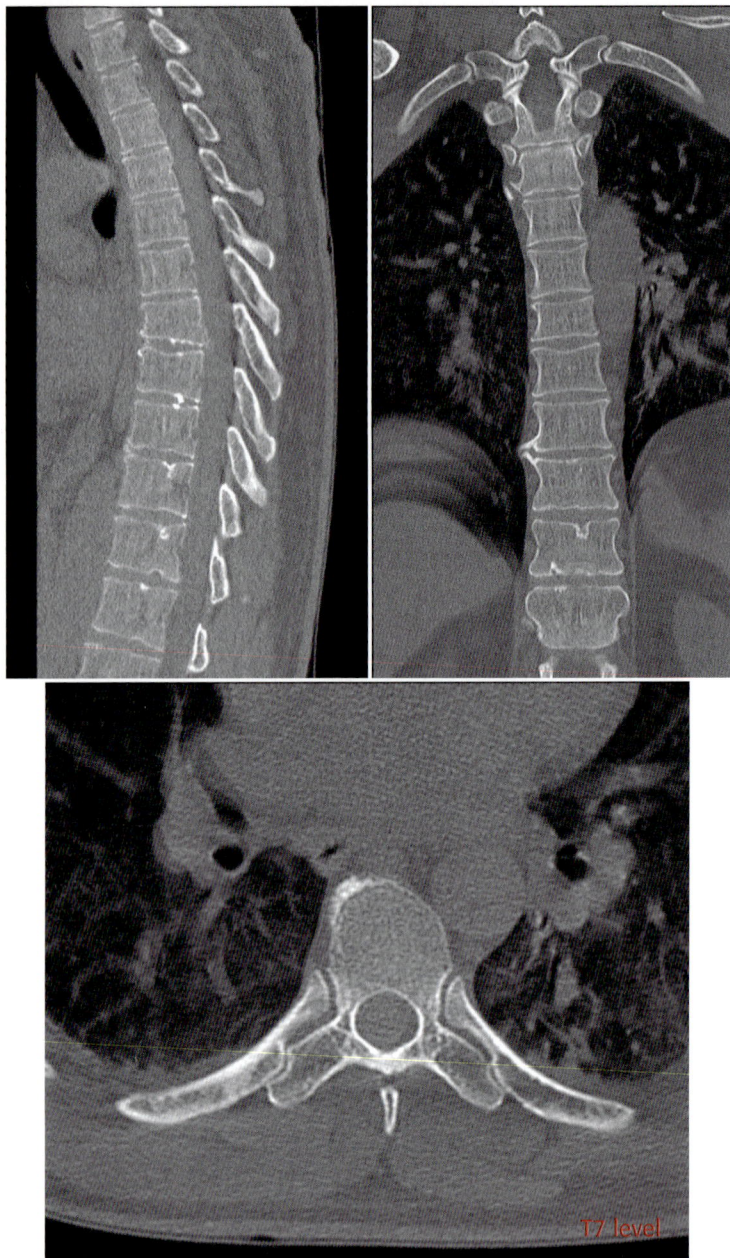

T7 level

Since falling down the stairs today, this 38-year-old man has complained of severe mid-thoracic back pain.

**Q**
Describe the injury pattern.

## A

There is anterior wedging of the body of a mid-thoracic vertebra. The height of the vertebral body posteriorly is maintained but there is around 20% loss of height anteriorly. The vertebral ring is intact. This is a typical compression fracture. There is generalised osteopaenia, which is a predisposing factor to vertebral compression fractures.

## Learning point

With a compression fracture, the anterior column fails under compression. The middle column remains intact and acts as a hinge. The posterior column is usually intact but with severe injuries it may partially fail in distraction (Denis, 1983).

Compression fractures may be anterior (anterior flexion mechanism) or lateral (lateral flexion mechanism) (Denis, 1983).

## PROBLEM 4.18

L4 level

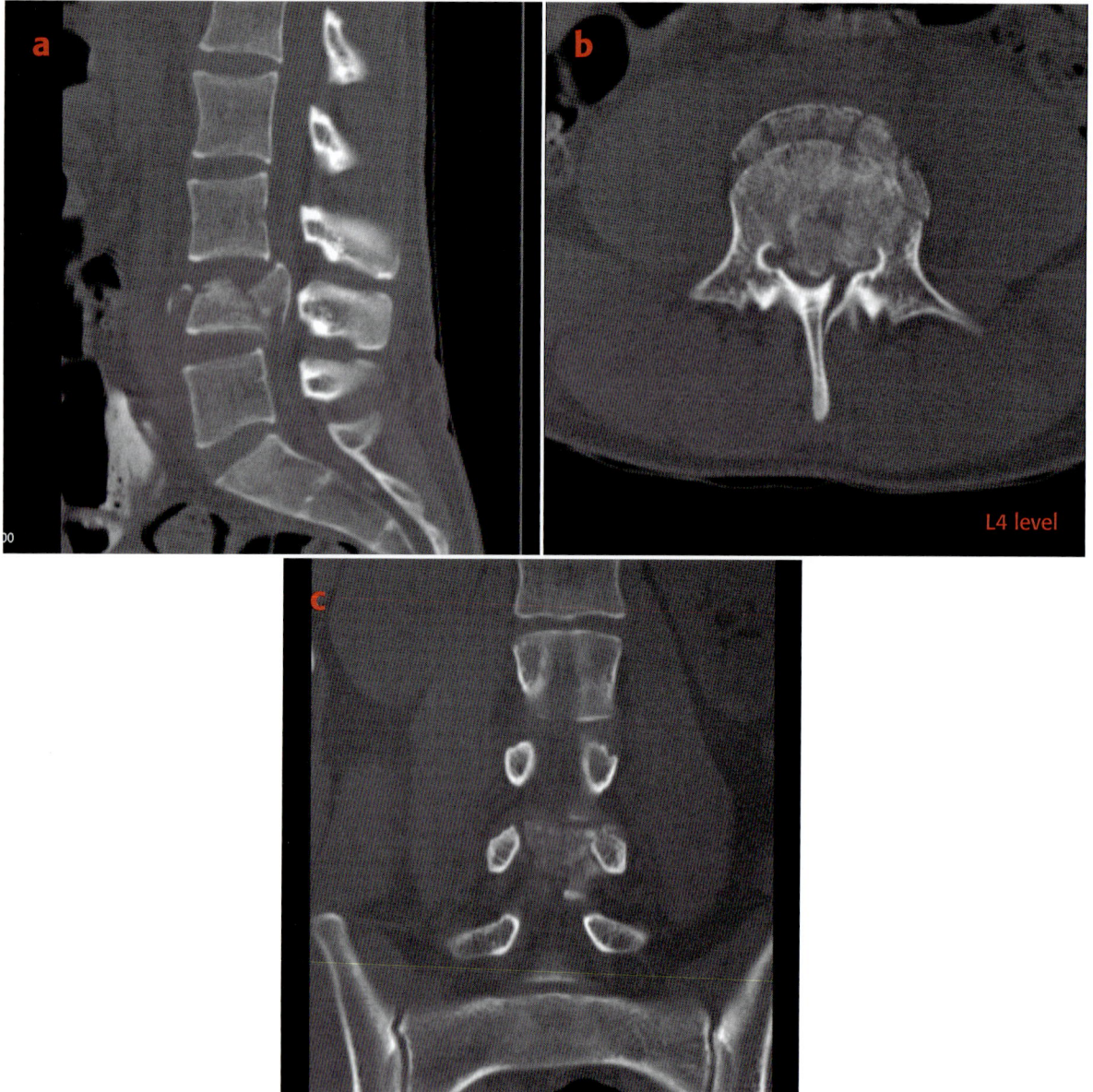

This 19-year-old man fell three metres off scaffolding while trying to attract the attention of his friend on the ground. He now has cauda equina syndrome.

**Q**

Describe the injury pattern.

## A

There is a comminuted fracture of the L4 vertebral body with significant loss of height of both anterior and posterior aspects of the vertebral body. There is an increase in the interpedicular distance (seen best in image c) with retropulsion of fragments into the vertebral canal, which is almost completely obliterated. There is a vertical fracture of the lamina. This pattern is typical of a burst fracture.

## LEARNING POINT

With burst fractures of the thoracolumbar spine, there is failure in compression of the anterior and middle columns, but not the posterior column. Failure in compression of the anterior column is shown by fracture of the cortex of the anterior vertebral body, which loses height. Failure in compression of the middle column is shown by similar findings in the posterior vertebral body. Characteristically, the pedicles are spread apart by the posterior vertebral body fracture. There is commonly a vertical fracture of the lamina, and splaying of the facet joints, without which there could not be significant widening of the interpedicular distance (Denis, 1983).

## PROBLEM 4.19

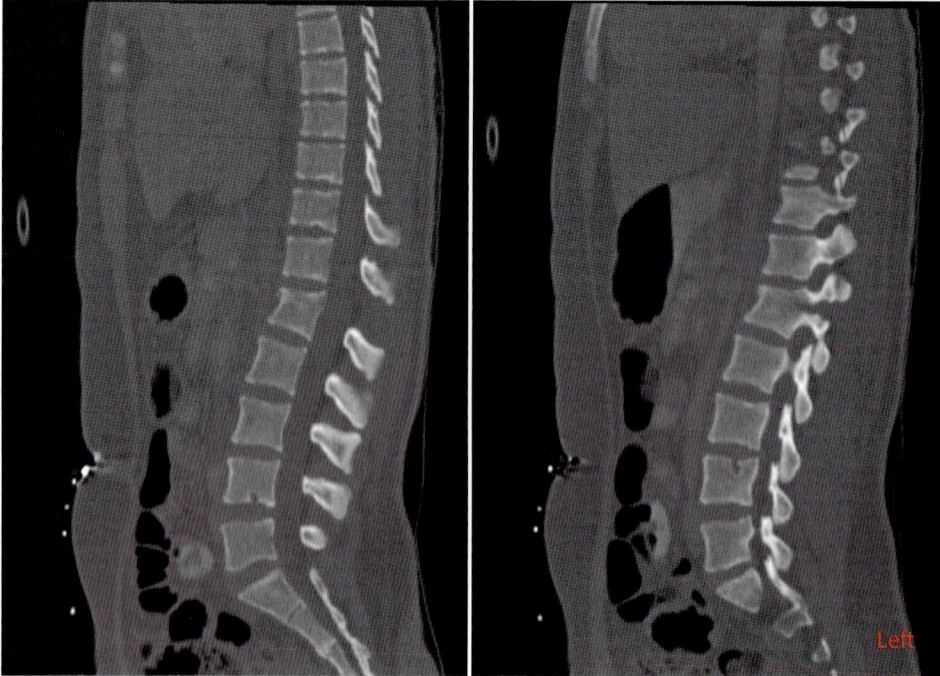

This 18-year-old woman was a back seat passenger in a car crash. In the emergency department, her GCS was 10 and she was moving all four limbs. Intubation was required for management of agitation.

## Q

1. Describe the injury pattern.
2. What other injuries is the patient at high risk of?

# A

1. There is marked widening of the interspinous interval at the T12/L1 level. A horizontal fracture line is seen through the vertebral body of L1, which extends through the pedicles and articular processes of L1, with widening of the fracture line posteriorly. There is no subluxation or dislocation. This is a "seat belt type" or "flexion–distraction" injury, in this case a "Chance" fracture. Schmorl's nodes are noted along the endplates of L4 but are of no clinical significance.

2. There is a high incidence (around 60%) of intra-abdominal injury in association with flexion–distraction injuries (Anderson, 1991).

## LEARNING POINT

With seat belt type (flexion distraction) injuries of the thoracolumbar spine, there is failure in distraction of the middle and posterior columns, with either no injury to the anterior column or minor compression. The injury may be through bone, through the ligaments or a combination of the two. When injury is through the bone at one level, it is known as a "Chance" fracture (Denis, 1983).

## PROBLEM 4.20

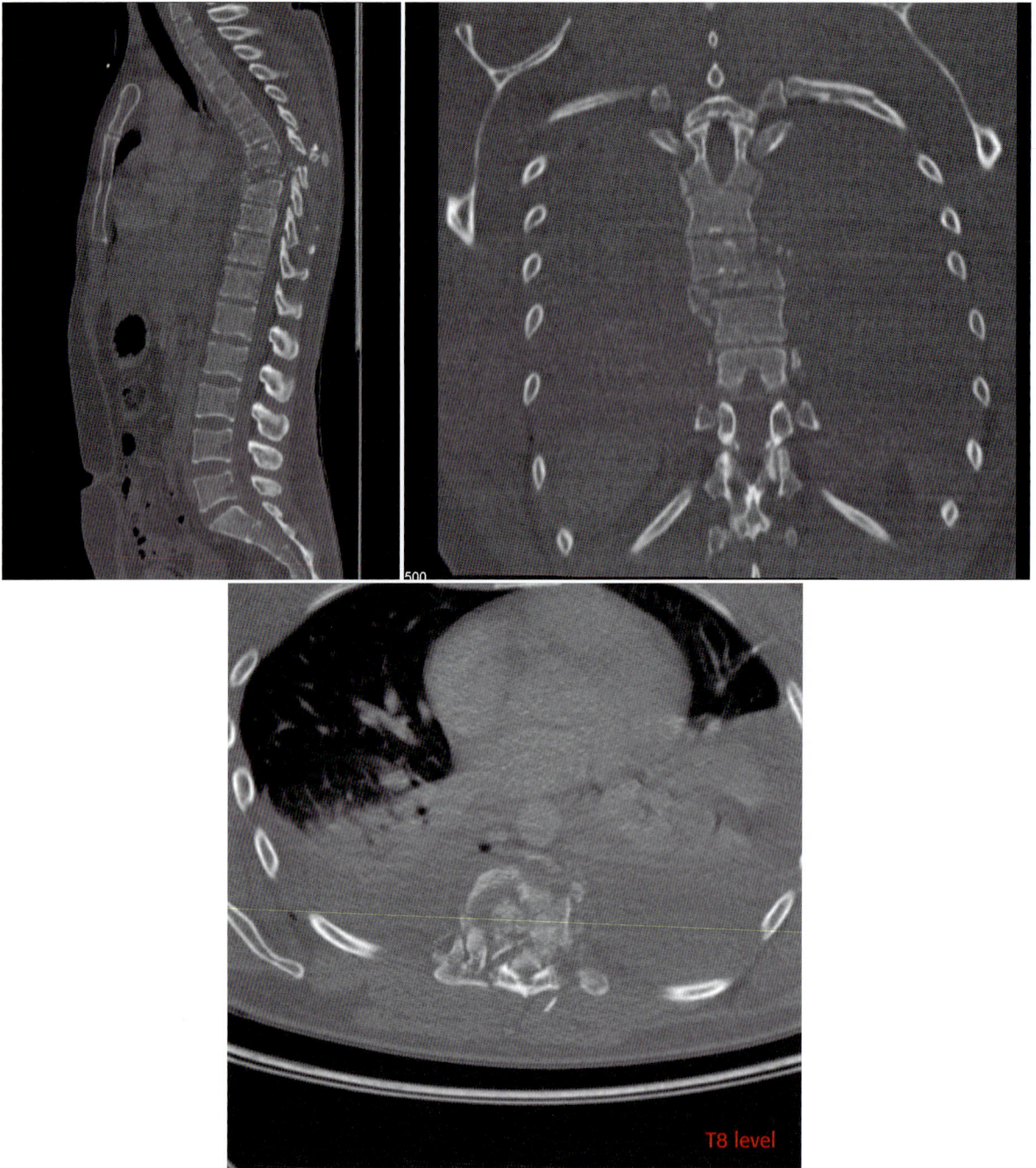

T8 level

This 26-year-old man was found to be paraplegic at the scene following a motorcycle crash.

**Q** Describe the injury.

# A

There is a flexion rotation fracture dislocation at the T7–T9 level. The body of T8 is severely comminuted with retropulsion of fragments into the spinal canal, which is almost completely obliterated. The bodies of T7 and T9 are anteriorly wedged. There is a kyphosis at the level of the lesion, with rotation and just under 50% lateral displacement. There is a fracture of the left fourth rib and bilateral pleural fluid. On the DVD, additional injuries may be seen, including multiple rib and transverse process fractures.

## LEARNING POINT

The main characteristic of a fracture dislocation injury is failure of all three columns, leading to translational deformity (subluxation or dislocation), which may be in the sagittal or coronal plane.

Fracture dislocations of the thoracic spine occur with high energy trauma. Other associated injuries should be actively sought.

## PROBLEM 4.21

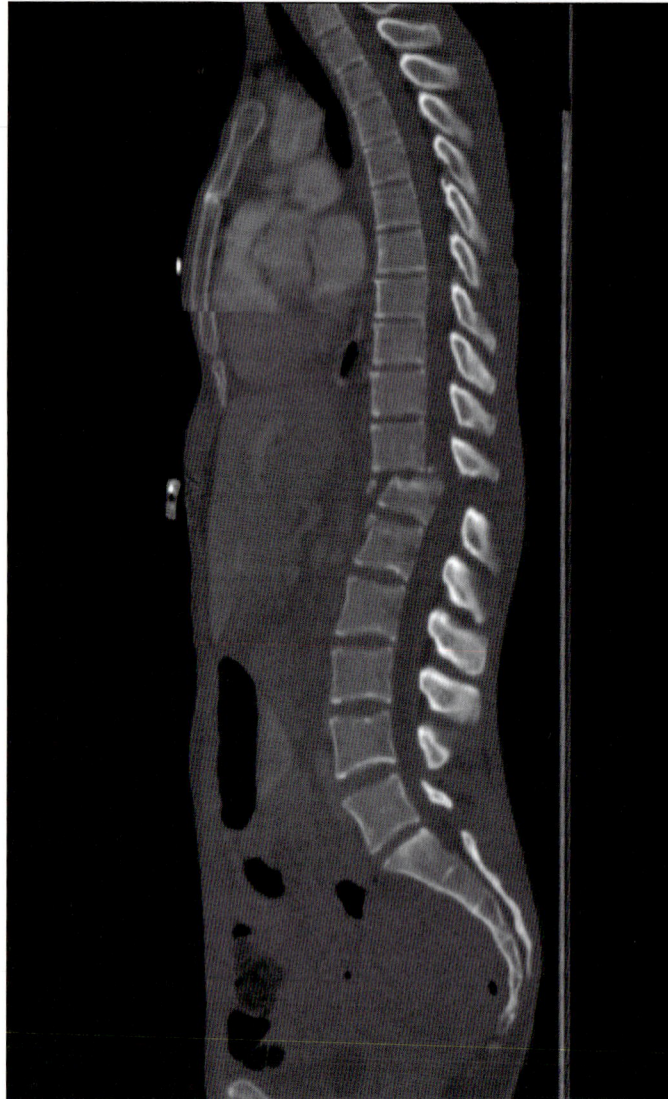

This 30-year-old woman was a restrained back seat passenger during a car crash. Prior to intubation, she was moving her arms but not her legs.

**Q**

Describe the injury pattern.

## A

There is a flexion–distraction dislocation at the T11/12 level. The body of T11 is shifted anteriorly on the body of T12. There is a bilateral posterior facet joint dislocation (seen on DVD) and marked widening of the interspinous interval at the T11/12 level. The body of T12 is compressed anteriorly, with some comminution of its superior endplate. There is also a minimally displaced fracture of the anterosuperior aspect of L1.

## LEARNING POINT

Fracture dislocations involve all three columns, making them extremely unstable injuries, commonly associated with neurological damage (Denis, 1983).

# PROBLEM 4.22

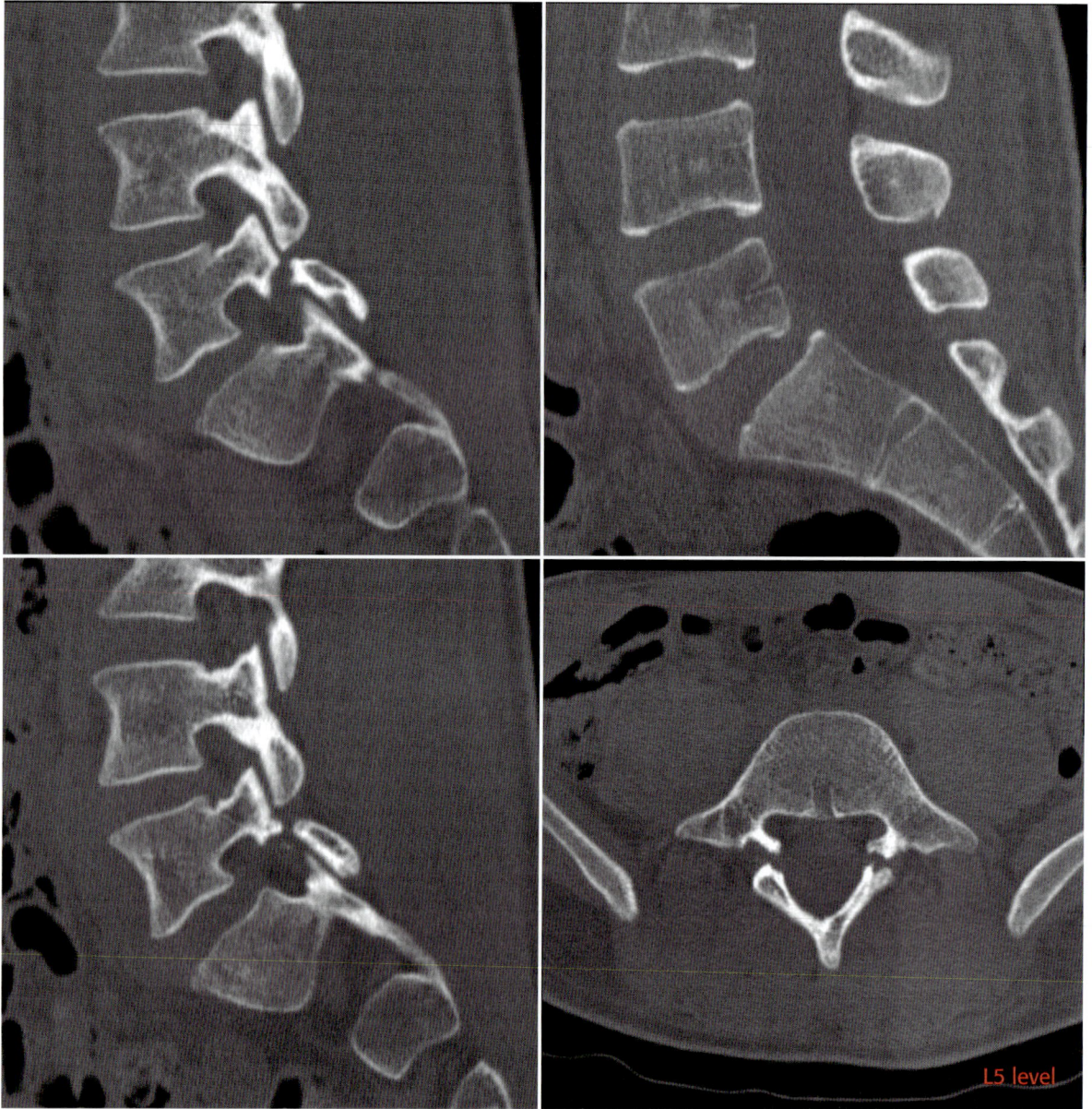

L5 level

This 28-year-old man was intubated and sedated for major chest trauma sustained in a high-speed car crash.

**Q** What is the abnormal finding on these images?

## A

There is discontinuity of the pars interarticularis of L5 bilaterally, associated with a small amount of anterior shift of L5 on S1. This process is chronic, as the parts of the bone adjacent to the disruption are corticated with marked sclerosis. This is consistent with minor spondylolisthesis caused by spondylolysis. It is unrelated to the recent traumatic episode.

## LEARNING POINT

Spondylolysis is a defect in the pars interarticularis of a vertebra. It may or may not be accompanied by the forward translation of one vertebra relative to another (spondylolisthesis). The L5/S1 interspace is the commonest site of spondylolisthesis (Froese, 2006).

# PROBLEM 4.23

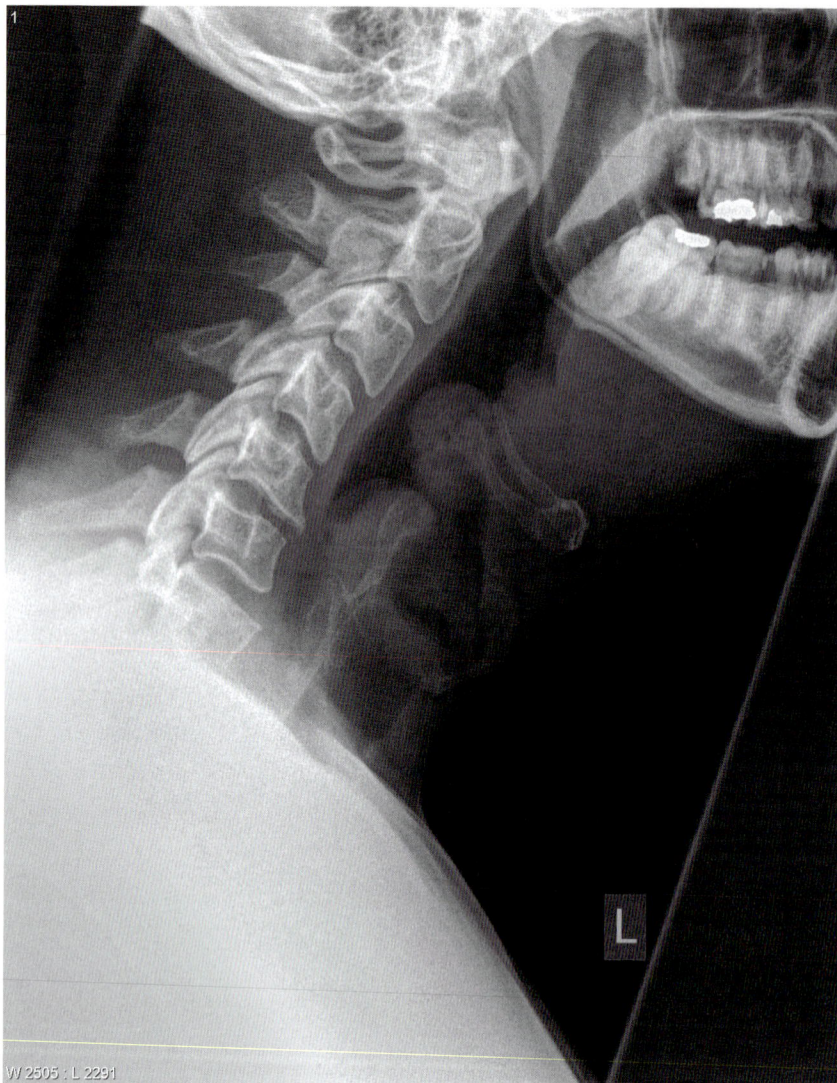

This 23-year-old man presented with fever, sore throat and stridor. You are called to the emergency department because of concerns about airway obstruction.

**Q**

What diagnosis does this image suggest?

# A

Posterior and slightly inferior to the hyoid bone, at the level of the laryngeal inlet, is a soft tissue mass extending into the anterior aspect of the airway. It has the appearance of the tip of a thumb. This appearance is typical of epiglottitis. A more inferior nodular opacity superimposed on the thyroid lamina is consistent with thickened, oedematous mucosa overlying the arytenoids and the aryepiglottic folds. The AP image on the DVD shows the incidental finding of bilateral cervical ribs.

## LEARNING POINT

Suspected adult epiglottitis is usually assessed by fibreoptic endoscopy or, if urgent intubation is required, by direct laryngoscopy. If fibreoptic endoscopy is not available, a lateral neck X-ray may help confirm the diagnosis.

If the patient is at risk of airway obstruction, any imaging undertaken before the airway is secured should be done in an area with resuscitation facilities, not unmonitored in the radiology department.

## PROBLEM 4.24

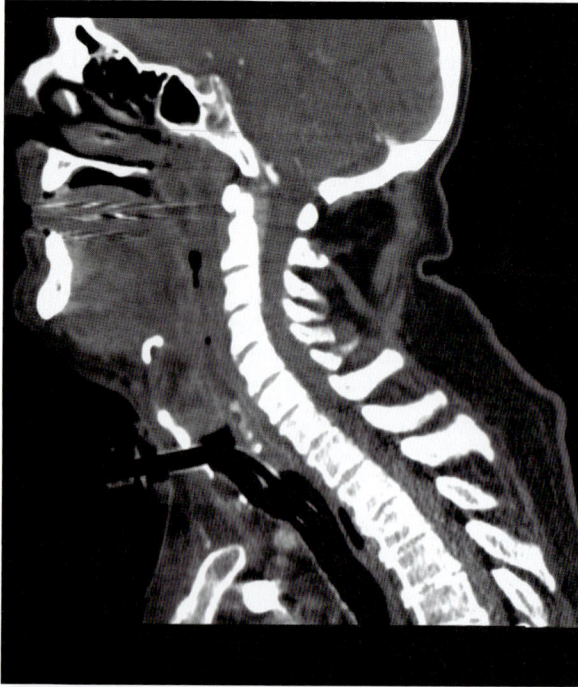

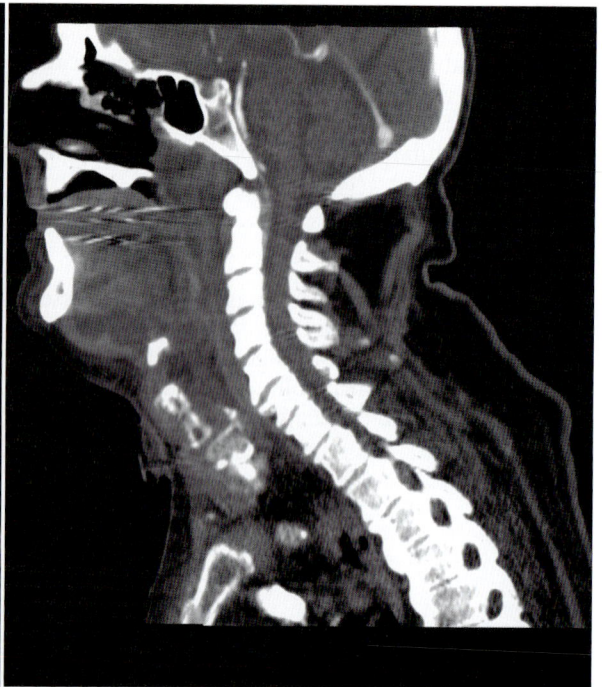

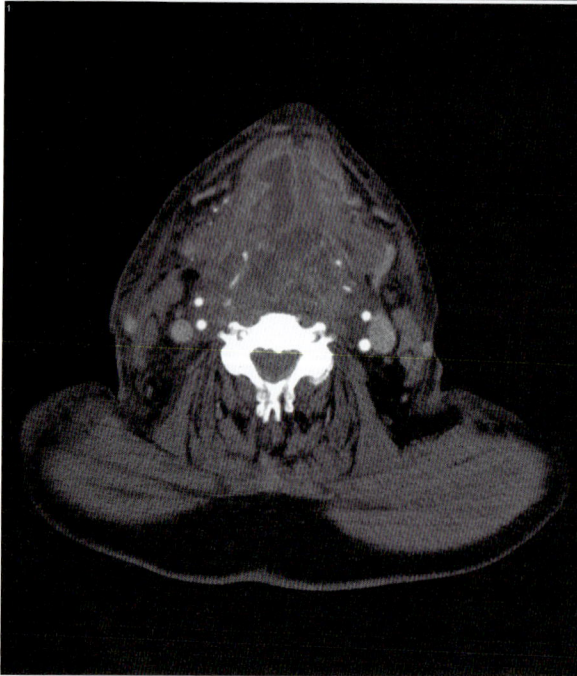

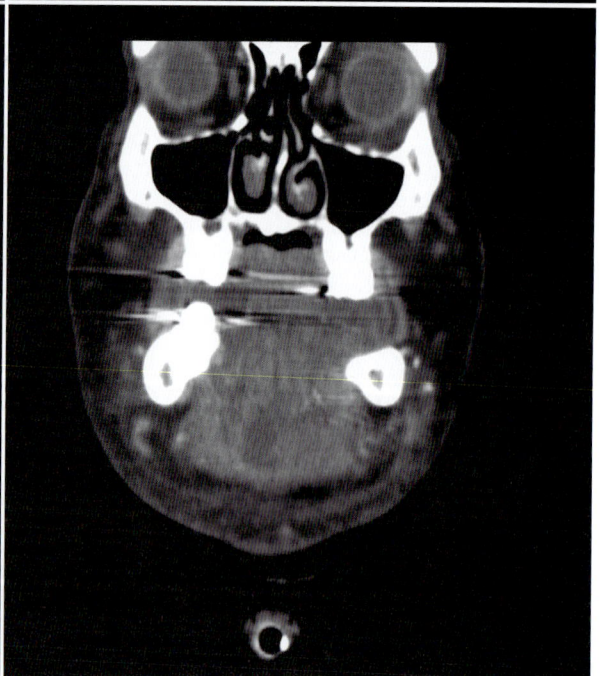

Emergency cricothyroidotomy was performed on this 66-year-old man for acute airway obstruction. The anterior neck was grossly swollen and inflamed. He was febrile with a neutrophil leucocytosis.

**Q**

What is the likely diagnosis?

# A

There is a hypodense, multilocular collection within the right submandibular space. The normal soft tissue planes are indistinct due to inflammatory changes. There is marked narrowing of the airway by swelling. A tracheostomy tube is in-situ.

These findings are consistent with Ludwig's angina, which is a severe soft tissue infection of the floor of the mouth.

## LEARNING POINT

In severe soft tissue infections of the neck, CT is useful to assess whether there are collections present that can be drained.

When infection causes significant upper airway obstruction, the airway should be secured prior to imaging. The CT scanning suite is not the best place to manage a difficult airway that becomes completely obstructed.

## PROBLEM 4.25

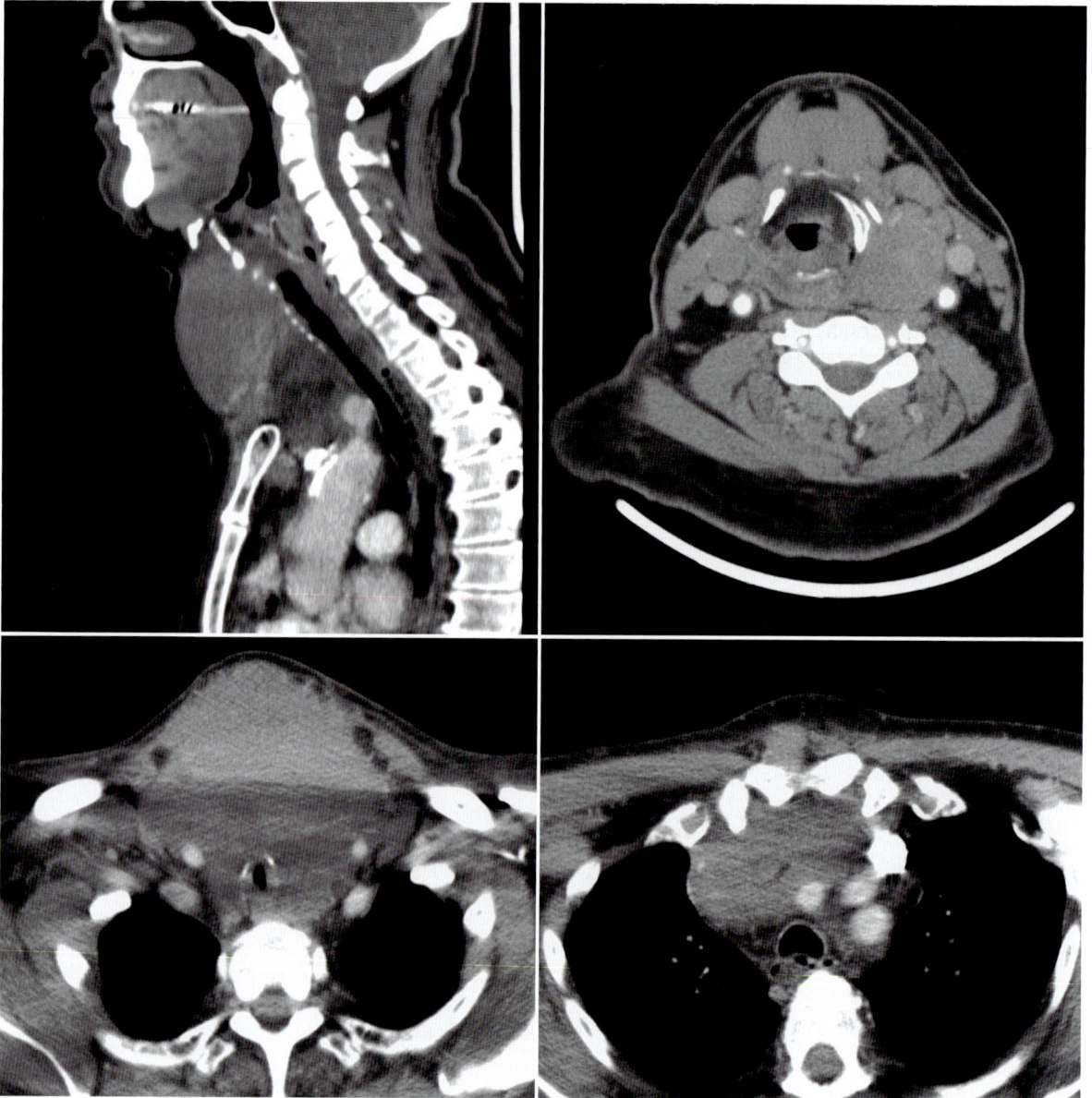

This 62-year-old man had obvious neck swelling with stridor at rest. He was noted to develop respiratory distress when supine.

**Q**
Suggest a differential diagnosis.

# A

There is a large, soft tissue mass in the anterior neck and upper mediastinum with associated lymphadenopathy. A normal thyroid gland is not seen. There is compression of the trachea and the veins of the neck and upper mediastinum. The right brachiocephalic vein is markedly compressed. The most likely explanations for these findings would be a lymphoma or a primary thyroid malignancy. Other possibilities would be multinodular goitre and autoimmune thyroiditis but these conditions would not explain the pathologically enlarged lymph nodes.

The apparent hypodensity in the lower mediastinum is caused by beam-hardening artefact from dense contrast in the left brachiocephalic vein.

## LEARNING POINT

Malignancy may present in an advanced state with compression of vital structures in the neck and/or upper mediastinum. When confronted with this clinical scenario, it should be remembered that some of the malignancies that present in this way are eminently curable. In particular, teratomas and lymphomas may be exquisitely sensitive to chemotherapy.

# PROBLEM 4.26

a — T2 Fat Sat

b — FSPGR — C3/4 level

c — T2 FSE — C3/4 level

d — T2 FSE — C3 level

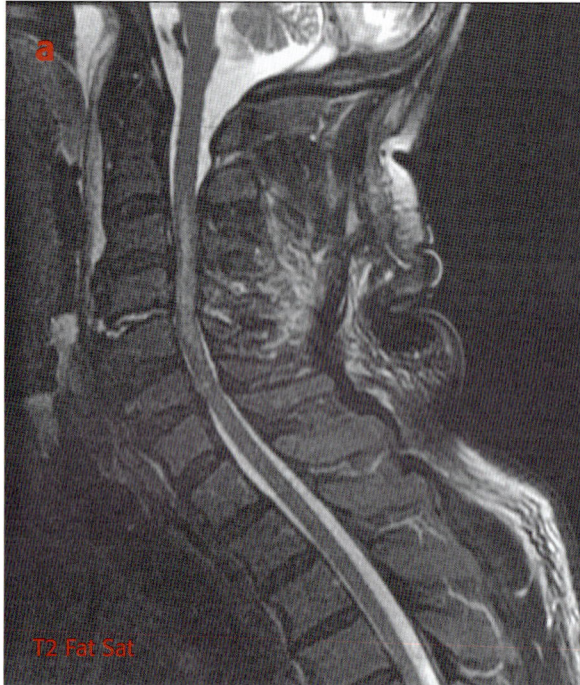

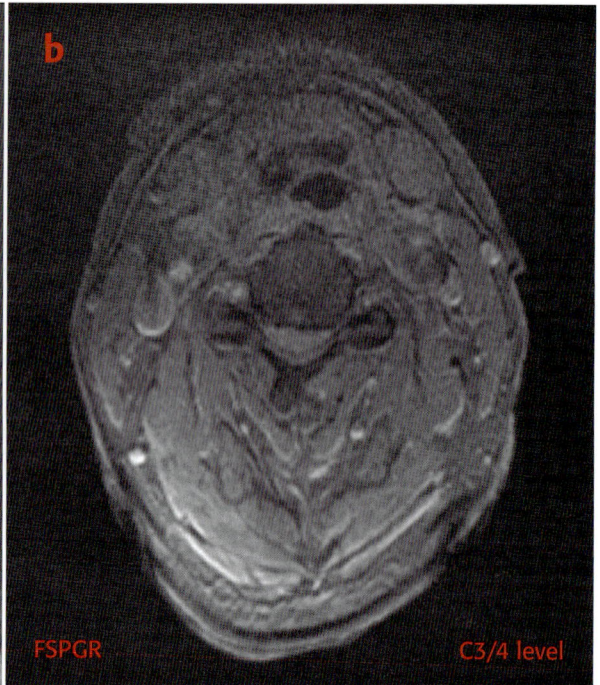

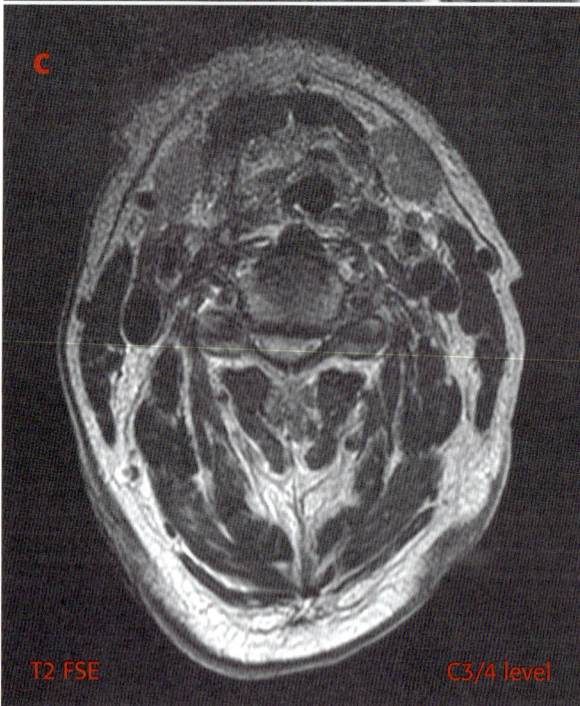

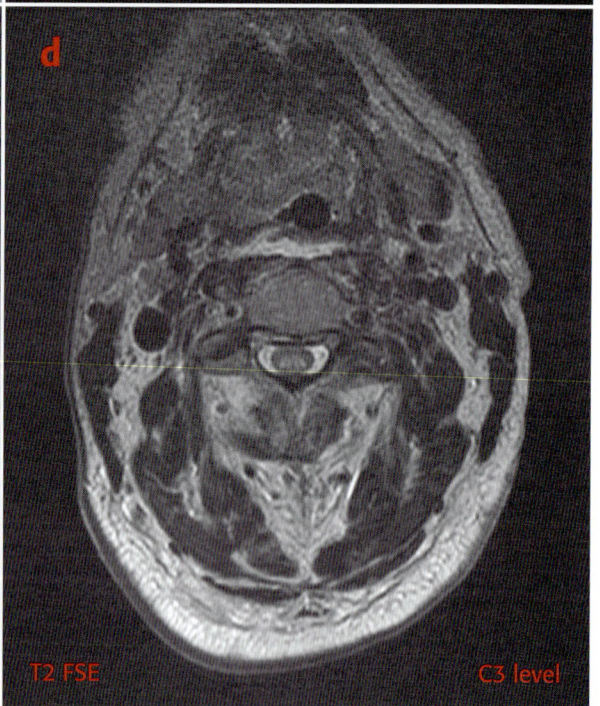

This 71-year-old man fell onto his face today. He now has clinical features of central cord syndrome. CT scan shows degenerative changes but no fractures.

**Q** Describe the injury.

## A

There is extensive oedema in the cord around the C3–5 level. Particularly at the C3/4 level, there is narrowing of the canal (images a, b and c). There is extensive osteophyte formation anteriorly. There is increased signal intensity in the C3/4 disc, and anterior to the anterior longitudinal ligament superior to this level. There is increased T2 signal intensity in the soft tissues adjacent to the spinous processes from C2 to C6. These features suggest a hyperextension injury.

## LEARNING POINT

Central cord syndrome may result from an extension injury due to cord compression between a hypertrophied spondylotic disc–osteophyte complex and a bulging ligamentum flavum, in the absence of any fractures.

## PROBLEM 4.27

T2

T1     C5 level

T2 GRE     C5 level

T1 Fat Sat + GD     C5 level

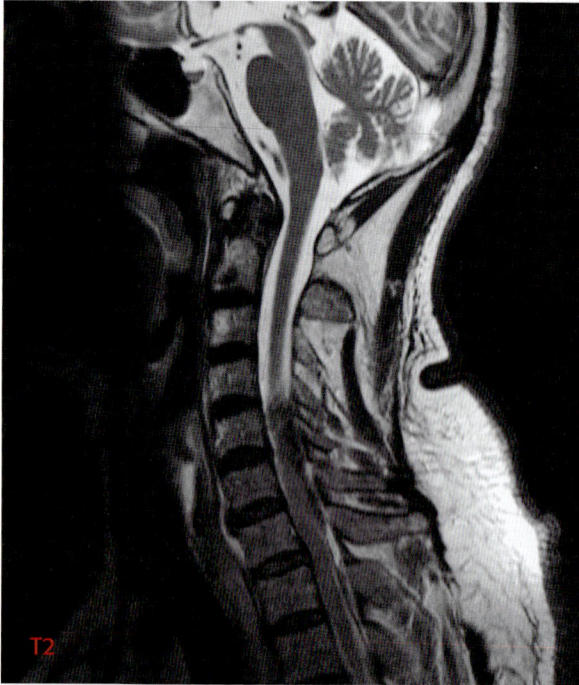

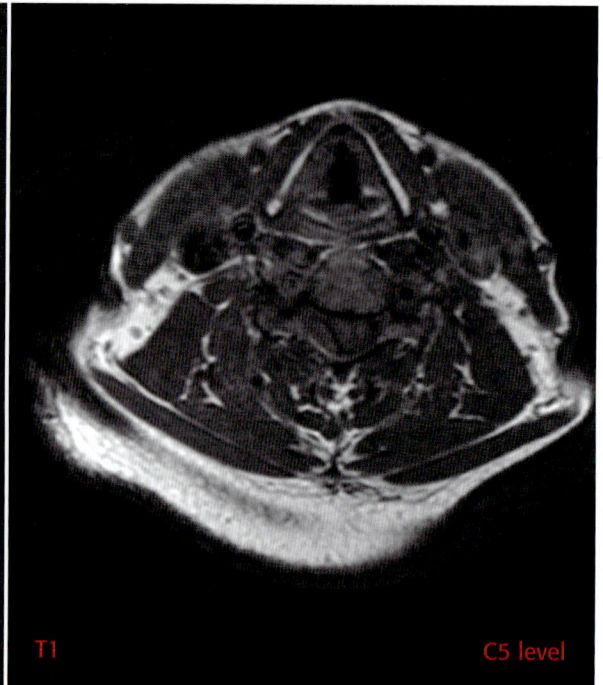

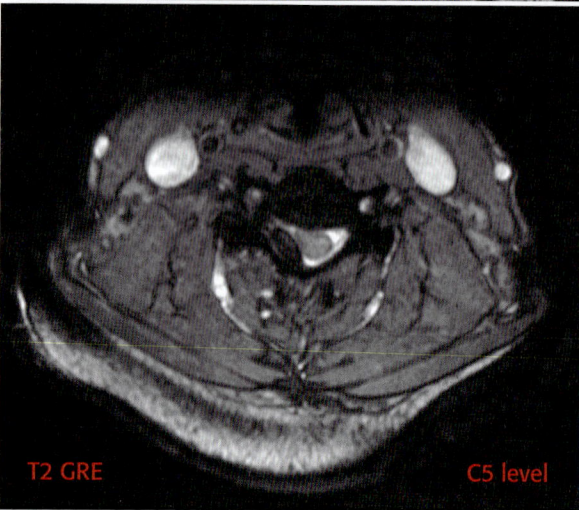

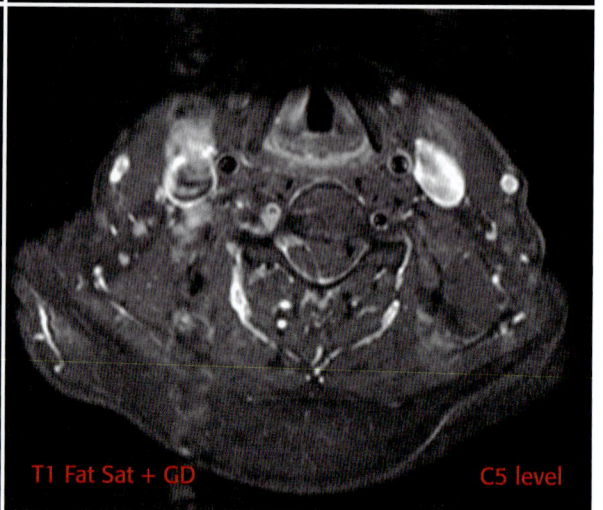

This 67-year-old man had rapid onset of quadri-paresis today, which is more marked on the right than the left and is accompanied by incomplete sensory loss at C6 and below.

**Q** What is the most likely reason for the neurological symptoms?

# A

There is a cervical epidural collection extending over several vertebral levels. Compared to the cord, it is T1 isointense and T2 hypointense.

There is peripheral enhancement on the post contrast sequence. The cord is displaced and compressed by the collection. These findings would be most consistent with an epidural haematoma.

## LEARNING POINT

MRI is the modality of choice for evaluating a spinal epidural haematoma, as it provides information regarding location, extent, degree of cord compression and acuteness of the haematoma.

Signal characteristics can vary but are isointense to the adjacent cord acutely, with conversion to hyperintensity in the subacute stage on T1-weighted images. On T2-weighted images, the majority of the signal abnormality is heterogeneously hypointense acutely and hyperintense subacutely. Gradient-echo may demonstrate blooming of haemorrhage.

A low T2 signal rim to the collection favours a haematoma over an abscess while peripheral linear post-contrast enhancement would favour an abscess over a haematoma. The clinical scenario and MR characteristics should allow accurate diagnosis in most cases.

See Chapter 6: Imaging modalities, p 375–6 for further explanation of terms.

# PROBLEM 4.28

MIP

T1 Fat Sat

T1 Fat Sat

T1 Fat Sat

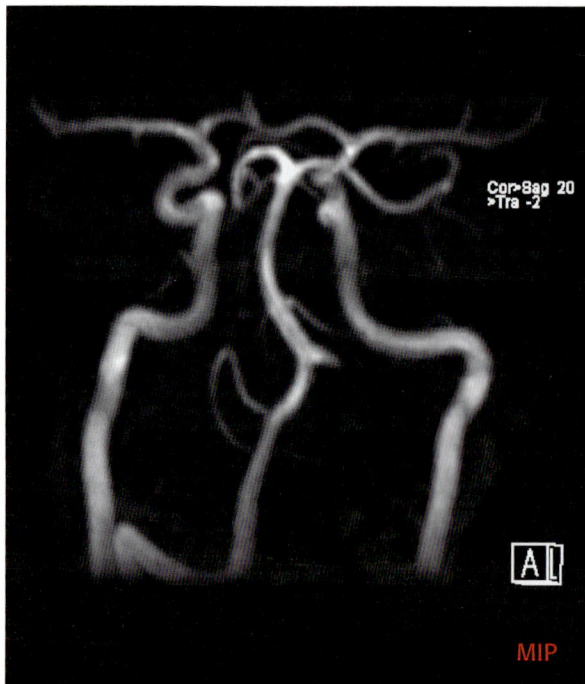

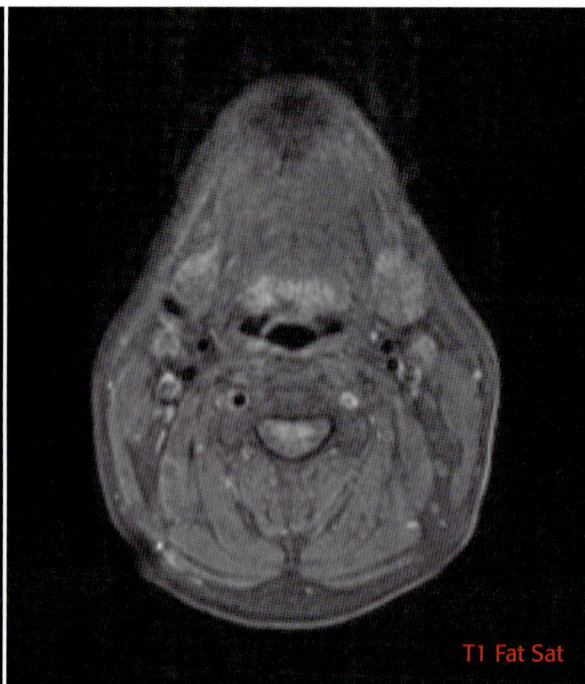

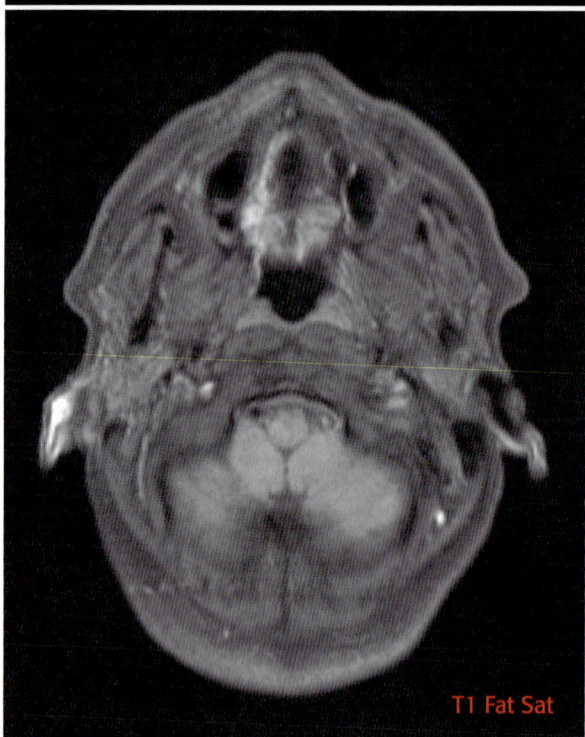

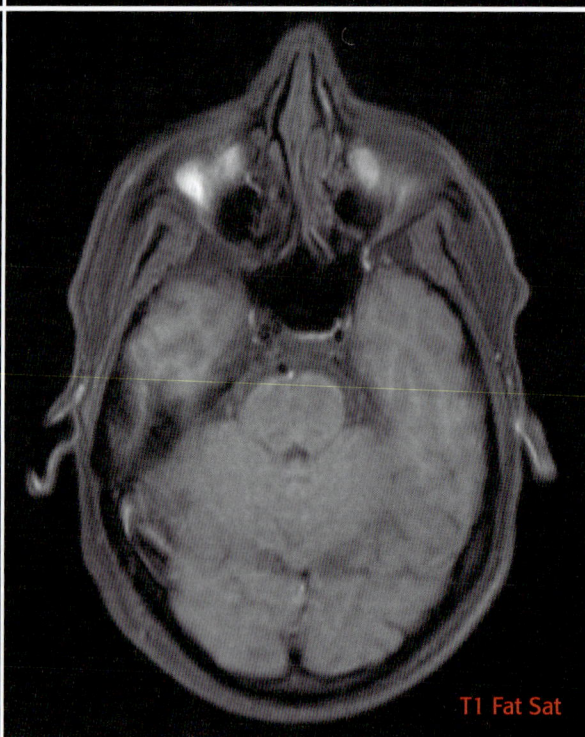

This 43-year-old-woman had her neck manipulated by her family doctor 24 hours ago. She now has vomiting, vertigo and nystagmus.

**Q**

What is the likely explanation of the symptoms?

## A

The axial T1 fat saturation images show absence of the normal flow void in the left vertebral artery. The absence of arterial flow in the left vertebral artery and its branch, the left posterior inferior cerebellar artery, is well demonstrated in the maximum intensity projection images.

See Chapter 6: Imaging modalities, p 375 for further explanation of terms.

## LEARNING POINT

Vertebral artery dissection can produce a wide spectrum of clinical manifestations from being asymptomatic to brain death. Lateral medullary syndrome may occur from posterior inferior cerebellar artery involvement.

# PROBLEM 4.29

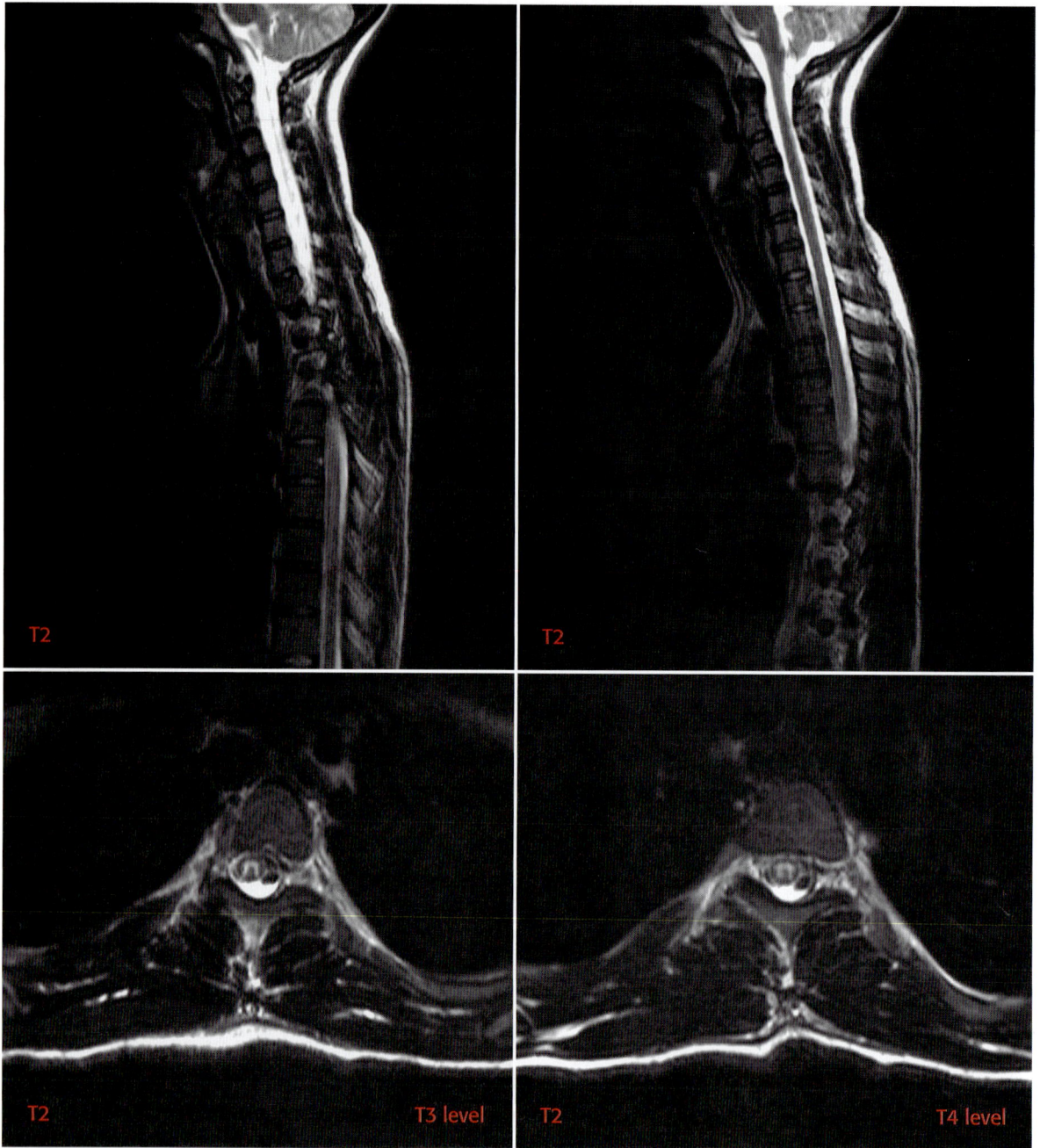

This previously well 21-year-old woman has developed paraplegia over the last 72 hours. She has a sensory level at T6.

**Q**
What is the most likely diagnosis?

# A

There is a long segment of increased T2 signal in the thoracic cord. There is no cord expansion. The spinal canal is not narrowed.

The most likely diagnosis is transverse myelitis. Other possible causes include cord ischaemia, infarction or multiple sclerosis. If the MRI of the head is normal, multiple sclerosis is unlikely. The MRI findings in cord ischaemia or infarction would be similar, but these diagnoses are unlikely without risk factors such as recent aortic surgery.

There is an incidental thoracic scoliosis, making it impossible to visualise the entire thoracic cord on one image.

The T2 hypointense areas seen within the CSF are due to CSF flow artefact.

## LEARNING POINT

Expansion and contraction of the intracranial vessels associated with the cardiac cycle results in pulsatile expansion and contraction of the brain. This produces to-and-fro movement of CSF, which may cause CSF flow artefacts on MRI. Signal intensity may be increased or reduced and the artefacts are typically seen in the lateral ventricles just superior to the foramen of Monro, the fourth ventricle and within the cervical and thoracic spinal canal.

## PROBLEM 4.30

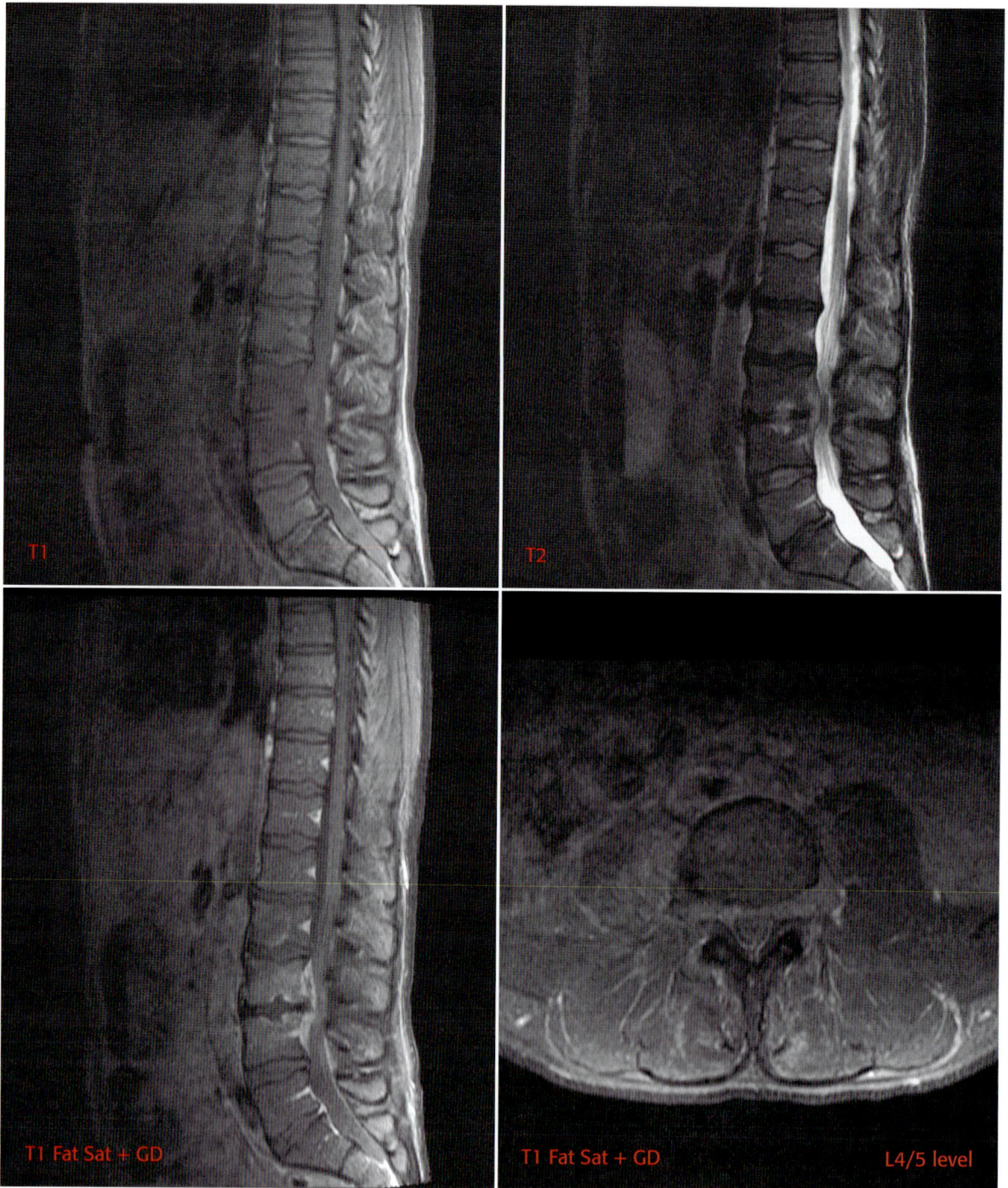

T1

T2

T1 Fat Sat + GD

T1 Fat Sat + GD                          L4/5 level

This 49-year-old man presented in septic shock. *Staphylococcus aureus* was isolated from blood cultures. No source of infection was apparent clinically.

**Q**

What source of sepsis is seen on these images?

# A

The T1 sagittal sequence demonstrates marrow oedema of the L3 and L4 vertebral bodies, which enhances on the post-contrast sagittal T1 fat saturated sequence. The intervening disc displays a bright T2 signal, consistent with oedema of the nucleus pulposus. No disc enhancement is seen. These findings, as well as loss of endplate definition, are consistent with discitis and osteomyelitis.

An anterior epidural lesion is noted at the L3/4 level, compressing the thecal sac. Within it are small non-enhancing areas, consistent with an epidural abscess.

There is abnormal enhancement of the psoas muscles bilaterally, which is more pronounced on the right and is consistent with inflammation. A non-enhancing central component would suggest an intramuscular abscess. Although no abscess is demonstrated on the images shown in the book, a small 4 mm abscess is shown on the post-contrast sequence in the DVD.

## LEARNING POINT

In the patient with staphylococcal bacteraemia with no obvious source, common occult sites of infection that may need surgical management include epidural abscess, psoas abscess and endocarditis.

## PROBLEM 4.31

a — No external pressure

b — External pressure applied

c — Pulse wave Doppler

d — Pulse wave Doppler

e — Needle insertion

f — Following guidewire insertion

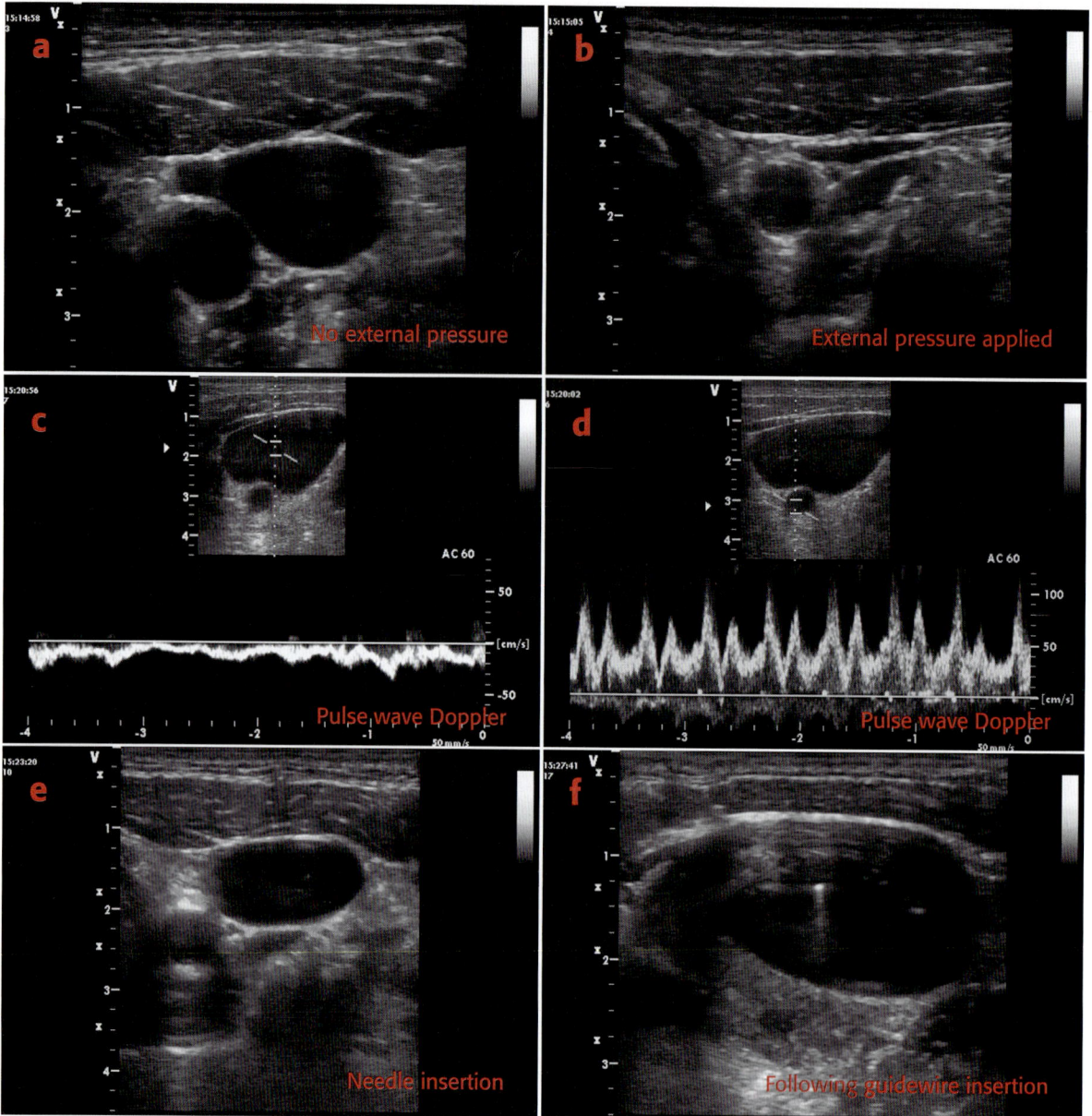

This 35-year-old man was admitted to ICU with abdominal sepsis. It was decided to insert a right internal jugular central venous catheter using real-time ultrasound guidance. These ultrasound images are shown in the order that they were obtained during the procedure.

## Q

1. What findings on these images identify which of the vessels is the vein?
2. Apart from the position of the vein, what other useful information have these images provided to the person undertaking cannulation?

# A

1. The findings which identify which of the vessels is the vein are:
   * The vein is thin walled and ovoid. The artery is thick walled and round (image a).
   * The vein collapses with external pressure, while the artery does not (image b).
   * Flow in the vein is continuous with pulse-wave Doppler (image c), while arterial flow is pulsatile (image d).

2. Other useful information these images provide to the person undertaking cannulation are:
   * The anatomical relation between the artery and the vein. In this patient, the vein lies in front of and to the right of the artery.
   * The vein is patent, of normal size, and suitable for cannulation.
   * Visualisation that the needle is directed towards the vein while it is being inserted (image e).
   * Confirmation that the guidewire is correctly placed within the vein (image f).

## LEARNING POINT

When central venous catheterisation is performed via the internal jugular vein, real-time ultrasound guidance (Maecken, 2007):

* shortens the time of the procedure
* reduces the number of failed attempts
* reduces the rate of complications

## REFERENCES

Allen BL, Ferguson RL, Lehmann TR, et al. A mechanistic classification of closed, indirect fractures and dislocations of the lower cervical spine. Spine 1982; 7(1): 1–27

Anderson LD, D'Alonzo RT. Fractures of the odontoid process of the axis. J Bone Joint Surg Am 1974; 56(8): 1663–74

Anderson PA, Montesano PX. Morphology and treatment of occipital condyle fractures. Spine 1988; 13(7): 731–6

Anderson PA, Rivara FP, Maier RV, et al. The epidemiology of seatbelt-associated injuries. J Trauma 1991; 31(1): 60–7

Denis F. The three column spine and its significance in the classification of acute thoracolumbar spinal injuries. Spine 1983; 8(8): 817–31

Froese BB. Lumbar spondylolysis and spondylolisthesis. emedicine. In Slipman CW, Talavera F, Foye PM, Allen KL, Cailleiet R, WebMD, 2006, Available: http://emedicine.medscape.com/article/310235-overview; accessed 7 May 2009

Maecken T, Grau T. Ultrasound imaging in vascular access. Crit Care Med 2007; 35(5 Suppl): S178–85

Matti MV, Sharrock NE. Anesthesia on the rheumatoid patient. Rheum Dis Clin North Am 1998; 24(1): 19–34

McConnel CT. The "open" exit foramen: A new sign of unilateral interfacetal dislocation or subluxation in the lower cervical spine. Emerg Radiol 1995; 2(5): 296–302

Platzer P, Jaindl M, Thalhammer G, et al. Clearing the cervical spine in critically injured patients: A comprehensive C-spine protocol to avoid unnecessary delays in diagnosis. Eur Spine J 2006; 15(12): 1801–10

Thumbikat P, McClelland MR. Acute injury to the spinal cord. Surgery (Oxford) 2007; 25(10): 413–19

Torretti J, Sengupta D. Cervical spine trauma. Indian J Orthopaed 2007; 41(4): 255–67

Truumees E. Os odontoideum. emedicine. In Riley LH, Talavera F, Shaffer WO, Patel D, Keenan MAE, WebMD, 2008, Available: http://emedicine.medscape.com/article/1265065-overview; accessed 7 May 2009

# CHAPTER 5

# LIMBS

## PROBLEM 5.01

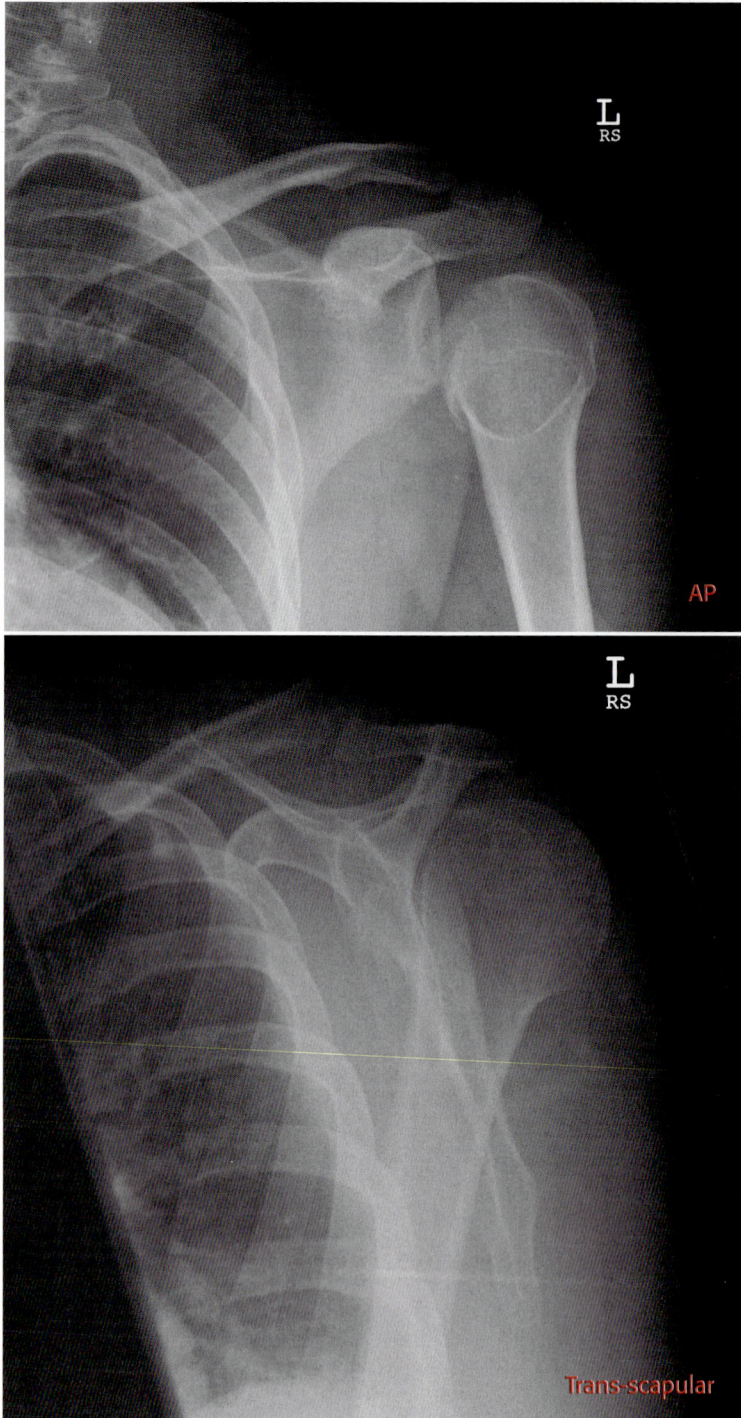

When this 40-year-old man was admitted to ICU with status epilepticus, some bruising was noticed around his left shoulder.

**Q** What problem do these images show?

# A

The AP view looks relatively normal although there are some subtle abnormalities. Due to internal rotation, the humeral head has a "light bulb" appearance, instead of a normal "hockey stick" appearance. The trans-scapular view clearly demonstrates a posterior dislocation of the shoulder. There is also an impaction fracture of the neck of the humerus.

## LEARNING POINT

Posterior dislocation of the shoulder is an uncommon injury, which is often missed. Classically, the history is one of seizures or electrocution but this injury may result from a fall on an outstretched arm. A clinical pointer towards this injury in the unconscious patient is that the arm is typically held adducted and in internal rotation and cannot be externally rotated from this position (Limb, 2005).

On the AP projection, the dislocated humeral head may appear to line up normally with the glenoid fossa. The abnormalities in this view are subtle, and often missed. The dislocation will be obvious in a trans-scapular view (Limb, 2005).

## PROBLEM 5.02

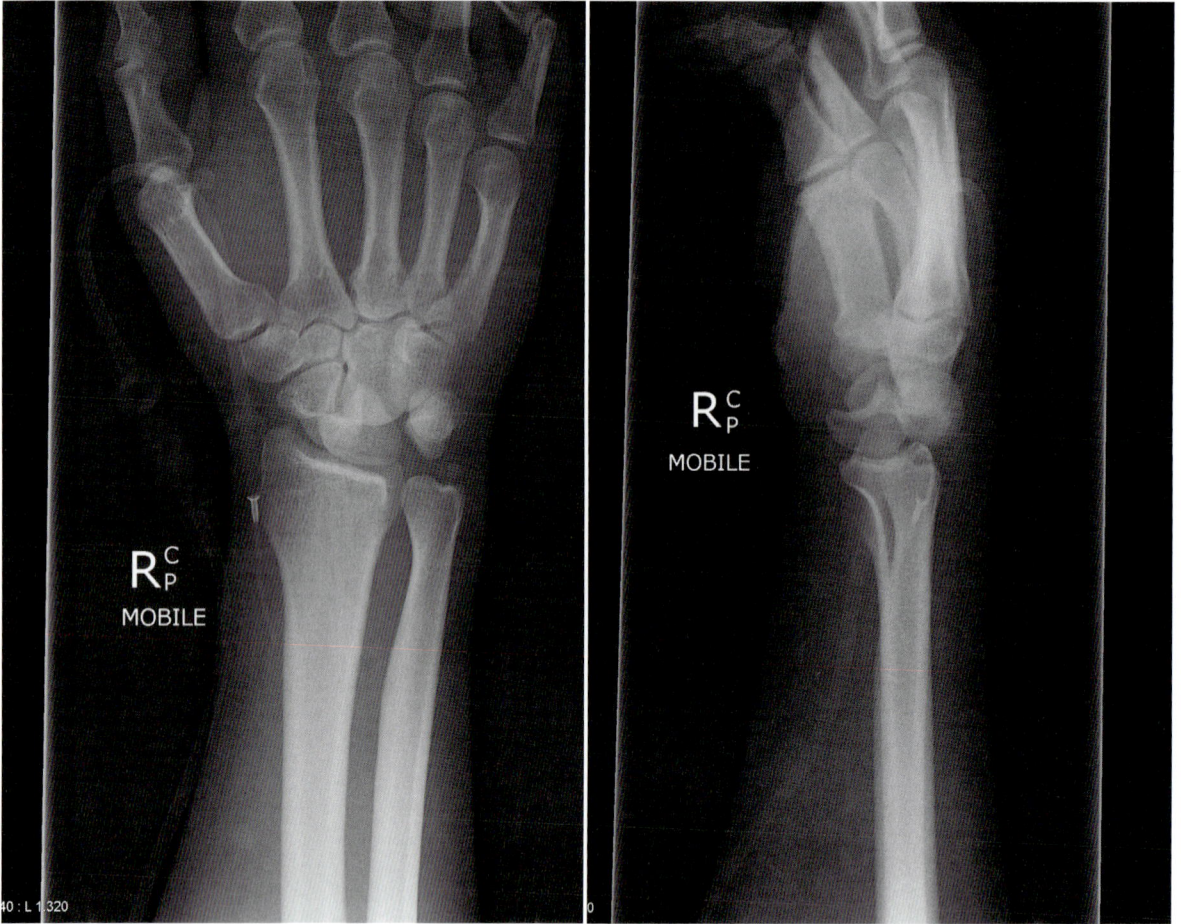

This 47-year-old man was an unrestrained passenger in a high-speed car crash and sustained multiple traumatic injuries. Bruising and swelling around the right wrist was noticed at ICU admission following an emergency laparotomy.

**Q**

What injury do these images show?

# A

On the AP view, the lunate (middle bone, proximal row of three carpal bones) appears triangular and overlaps the other carpal bones. There is loss of the normal smooth carpal arcs of the proximal and distal articular surfaces. On the lateral view, the lunate has rotated so that its concave surface (usually articulated with the capitate) faces somewhat anteriorly. The lunate retains its normal relation to the distal radius, while the capitate and other carpal bones are dislocated posteriorly. These findings are typical of a perilunate dislocation (Kozin, 1998). The ulnar styloid tip is also fractured.

## LEARNING POINT

Perilunate dislocations are commonly missed, even when wrist X-rays are obtained. In the unconscious patient who cannot complain of pain, there may be no obvious abnormality on clinical examination. Delayed treatment may result in significant long-term functional limitation due to arthritis or median nerve palsy (Kozin, 1998).

## PROBLEM 5.03

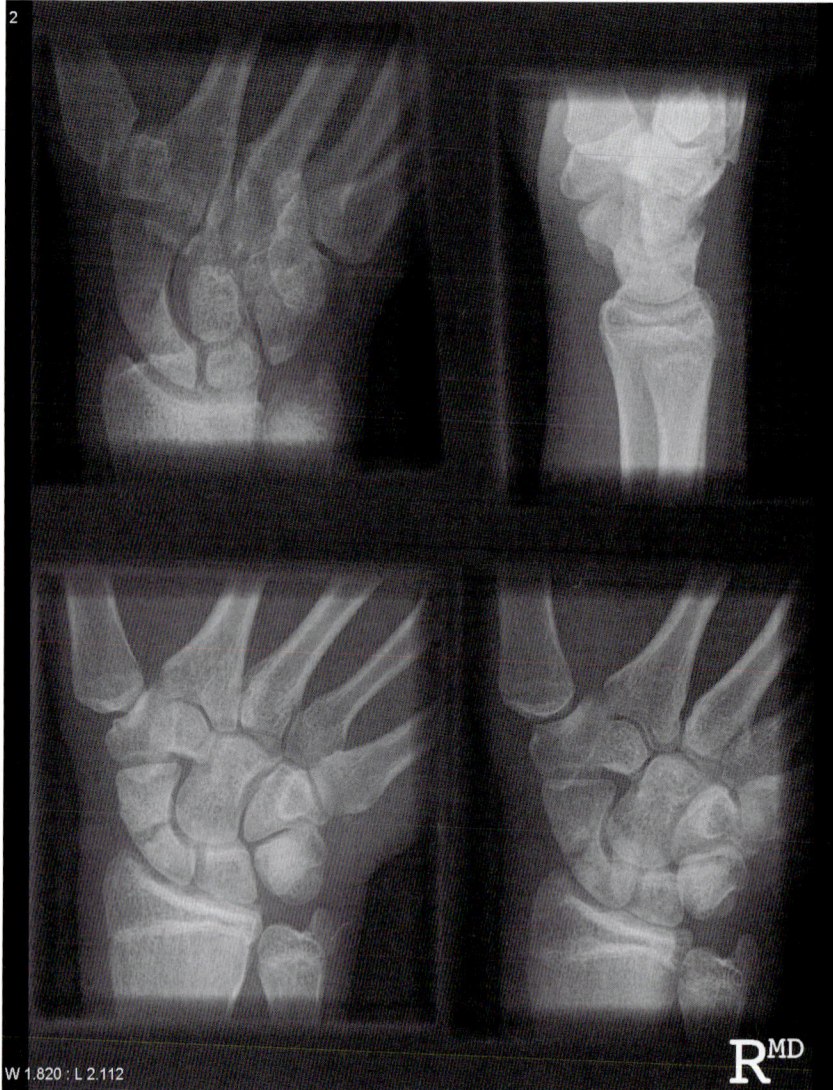

This 17-year-old man sustained major chest and abdominal trauma in a high-speed car crash. His right wrist was swollen and tender.

**Q** What injury is seen on these images?

## A

There is an undisplaced fracture through the waist of the scaphoid.

## LEARNING POINT

Initial plain X-rays often miss scaphoid fractures, especially when acquired only in an AP projection. An AP view in ulnar deviation demonstrates these fractures to a better advantage. CT and MR scans have a much higher sensitivity than plain X-ray for this injury.

When patients survive major trauma without neurological injury, long-term functional limitations are determined mainly by orthopaedic injuries. Missing a seemingly minor injury in a patient with life-threatening chest and abdominal injuries may result in significant long-term morbidity.

## PROBLEM 5.04

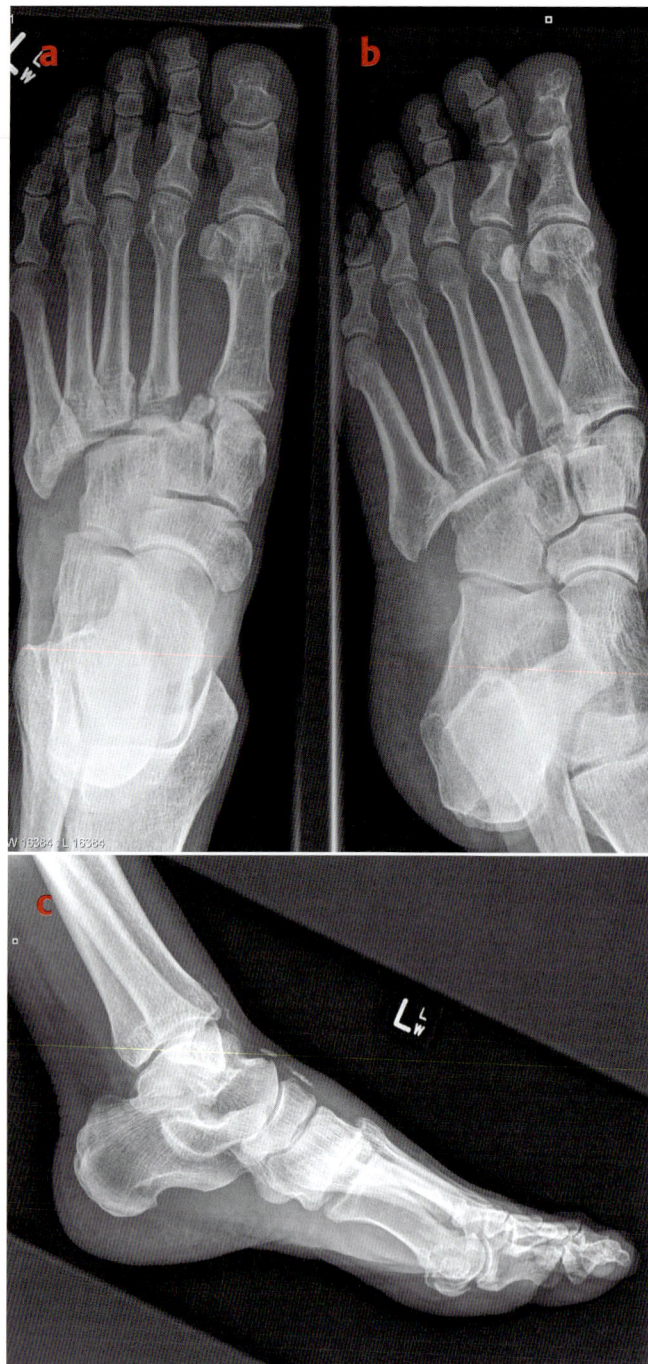

This 70-year-old man was in a high-speed car crash and is ventilated because of chest injuries. On the ward round, it is noted that there is swelling of the foot and bruising of the medial side of the plantar aspect of the midfoot.

**Q**

What injury is shown on these images?

# A

In the AP view (image a):

- the second to fifth metatarsals are displaced laterally
- the medial borders of the second metatarsal and the middle cuneiform do not align, due to lateral shift of the metatarsal
- the space between the first and second metatarsals is widened (normal < 2 mm)
- the base of the second metatarsal is fractured, and a "fleck" sign is present (best appreciated on the DVD images). The fleck sign is an avulsion fragment adjacent to the base of the first metatarsal, pathognomonic of a Lisfranc fracture

In the oblique view (image b), there is lateral displacement of the second to fifth metatarsals resulting in loss of alignment of:

- the lateral borders of the lateral cuneiform and the third metatarsal
- the medial borders of the fourth metatarsal and the cuboid

In the lateral view (image c):

- the second metatarsal is displaced dorsally in relation to the middle cuneiform

These findings are typical of a Lisfranc injury. Incidental calcification of the dorsalis pedis artery is noted.

# LEARNING POINT

The Lisfranc ligament links the medial cuneiform to the base of the second metatarsal. When it is disrupted, the lateral four metatarsals can sublux laterally in relation to the tarsal bones and the first metatarsal (Sands, 2004).

Since the natural history of an untreated Lisfranc injury is very poor, the diagnosis is important to make. Clinical findings may include midfoot swelling (especially dorsal), with pain to palpation in the tarsometatarsal area and ecchymosis on the medial side of the plantar aspect of the midfoot (Sands, 2004).

## PROBLEM 5.05

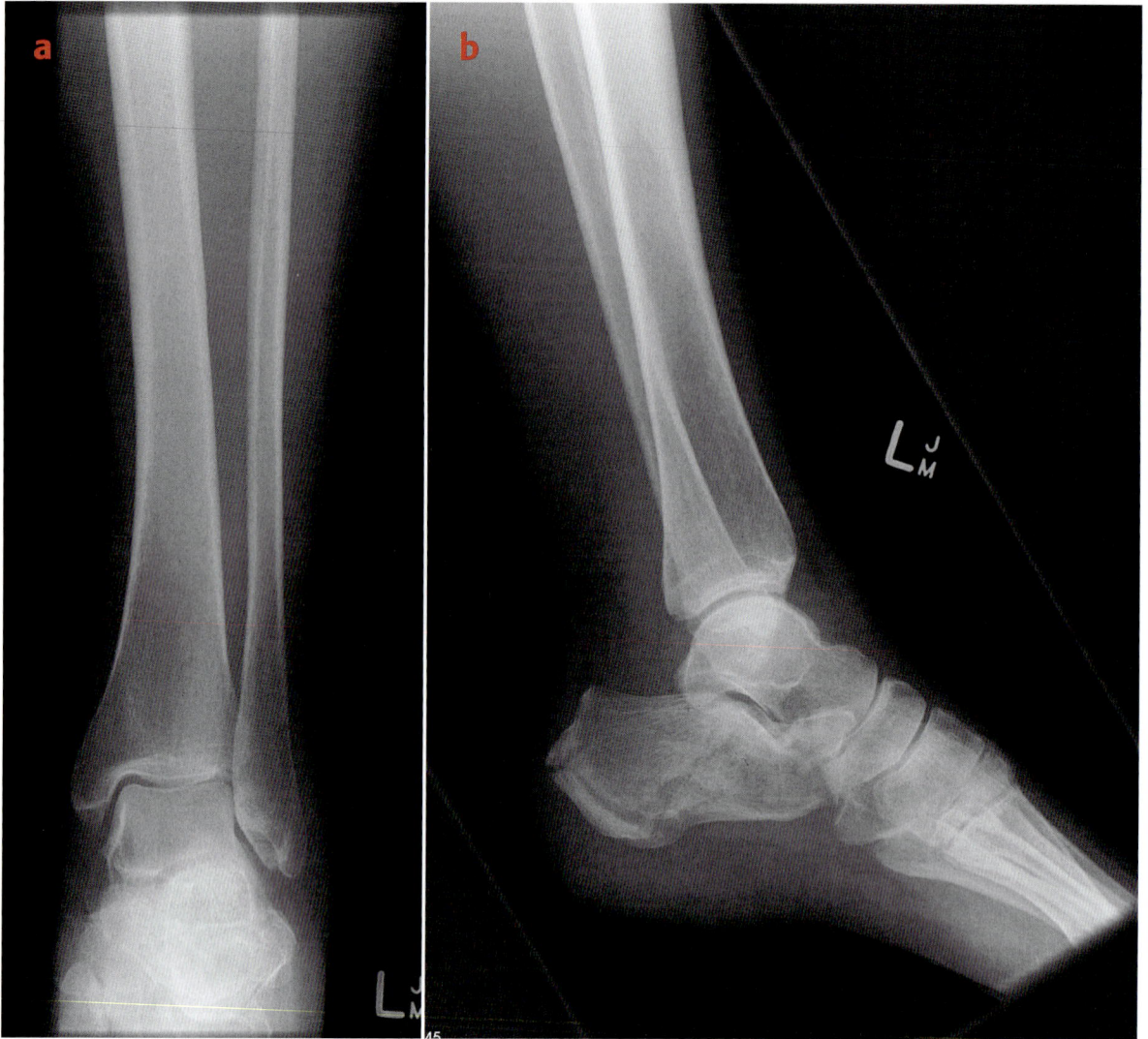

This 45-year-old woman was working on a construction site. She fell six metres and was unconscious at the scene. On arrival at the emergency department, she was intubated because of agitation and confusion. The CT head scan shows minor frontal cerebral contusion. Swelling and bruising around her left ankle and proximal foot were noted at the time of admission to intensive care.

**Q**

Describe the injury.

# A

There is a comminuted fracture of the calcaneus, best seen on the lateral view (image b). It appears to involve the subtalar joint.

## LEARNING POINT

When a calcaneal fracture results from a fall from a significant height, it is often associated with other injuries produced by axial compression forces. These include contralateral calcaneal fracture, vertical shear fracture of the pelvis and spinal burst fracture.

## PROBLEM 5.06

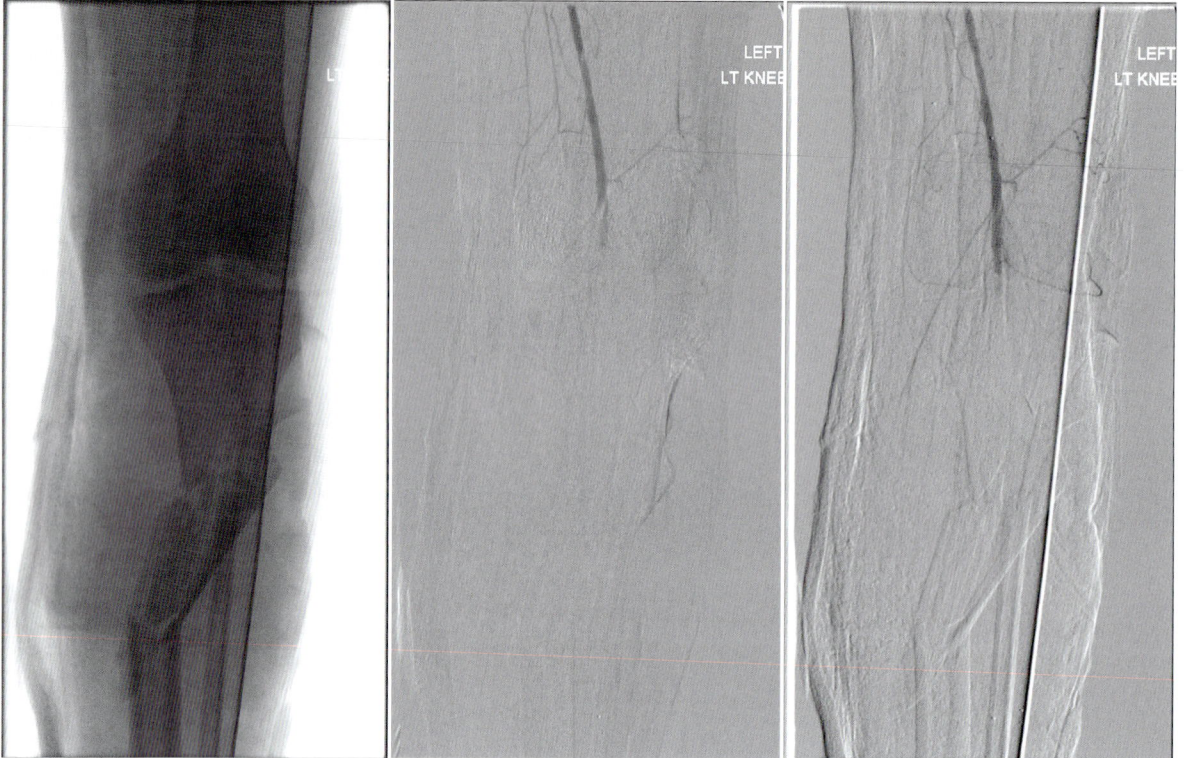

This 35-year-old pedestrian was struck by a car, injuring his left leg. His left foot is pale, with no pulses and abnormal sensation.

**Q**
Describe the findings on this digital subtraction angiogram.

## A

There are comminuted fractures of the tibia and fibula, with significant deformity at the fracture sites. Normal contrast opacification of the arterial system is seen down to the level of the popliteal artery but there is an abrupt cut off at this level. The vessels distal to this level are not seen. These findings are consistent with a traumatic occlusion of the popliteal artery.

## LEARNING POINT

When major limb fractures are present, the integrity of the circulation distal to the fracture should be carefully examined. If the circulation is compromised, the first step is to reduce any dislocation or gross deformity. If this does not correct the problem, then vascular reconstruction may be required.

CT angiogram or digital subtraction angiogram are the best modalities to assess vascular integrity following trauma.

# PROBLEM 5.07

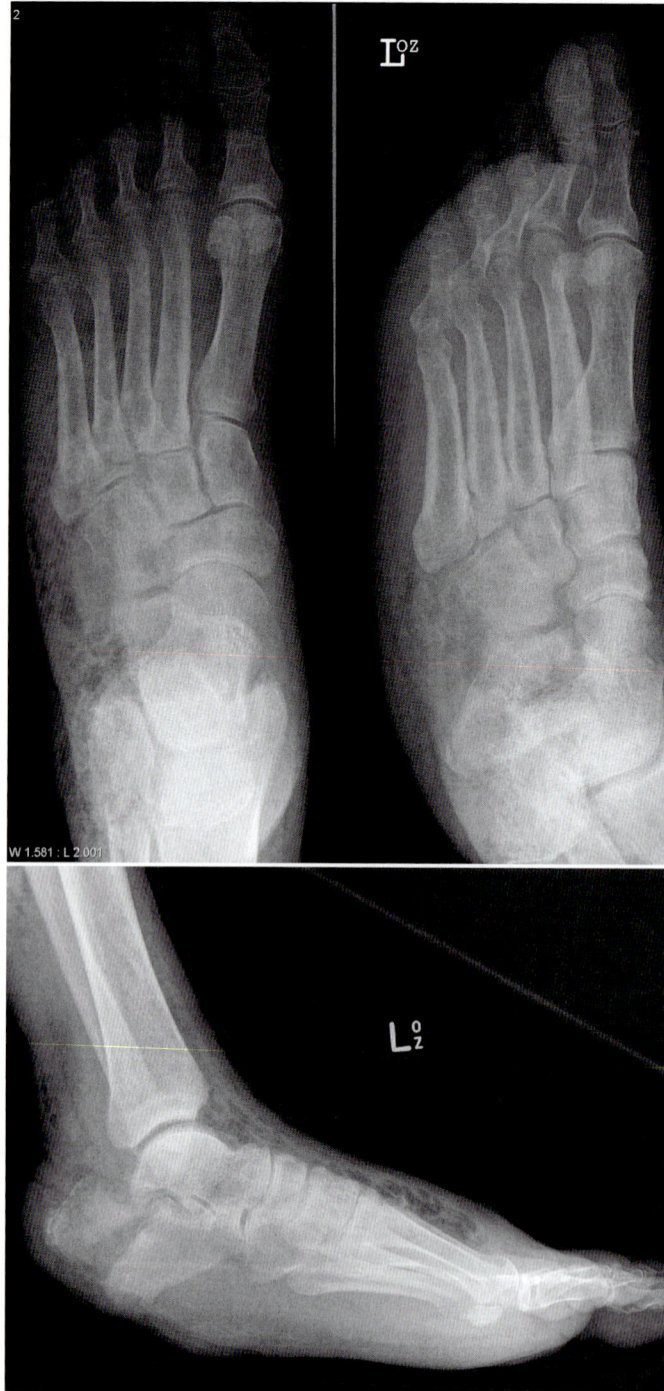

Two days ago, this 60-year-old man fell off a ladder and sustained an open injury to the left heel. He is now complaining of severe pain over his entire foot.

## Q

What problems do these images suggest?

## A

There is a fracture of the calcaneum. Gas can be seen within the soft tissues of the foot and lower leg, particularly on the dorsal and lateral aspect of the foot. The Achilles tendon is outlined by gas. The distribution of gas is far more extensive than could be attributed to air entering the tissues from an open wound, and is strongly suggestive of gas gangrene.

## LEARNING POINT

With early surgical debridement and prophylactic antibiotic therapy for open wounds, severe clostridial soft tissue infections are now rare. MRI has a role in determining the extent of severe soft tissue infection but should not delay surgery.

## PROBLEM 5.08

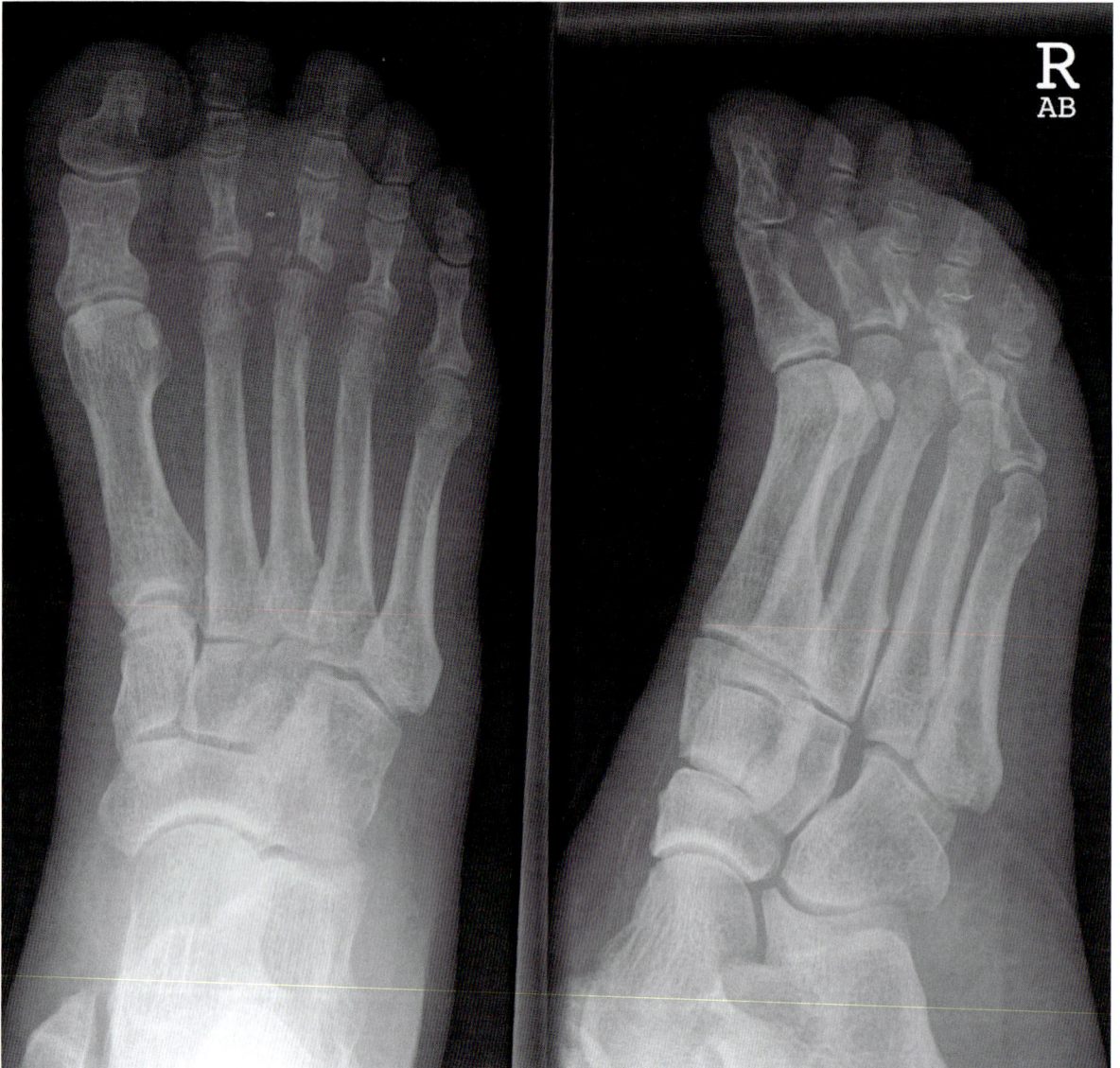

This 50-year-old man presented to the emergency department with septic shock. He gave a history of six weeks of pain and swelling in the sole of his right foot, at the base of the second and third toes. On examination, this region was swollen, tender and erythematous.

**Q**
What problem do these images suggest?

## A

There is a small, metallic foreign body just distal to the metatarsophalangeal joint, between the proximal phalanges of the second and third toes. The adjacent soft tissues are markedly swollen. Multiple lucencies are seen within the second and third proximal phalanges with cortical erosion. This process extends into the third metatarso-phalangeal joint which is widened. Cortical erosion is also seen in the middle phalanx of the right third toe. These findings are consistent with cellulitis and osteomyelitis caused by a foreign body. Vascular calcification suggests that arterial insufficiency could be a contributing factor.

## LEARNING POINT

Osteomyelitis may be due to haematogenous spread (common in children) or to direct spread from a contiguous focus of infection (common in adults). Foci of infection from which direct spread commonly occurs include open fractures, diabetic wound infections or surgical treatment of closed injuries (Pineda, 2006).

Plain X-rays are often normal in early acute osteomyelitis. As the disease progresses, findings may include (Dahnert, 2007; Pineda, 2006):

- localised soft tissue swelling adjacent to the affected area
- features of bone destruction, such as cortical erosions or radiolucent areas within the bone
- joint involvement (septic arthritis is common)
- periosteal new bone deposition
- detached segments of necrotic bone known as sequestra

Bone scintigraphy scans and MRI are highly sensitive for detecting early osteomyelitis. MRI provides additional information about the extent of the infection and involvement of adjacent soft tissues. CT is less sensitive for early disease but may provide addition information about bony anatomy (Pineda, 2006).

# PROBLEM 5.09

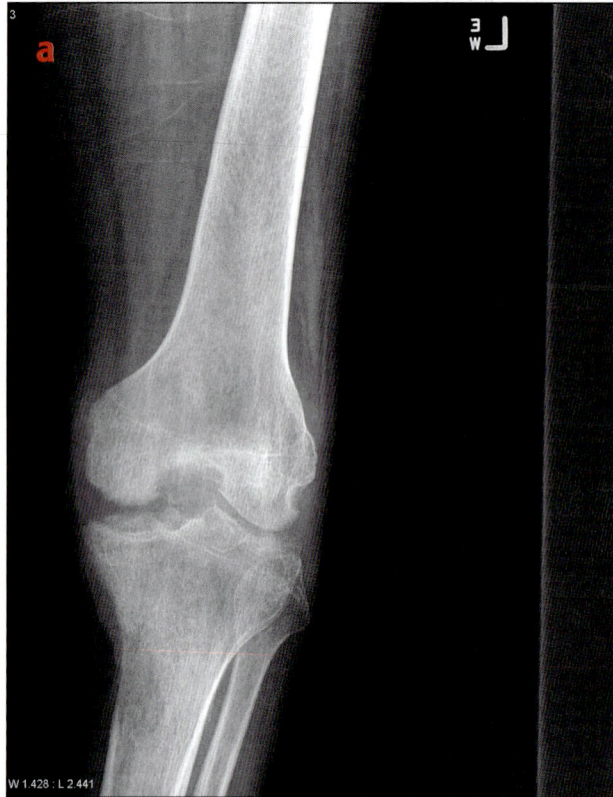

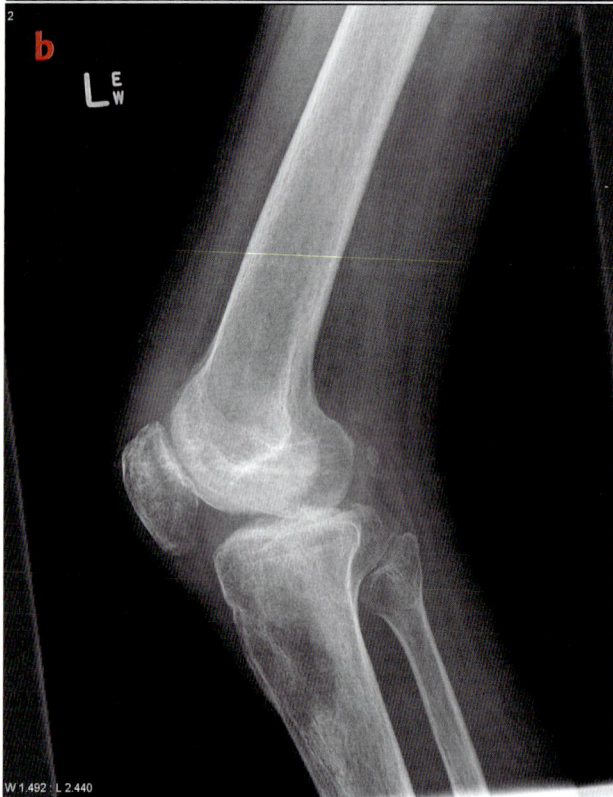

This 57-year-old man fell off his pushbike two months ago. He sustained a wound on the medial aspect of his upper left leg that required debridement and hospitalisation for two weeks. Last week, he developed pain in his left knee and now cannot weight bear on his left leg. He has been admitted to the emergency department with septic shock.

## Q

What diagnosis is suggested by these images?

## A

On the AP view (image a), there is widening of the joint space, seen best on the medial aspect of the joint. On the lateral view (image b) there is fluid in the suprapatellar pouch. These findings are typical of knee joint effusion.

On the medial aspect of the knee joint, there is erosion of the subchondral cortex of the tibia and femur, and blurring of the joint margins. In this clinical context, this is highly suggestive of septic arthritis. There is a lucent area in the proximal tibial shaft, with overlying soft tissue abnormality, suggestive of osteomyelitis.

## LEARNING POINT

In early septic arthritis, X-rays are usually normal but may show a joint effusion. Joint space narrowing due to destruction of articular cartilage and osteopaenia around the joint may develop rapidly. Erosion of the articular cortex and reactive bone sclerosis occur after 8–10 days (Dahnert, 2007; Wilson, 2004).

On plain X-ray, effusions are readily seen in the knee and the elbow but are much less apparent in other joints. An effusion in the elbow is indicated on plain X-rays by the appearance of triangular radiolucencies anterior and posterior to the distal humerus (often called "sail signs"). These represent intra-articular fat pads that have been displaced by the effusion.

# PROBLEM 5.10

Axial T1

Axial T1 Fat Sat + GD

Axial T2 Fat Sat

Axial T2 Fat Sat

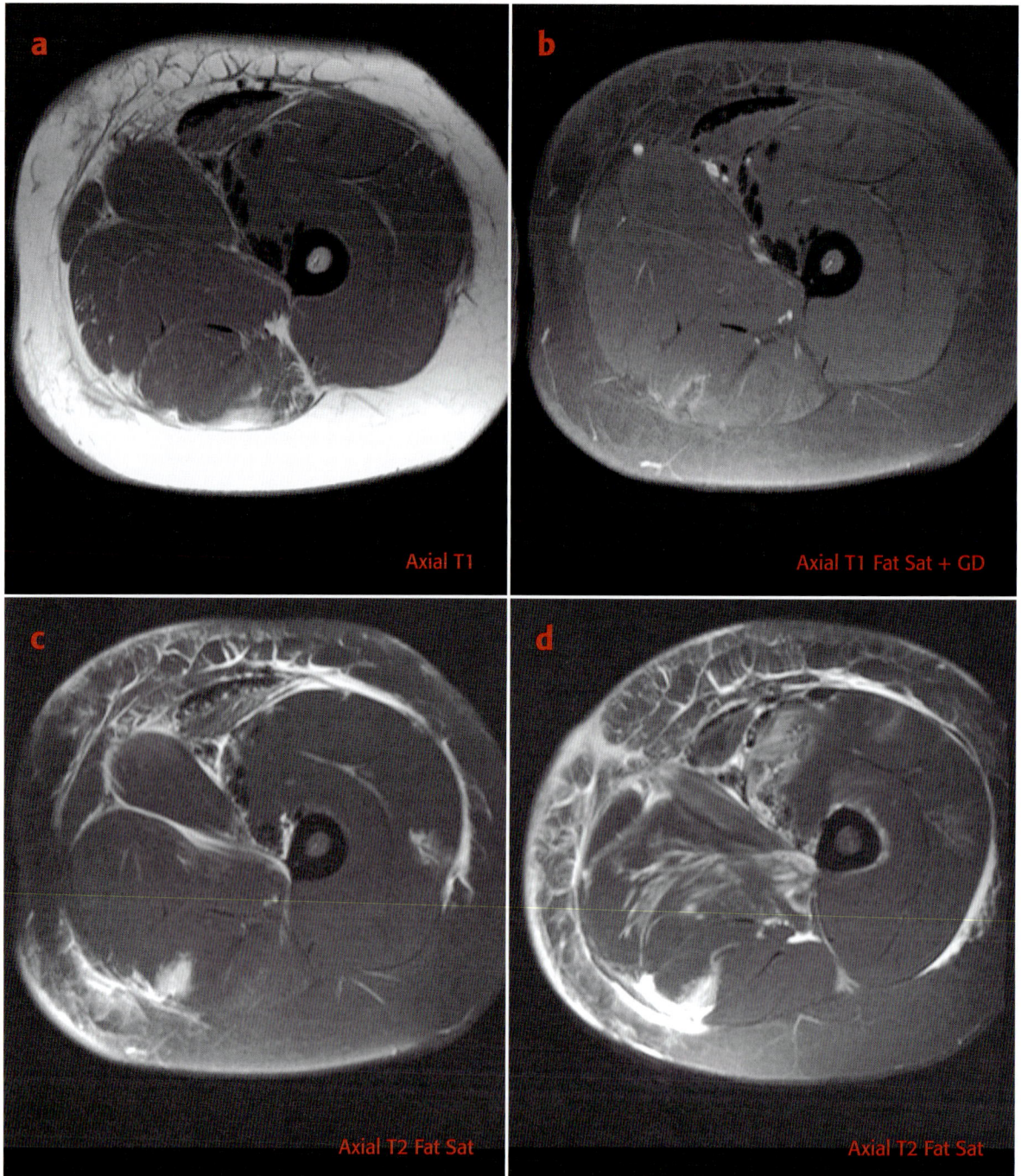

This 25-year-old man gave a history of a painful black area the size of a small coin developing on the skin of the anteromedial aspect of his left thigh last night. When he woke this morning, he felt unwell. The skin lesion was larger and had developed blisters. He now has septic shock and acute renal failure.

## Q

What diagnosis do these images suggest?

# A

Intermuscular and intramuscular gas is present, which is seen as areas of low signal on all three sequences. The axial T1 image shows skin thickening (best seen posteromedially) and subcutaneous fat stranding (best seen anteriorly). The axial T2 Fat Saturation images show extensive oedema of the skin and subcutaneous tissues. On image c, the oedema involves the fascial planes and a few small areas of muscle. On image d, there is more extensive muscle involvement. On the post-GD contrast sequence a small area of intramuscular contrast enhancement is seen (image b), corresponding to an area of oedema (image c) on the T2 sequence. These findings are typical of necrotising fasciitis.

# LEARNING POINT

Necrotising fasciitis is characterised clinically by necrotic or blistering skin lesions with systemic illness and pain out of keeping with the physical signs. Large areas of soft tissue and muscle are often involved. Early aggressive debridement and broad-spectrum antibiotics are required. The role of imaging in this condition is limited, as the priority is urgent surgical intervention. In the occasional case where imaging is required, MRI is the modality of choice.

# PROBLEM 5.11

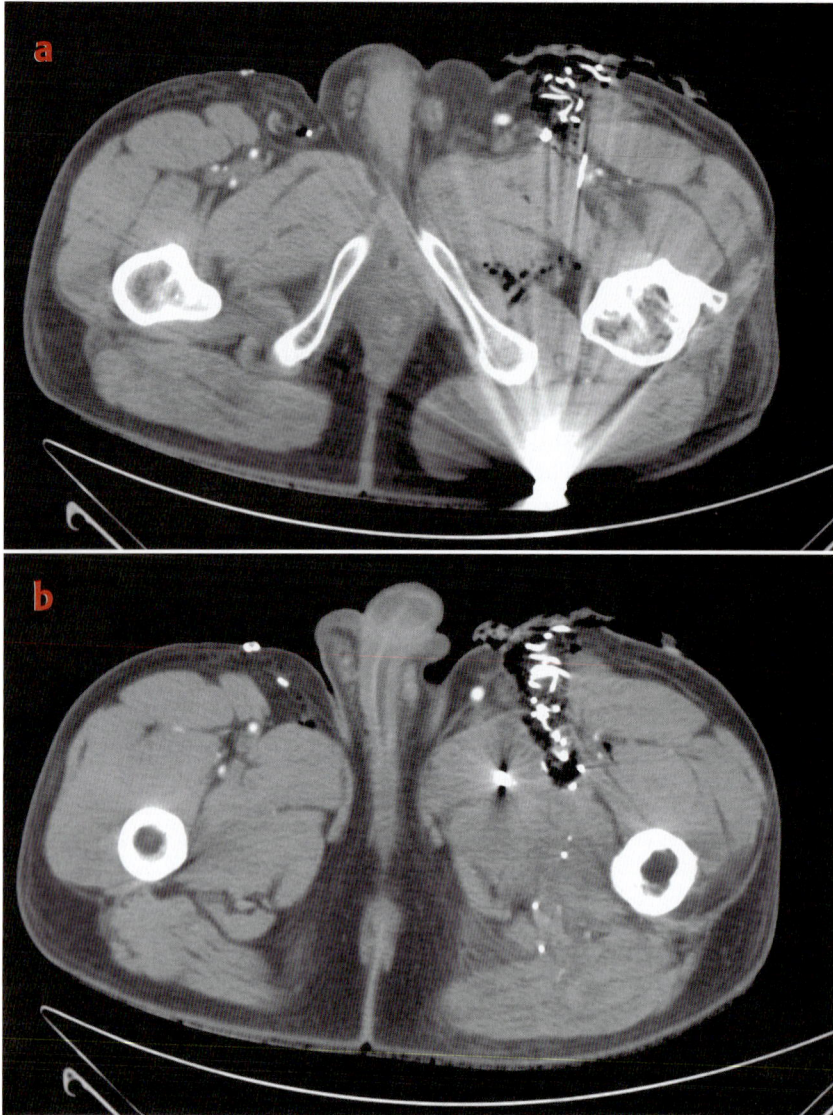

This 45-year-old man was shot in the upper thigh during an armed robbery. On arrival at hospital, he was immediately taken to the operating theatre for exsanguinating haemorrhage. A saphenous vein reconstruction of his femoral artery was performed and the wound was packed. These images were obtained following the operation.

**Q**

Describe the findings on these images.

# A

There is a wound on the anterior aspect of the left thigh, which contains packing. There are multiple metallic foreign bodies scattered through the soft tissue of the thigh. The largest of these is in the subcutaneous tissue overlying the left gluteus maximus muscle. Haematoma of the left gluteus maximus and the adductor muscles is denoted by attenuation of intramuscular fat planes (image b). There is surgical emphysema in the deep tissues. Surgical clips are seen on the anterior aspect of the right thigh, consistent with the saphenous vein donor site. There is flow in the left femoral arterial graft. The patency of the graft is confirmed in the full set of images on the DVD.

## LEARNING POINT

With gunshot wounds, it is common that there will be significant tissue damage at sites remote from the linear track between entry and exit wounds.
- Transfer of kinetic energy from a bullet may result in tissue disruption significantly greater than the diameter of the projectile would suggest.
- Bullets often fragment with impact and each fragment may damage the tissues through which it traverses.

## PROBLEM 5.12

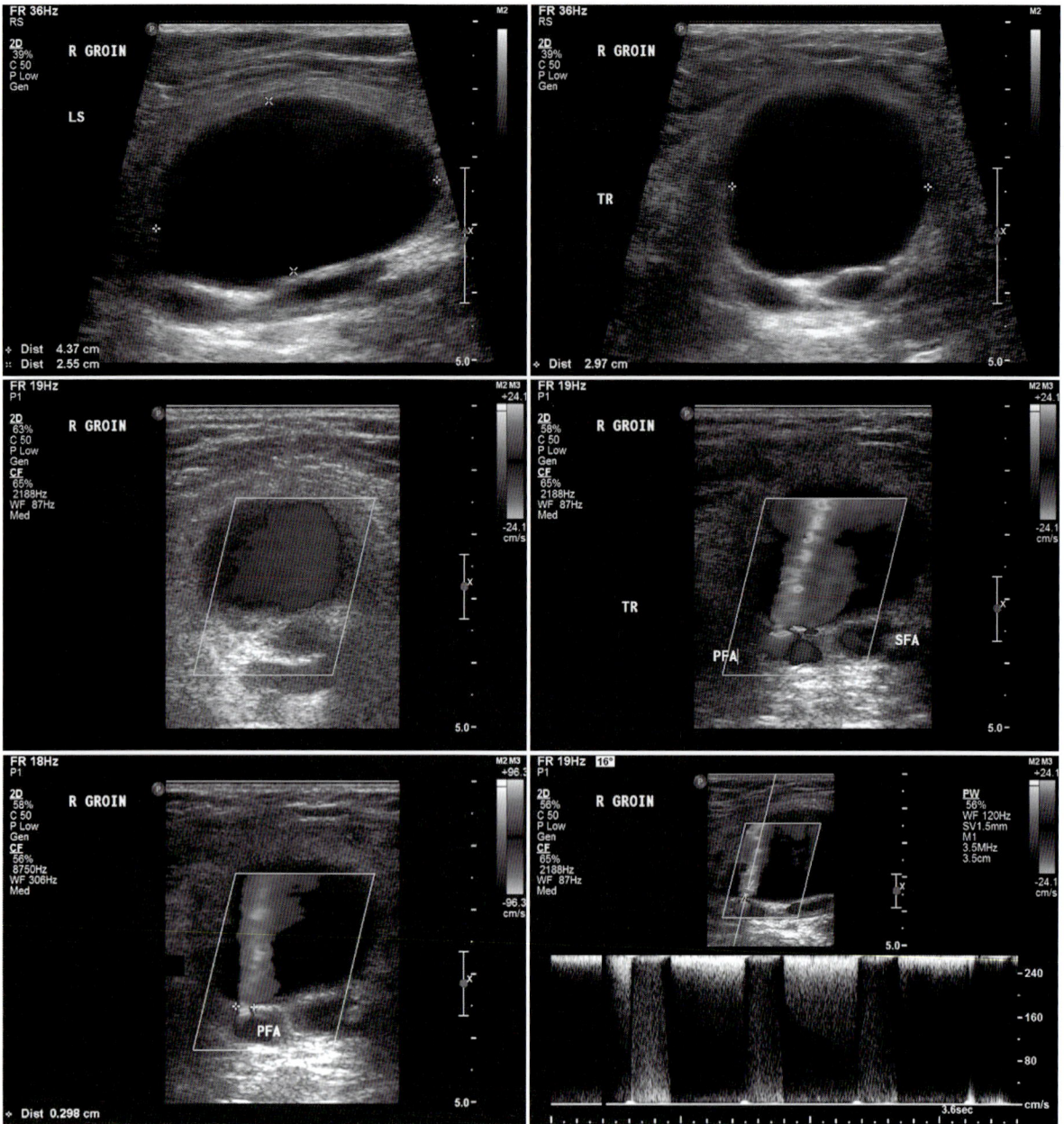

This 60-year-old woman underwent elective coronary angiography with angioplasty and stenting one week ago. The procedure was uneventful and she continues to take aspirin. She now presents with a pulsatile mass in the right groin, adjacent to the catheter insertion site.

**Q**

What problem do these images of a duplex scan of the right groin demonstrate?

## A

There is an echo free cavity measuring 4.37 × 2.55 × 2.97 cm in the right groin, adjacent to the profunda femoris artery. Swirling colour flow is recorded within the cavity and there is high-velocity colour flow within a tract between the cavity and the artery. The width of the communication between the artery and the cavity is small in relation to the size of the artery, and to-and-fro flow is demonstrated on the Doppler waveform in this region. These findings are typical of a pseudo-aneurysm and, in this clinical context, represent a complication of the cardiac catheterisation.

## LEARNING POINT

A pseudoaneurysm is a pulsatile haematoma that communicates with an artery through a disruption in the arterial wall (Kronzon, 1997). Pseudoaneurysm complicates 0.1–0.2% of diagnostic coronary angiograms and 1–2% of cardiac interventional procedures that use a femoral arterial access site. It is more common when the puncture site is at, or distal to, the bifurcation of the common femoral artery (Lenartova, 2003).

## PROBLEM 5.13

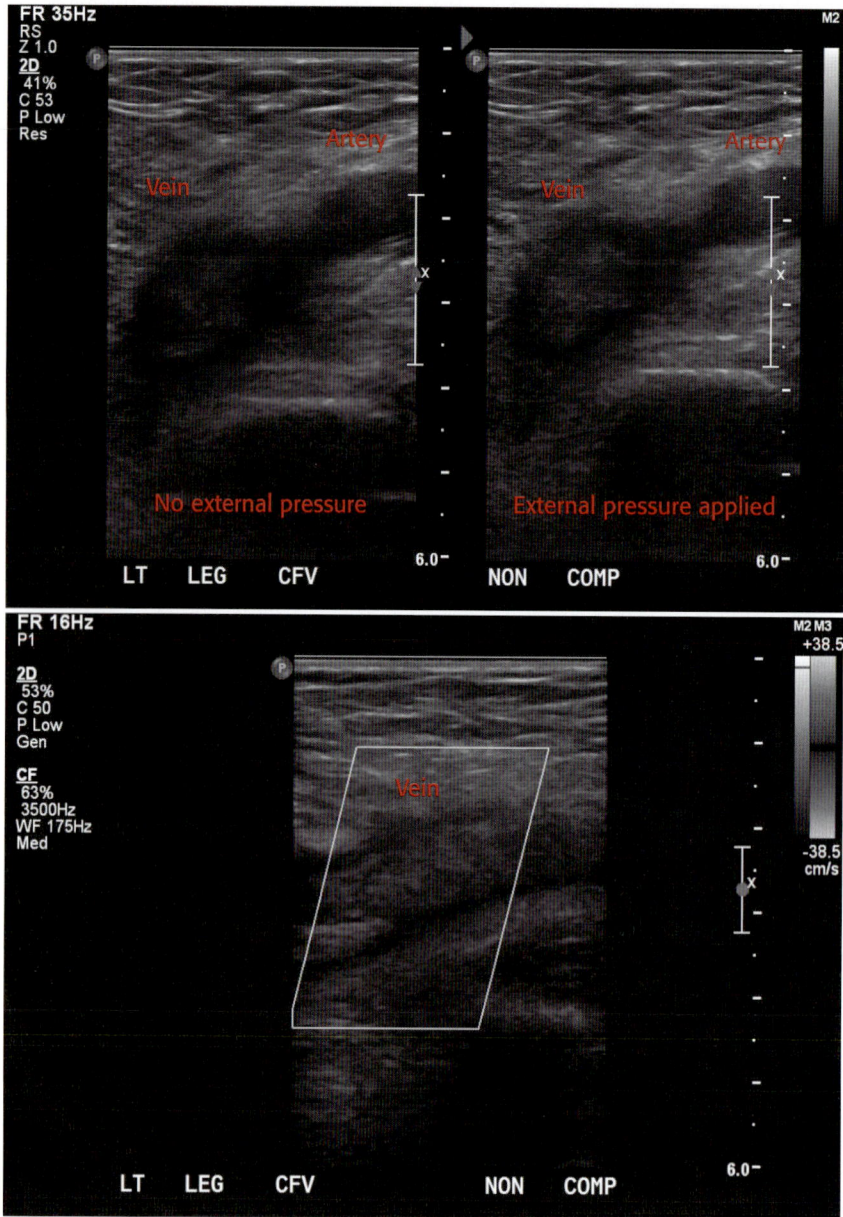

This 45-year-old man was in a car crash eleven days ago. He sustained injuries to his chest and abdomen, as well as a left tibial fracture, which was treated with open reduction and internal fixation. He continues to require mechanical ventilation. On the ward round today, his left leg was found to be much more swollen than yesterday.

**Q**

What are the findings on these ultrasound images of the left common femoral vein?

# A

The lumen of the common femoral vein is filled with a strongly echogenic mass. The vein is not compressed when external pressure is applied.

There is no flow seen within the vein on colour Doppler imaging. These findings are typical of a common femoral vein thrombosis.

## LEARNING POINT

Duplex ultrasonography combines 2D imaging and colour Doppler imaging and is the investigation of choice for suspected deep venous thrombosis (DVT). It allows correct diagnosis of other conditions that may mimic DVT, such as Baker's cyst, calf haematoma and popliteal artery aneurysm. When assessing for DVT in the lower limb, it is less sensitive in the calf than for more proximal veins. Significant limitations are that ultrasound may not image the iliac veins well, it may be impractical to study patients in plaster casts and it is of little value for detecting a new thrombosis in a post-phlebitic limb (Orbell, 2008).

Alternative imaging techniques include:
- indirect CT contrast venography: intravenous (IV) contrast is injected at a site away from the affected limb. This can be performed at the same time as CT pulmonary angiography, without the need for additional contrast (Orbell, 2008).
- direct CT contrast venography: IV contrast injection into affected limb
- MRI venography
- contrast venography: IV contrast is injected into the affected limb

## REFERENCES

Dahnert W, ed. Radiology review manual. 6th edn. Philadelphia: Lippincott Williams and Wilkins; 2007.

Kozin SH. Perilunate injuries: Diagnosis and treatment. J Am Acad Orthop Surg 1998; 6(2): 114–20

Kronzon I. Diagnosis and treatment of iatrogenic femoral artery pseudoaneurysm: a review. J Am Soc Echocardiogr 1997; 10(3): 236–45

Lenartova M, Tak T. Iatrogenic pseudoaneurysm of femoral artery: Case report and literature review. Clin Med Res 2003; 1(3): 243–7

Limb D, McMurray D. Dislocation of the glenoid fossa. J Shoulder Elbow Surg 2005; 14(3): 338–9

Orbell JH, Smith A, Burnand KG, et al. Imaging of deep vein thrombosis. Br J Surg 2008; 95(2): 137–46

Pineda C, Vargas A, Rodriguez AV. Imaging of osteomyelitis: current concepts. Infect Dis Clin North Am 2006; 20(4): 789–825

Sands AK, Grose A. Lisfranc injuries. Injury 2004; 35 (Suppl 2): SB71–6

Wilson DJ. Soft tissue and joint infection. Eur Radiol 2004; 14 (Suppl 3): E64–71

# CHAPTER 6

# IMAGING MODALITIES

# PLAIN X-RAYS

X-rays are a form of electromagnetic radiation. They can be generated in the vacuum within an X-ray tube by bombarding a tungsten target (anode) with electrons from a filament of tungsten wire (cathode). The electrons are accelerated towards the target by the high potential difference between the anode and cathode (Long, 2006).

The path of the X-ray beam is from the beam source (X-ray tube), through the tissues being imaged, to an image receptor. The image receptor may be either a traditional film-based system or a filmless computed radiography system. The film-based system consists of a film holder (cassette), an intensifying screen coated with phosphor, which fluoresce when exposed to X-rays, and the film. The film is developed after image acquisition and then viewed directly. The computed radiography system consists of a sealed cassette containing phosphor material. After image acquisition, the cassette is scanned with a laser system and viewed on the computer screen of a Picture Archiving and Communication System (Long, 2006; Novelline, 2004).

The attenuation of X-rays by tissues depends on both their density and thickness. X-rays often pass through multiple tissues and the image formed represents the sum of all the densities interposed between the beam source and the image receptor. The appearance of tissues on images allows them to be classified into the four basic radiographic densities of air, fat, water (or soft tissue) and bone (Erkonen, 2005).

Tissues must be of different density for the boundary between the two tissues to be seen on an X-ray image. Consider the boundary between the heart and the lung. On the plain X-ray image, this boundary is normally seen as a distinct cardiac border because the water density heart lies against the air density lung. Consolidated lung has water density. Therefore, if the lung adjacent to the heart becomes consolidated, the cardiac border becomes indistinct and may not be apparent on the image. Similarly, air filled bronchi cannot be seen within normal air density lung but, if the lung becomes consolidated, the bronchi may be seen as air bronchograms.

As the X-ray beam travels from the beam source to the image receptor, its cross-sectional area increases and its intensity reduces in keeping with the inverse square law. Because the object being imaged is closer to the beam source than the image receptor, the image is magnified. The magnification depends on both the distance from object to image receptor and the distance from beam source to image receptor (Long, 2006). Chest X-ray images are usually obtained with the beam directed in a posteroanterior (PA) direction and the image receptor placed against the front of the chest. Mediastinal structures are located anteriorly, close to the image receptor, so there is minimal magnification of these structures. With portable X-ray imaging, the beam is directed in an antero-posterior (AP) direction and the image receptor placed against the back of the chest. As the mediastinal structures are now further from the image receptor, there is significant magnification of them, which produces apparent widening on the AP image. This appearance may be compounded by gravitational effects. The PA image is acquired in the erect position, so gravity narrows and elongates the mediastinum. The AP image is often acquired with the patient supine, in which case this effect is absent.

# ULTRASOUND

## Tissue imaging

Pulses of ultrasound are generated by a piezoelectric crystal and enter the body, travelling at a velocity of approximately 1540 ms$^{-1}$ in soft tissues. Ultrasound pulses are reflected from tissue interfaces and the reflected pulse returns to the crystal, where it generates an electrical signal. Image generation is based on the time delay between sending the pulse and receiving reflections from the tissue interfaces. Deeper structures have a longer time delay than superficial structures. The time delay between transmitting the pulse and receiving the reflected signal, and the assumed velocity of ultrasound in the tissues, is used to calculate the depth (Anderson, 2007).

With M-mode ultrasound, the ultrasound pulse is directed along a single line through the structures of interest. The display shows tissue depth on the y-axis and time on the x-axis. The brightness of any point on the display is determined by the intensity of the corresponding reflected signal. M-mode allows a rapid sampling frequency, providing good temporal resolution of rapidly moving structures (Anderson, 2007).

2D ultrasound images may be generated by either a phased array or a linear array transducer. With a phased array transducer, the beam is swept across a tomographic plane to produce a sector-type image. Each sweep of the ultrasound beam generates an image and the frequency of the sweeps determines the image frame rate on the video display. With a linear array transducer, multiple parallel beams in a tomographic plane produce a rectangular image. With both transducer types, the display shows the tomographic plane with the brightness of any point determined by the intensity of the corresponding reflected signal (Feigenbaum, 2005; Otto, 2004).

Standard ultrasound imaging is based on the fundamental frequency generated by the transducer. As the ultrasound wave propagates through the tissues, harmonic frequencies are generated, which may be used to generate images that are often superior to standard images (Otto, 2004)

The frequency of the transmitted pulse is important in determining image quality. Image resolution is better with high frequencies, while depth of penetration is better with low frequencies. There is a trade off between these two factors. In general, superficial structures are best imaged with high frequencies, while deeper structures are best imaged with low frequencies (Anderson, 2007).

A basic artefact of ultrasound tissue imaging is acoustic shadowing. This is where an intensely echogenic structure blocks propagation of the ultrasound wave, producing an echo-free shadow distal to the structure. This artefact may be useful (e.g. giving a characteristic appearance with echogenic gallstones) or interfere with image generation (e.g. image degradation deep to bone or gas) (Otto, 2004).

## Doppler ultrasound

When ultrasound waves are reflected from an interface moving towards the transducer, there is an increase in frequency of the waves. The opposite is true when the interface is moving away. This is a manifestation of the Doppler effect, easily exemplified by the fall in frequency of the sound from the siren of a passing ambulance. Doppler ultrasound may be used in a continuous wave (CW) or pulsed wave (PW) modality. These are often used to examine blood flow, with the interface being the red blood cell membrane (Anderson, 2007).

With CW Doppler, the ultrasound beam is directed along a single line. The transducer generates a continuous wave of ultrasound at a set frequency and records the reflected signal. The peak change in frequency between the generated and reflected frequency measures the maximum velocity directed towards (or away from) the transducer. This technique allows assessment of the maximum velocity with no limitation on how high this is, but lacks spatial resolution. The maximum velocity could have been generated anywhere along the beam path. Conventionally, the display shows movement towards the transducer as a positive velocity above the baseline and away from the transducer as a negative velocity below the baseline (Anderson, 2007).

With PW Doppler, a small window is set as the area of interest. The ultrasound beam is again directed along a single line through the area of interest. The transducer generates pulses of ultrasound at a set frequency and records the reflected signal, assessing the change in frequency between the two. This time, however, recording of the signal only takes place at the time delay corresponding to the depth of the area of interest, so the velocity recorded is the velocity of that area only. Thus, pulsed wave Doppler gives spatial resolution while CW Doppler does not. PW Doppler is usually set up using 2D ultrasound so that the area of interest can be visualised and the window set accordingly. There is a limitation imposed by the PW nature of this technique. The changes in frequency used to generate velocity information become ambiguous if they are greater than half the pulse repetition frequency (Nyquist limit). This means that PW Doppler can only be used to examine relatively low blood flows, while assessment of high velocity turbulent jets requires CW techniques (Anderson, 2007).

The technique of PW Doppler may be extended to multiple areas of interest. This allows a colour flow map to be generated and superimposed on a 2D ultrasound image of the anatomical structures. This technique is termed colour flow imaging. Conventionally, blue is used to display flow away from the transducer and red for flow towards it. This can be remembered with the mnemonic: BART (Anderson, 2007).

# COMPUTED TOMOGRAPHY

In the current generation of CT scanners, the X-ray tube rotates in a circle around the patient while the patient is moved continuously through the gantry. The X-ray tube follows a helical path relative to the patient. Multiple rows of detectors are located in the gantry opposite the X-ray tube, allowing rapid data acquisition. At the time the scan is performed, the technician sets a range of parameters suitable for the examination being conducted and these parameters define the resolution of the scan (Hofer, 2005).

The raw dataset acquired is used to reconstruct a matrix of voxels (cuboid volume elements). Each voxel is assigned a value calculated from the attenuation of the X-rays passing through it. This value corresponds to the average density of the tissue in the voxel. The voxels are arranged in a series of slices, that are 1 voxel thick. These slices can then be displayed as a 2D image with the brightness of each pixel dependent on the attenuation value of the corresponding voxel (Hofer, 2005).

Conventionally, the basic axial 2D image is displayed as if the patient is supine and the observer

| TABLE 6.1: Typical densities of a range of tissues, in Hounsfield units. Adapted from Hofer, 2005. ||
|---|---|
| **Tissue** | **Density (HU)** |
| Bone (compact and spongy) | > 100 |
| Clotted blood | 80 ± 10 |
| Blood | 55 ± 5 |
| Solid abdominal organs | 30–80 |
| Liver | 65 ± 5 |
| Spleen/muscle/lymphoma | 45 ± 5 |
| Exudate | 25 ± 5 |
| Transudate | 18 ± 2 |
| Fat/connective tissue | −15 ± 65 |
| Fat | −90 ±10 |
| Water density fluids | 0–10 |

is standing at the patient's feet. The patient's right side is on the left-hand side of the screen and vice versa; anterior is on top of the screen and posterior at the bottom. To gain an appreciation of the 3D nature of the anatomy, images are scrolled through on a computer screen, allowing structures such as blood vessels to be followed as they pass between slices (Hofer, 2005).

The attenuation value of a voxel is related to the average density of the tissue in it. When a single structure does not occupy the full volume of a voxel, partial volume effects occur, which may result in poor definition of the borders of a structure. This explains the poor definition of sites such as the poles of the kidney (Hofer, 2005).

The density of a structure on the CT scan can be measured. This can provide useful diagnostic information, such as allowing a pleural effusion to be distinguished from a haemothorax. Care must be taken to include several voxels in the region of interest to avoid errors due to statistical fluctuations and to avoid partial volume effects. Density is measured in Hounsfield units (HU), a scale where water is 0 HU and air is -1000 HU. Typical densities for tissues are given in Table 6.1. The density of almost all soft tissue organs lie in the 10–90 HU range (Hofer, 2005).

A modern computer screen can display 256 shades of grey but the human eye can only distinguish approximately 20. If the full range of tissue densities (-1000 to +1000 HU) were to be displayed on the computer screen, it would not be possible to distinguish between many tissues of interest. For this reason, it is necessary to display only a small range (window) of densities, centred on the density level of the tissue being examined. Typical windows used are "soft tissue", "bone", "lung" and "brain".

In addition to the axial 2D reconstruction, it is possible to generate other reconstructions from the raw dataset, which help appreciate the anatomy in three dimensions. This post processing is done after the patient leaves the CT suite. Multiplanar reconstruction (MPR) simply reconstructs the raw dataset into a new matrix of voxels, with the slices arranged in a different plane. Typical planes are axial, sagittal and coronal. Oblique reformats may also be performed in any plane (Pavone, 2001).

Maximal Intensity Projection (MIP) is used to depict 3D "voxel" information on a 2D image. For each pixel, the value to be displayed is calculated by evaluating each of the voxels lying along a line perpendicular to the screen (analogous to the viewer's line of sight), and displaying the maximum voxel value on the line. The angle of view may be changed by rotating the image, giving a further 3D perspective. This technique is useful for displaying contrast enhanced blood vessels both on CT and MRI (Pavone, 2001).

Surface-shaded display shows the surface of a structure that has been defined by having density above a set value of Hounsfield units. The appearance is enhanced by a hypothetical source of light that the computer uses to create shading. The image generated may be rotated, allowing the entire surface of the structure to be examined. This technique is useful for displaying bony structures (Pavone, 2001).

Volume rendering is a more complex and computationally costly method of displaying 3D information. A wide variety of applications include CT angiography and virtual colonoscopy (Pavone, 2001).

CT scans are often combined with the intravenous injection of an iodinated contrast medium. Contrast administered intravenously distributes rapidly throughout the extracellular space (except for the central nervous system) and is excreted by the kidneys. The time between intravenous contrast injection and data acquisition determines the pattern of contrast enhancement. As the time from injection progresses, contrast is seen within the arteries (arterial phase), then the tissues (late venous phase), then in the urinary collecting system (delayed phase). Intravenous administration of iodinated contrast media is associated with dose-dependant nephrotoxicity, particularly in patients with impaired renal function (Adam, 2008).

# MAGNETIC RESONANCE IMAGING

Protons have charge and spin, hence act as small magnets. When they are exposed to a strong magnetic field they tend to align with the magnetic field and their axes of rotation wobble at the same frequency (Larmor frequency). The wobbling of the axes of rotation of the individual protons are out of phase with one another. If they are then exposed to a strong radiofrequency (RF) pulse of an appropriate frequency, their alignment will change and the wobbling of the axes of rotation of the protons will move into phase. When the RF pulse stops, the protons release energy as radio frequency waves (the signal) then move back into alignment with the magnetic field and the wobbling of the axes of rotation once again becomes out of phase. The rate of return to the baseline state is characterised by two independent processes, each with their own time constant. T1 is the "longitudinal relaxation time constant" and relates to the rate at which the protons move back into alignment with the magnetic field. T2 is the "transverse relaxation time constant" and relates to the rate at which the wobbling of the axes of rotation move out of phase (Schild, 1990).

The preceding paragraph describes the basic principles of MRI, but the practical application is considerably more complex. Sequences use multiple RF pulses, with varying frequency, direction, and other parameters, in order to generate images with different characteristics. A detailed explanation of how these images are generated is beyond the scope of this book but a simplified overview may be helpful. One issue is that different MRI manufacturers use different names to describe very similar sequences. MRI sequences may be categorised into four broad groups.

## (1) Spin echo sequences

These are the most frequently used sequences. They include the standard T1-weighted, T2-weighted and proton density (PD) images.

With a PD image, the effects of T1 and T2 are eliminated so the intensity of signal depends on the density of protons in the tissue (Blink, 2004).

The intensity of the signal in a T1-weighted image depends on both the density of protons in the tissue and the T1 value of the tissue. Tissues in which the protons are tightly bound (e.g. fat) are associated with short T1 values (high intensity on image), while tissues in which the protons are loosely bound (e.g. CSF) are associated with long T1 values (low intensity on image) (Schild, 1990).

The intensity of the signal in a T2-weighted image depends on both the density of protons in the tissue and the T2 value of the tissue. Mobile fluid environments (e.g. CSF) are associated with long T2 values (high intensity on image), while less mobile fluid environments (e.g. white matter) are associated with short T2 values (low intensity on image). Lesions in the CNS that have high water content or have disruption of the structure of the tissue at a cellular level will have a high T2 signal (Schild, 1990).

Fast spin echo (FSE) allows rapid image acquisition, thereby minimising movement artefact and gives a different contrast pattern to other sequences (Blink, 2004). It is useful for examining the spinal cord in trauma, assessing for oedema or haematoma.

Fat-suppressed images may be obtained for T1- and T2-weighted sequences. This is useful for imaging bony structures, where fat from marrow may obscure pathology.

## (2) Gradient echo (GRE) sequences

With these sequences, there is rapid image acquisition and images may be T1-weighted, T2-weighted or PD (Blink, 2004).

The fast spoiled gradient echo (FSPGR) sequence is highly sensitive for detecting tissue containing iron or calcium, which will both produce a markedly hypointense signal. It is useful for assessing haematoma or examining the bones.

## (3) Inversion recovery sequences

Two sequences commonly used are (Blink, 2004):
- Fluid attenuated inversion recovery (FLAIR) sequence, which eliminates the signal from CSF. It is sensitive to oedema and inflammation.
- Short T1 inversion recovery (STIR) sequence, which eliminates the signal from fat tissue. This is useful when high signal from fat in the marrow may obscure pathology such as subtle traumatic bone marrow oedema.

## (4) Diffusion weighted imaging (DWI)

DWI assesses the movement of protons due to diffusion over a short time. If there is restricted diffusion, the signal is of high intensity. If there is unrestricted diffusion (e.g. CSF), there is low intensity signal. Unfortunately, the signal on DWI is not just produced by the diffusion characteristics, but also changes in parallel with the T2 and PD of the tissue. To eliminate these confounders, an apparent diffusion coefficient (ADC) map is generated. The ADC signal is low with true restricted diffusion. Using a combination of these sequences, vasogenic oedema (intensity high on T2, high on DWI and high on ADC map) may be distinguished from cytotoxic oedema (intensity high on T2, high on DWI, and reduced on ADC map) (Mikulis, 2007).

## Gadolinium contrast

Gadolinium (Gd) is a paramagnetic substance that acts as a contrast agent by markedly shortening T1 when it is present. Gd-based contrast distributes throughout the extracellular fluid, and does not cross the normal blood–brain barrier. In pathological conditions in which the blood–brain barrier breaks down, there is marked hyper-intensity (enhancement) of affected areas on T1-weighted images (Roberts, 2007).

Gd administration may be combined with a fat-suppressed sequence ('Fat sat'), which eliminates the normally bright T1 signal from the protons in fat. This may be useful in the diagnosis of infections such as epidural abscess or neoplasia.

In patients with both acute and chronic renal failure (GFR < 30 mL/min), Gd contrast administration is associated with nephrogenic systemic fibrosis and should be avoided if possible (Bhave, 2008). There is some evidence that Gd contrast may have nephrotoxic effects (Perazella, 2007).

## MRI sequences for neurological imaging

The exact sequences used will vary depending on the clinical question and the region of the body being examined. A range of sequences are chosen that provide complementary information. Sequences that are commonly used for imaging the brain and spinal cord are described below.

## MRI sequences for brain imaging

- Axial T1-weighted spin echo (T1): shows fluid signal hypointense to that of normal brain. Subacute blood, proteinaceous material and fat signal are hyper-intense relative to the brain.
- Axial T2 FLAIR: nulls the normally bright T2 signal of CSF (becomes black), while other parenchymal fluid appears bright (as in oedema or tumour).
- Axial DWI and ADC: depict restricted diffusion in acute infarcts, abscesses and some hypercellular neoplasms. These sequences are used to look for acute infarcts.
- Axial gradient echo: is highly sensitive for blood, which appears markedly hypo-intense in signal. It generally overestimates the actual haematoma size (blooming effect).

## MRI sequences for spinal cord imaging

- T1- and T2-weighted spin echo with and without fat suppression. Fat suppression improves the ability to assess inflammatory processes in fatty tissues. T1 sequences highlight the normally slightly hyperintense vertebral marrow, so with oedema (fractures, tumours or infections), the marrow becomes darker (hypointense). On T2 sequences, the CSF is bright (myelographic effect), as is any marrow oedema. T2 sequences are good for depicting cord injury.
- Axial Gradient echo as FSPGR to assess for haematoma, and optimise visualisation of bony structures.

## REFERENCES

Adam A, Dixon AK, Grainger RG, et al (eds). Grainger & Allison's diagnostic radiology. A textbook of medical imaging. Philadelphia; Elsevier: 2008

Anderson B. Echocardiography: The normal examination and echocardiographic measurements. Brisbane: MGA Graphics; 2007

Bhave G, Lewis JB, Chang SS. Association of gadolinium based magnetic resonance imaging contrast agents and nephrogenic systemic fibrosis. J Urol 2008; 180(3): 830–5; discussion 835

Blink EJ. An easy introduction. Basic MRI physics for anyone who has not a degree in physics. Available: http://www.mri-physics.com; accessed 7 May 2009

Erkonen WE. Chapter 1: Radiography, computed tomography, magnetic resonance imaging, and ultrasonography: Principles and indications. In: Erkonen WE, Smith WL, eds. Radiology 101. The basics and fundamentals of imaging. 2nd edn. Philadelphia: Lipincott Williams and Wilkins; 2005: 3–15

Feigenbaum H, Armstrong WF, Ryan T. Chapter 2: Physics and instrumentation. In: Feigenbaum H, Armstrong WF, eds. Feigenbaum's echocardiography. 6th edn. Philadelphia: Lippincott Williams and Wilkins; 2005: 11–45

Hofer M, ed. CT teaching manual. A systematic approach to CT reading. New York: Thieme Medical Publishers; 2005

Long BW, Frank ED, Ehrlich RA, eds. Radiography essentials for limited practice. 2nd edn. St. Louis: Saunders; 2006

Mikulis DJ, Roberts TP. Neuro MR: Protocols. J Magn Reson Imaging 2007; 26(4): 838–47

Novelline RA, ed. Squire's fundamentals of radiology. Cambridge: Harvard University Press; 2004

Otto CM, ed. Textbook of clinical echocardiography. 3rd edn. Philadelphia: Saunders; 2004

Pavone P, Luccichenti G, Cademartiri F. From maximum intensity projection to volume rendering. Semin Ultrasound CT MR 2001; 22(5): 413–19

Perazella MA, Rodby RA. Gadolinium use in patients with kidney disease: A cause for concern. Semin Dial 2007; 20(3): 179–85

Roberts TP, Mikulis D. Neuro MR: Principles. J Magn Reson Imaging 2007; 26(4): 823–37

Schild HH, ed. MRI made easy (well almost). Berlin: Nationales Druckhaus; 1990

# Appendix

## AMERICAN ASSOCIATION FOR THE SURGERY OF TRAUMA ORGAN INJURY SCALE – SPLEEN, LIVER AND KIDNEY*

### SPLEEN

| Grade | Injury Type | Description of Injury |
|-------|-------------|-----------------------|
| I | Haematoma | Subcapsular (< 10% surface area) |
| | Laceration | Capsular tear (< 1cm parenchymal depth) |
| II | Haematoma | Subcapsular (10% to 50% surface area); intraparenchymal (< 5 cm in diameter) |
| | Laceration | Capsular tear (1–3 cm parenchymal depth that does not involve a trabecular vessel) |
| III | Haematoma | Subcapsular (> 50% surface area or expanding); ruptured subcapsular or parenchymal haematoma; intraparenchymal haematoma (≥ 5 cm or expanding) |
| | Laceration | > 3 cm parenchymal depth or involving trabecular vessels |
| IV | Laceration | Laceration involving segmental or hilar vessels producing major devascularisation (> 25% of spleen) |
| V | Haematoma | Completely shattered spleen |
| | Laceration | Hilar vascular injury devascularises spleen |

### LIVER

| Grade | Injury Type | Description of Injury |
|-------|-------------|-----------------------|
| I | Haematoma | Subcapsular (< 10% surface area) |
| | Laceration | Capsular tear (< 1cm parenchymal depth) |
| II | Haematoma | Subcapsular (10% to 50% surface area); intraparenchymal (< 10 cm in diameter) |
| | Laceration | Capsular tear (1–3 cm parenchymal depth, < 10 cm in length) |
| III | Haematoma | Subcapsular (> 50% surface area of ruptured subcapsular or parenchymal haematoma); intraparenchymal haematoma (> 10 cm or expanding) |
| | Laceration | > 3 cm parenchymal depth |
| IV | Laceration | Parenchymal disruption involving 25–75% hepatic lobe or 1–3 Couinaud's segments |
| V | Laceration | Parenchymal disruption involving > 75% of hepatic lobe or > 3 Couinaud's segments within a single lobe |
| | Vascular | Juxtahepatic venous injuries (i.e. retrohepatic vena cava / central major hepatic veins) |
| VI | Vascular | Hepatic avulsion |

## KIDNEY

| Grade | Injury Type | Description of Injury |
|---|---|---|
| **I** | Contusion | Microscopic or gross haematuria, urologic studies normal |
| | Haematoma | Subcapsular, non-expanding without parenchymal laceration |
| **II** | Haematoma | Non-expanding perirenal haematoma confined to renal retroperitoneum |
| | Laceration | < 1.0 cm parenchymal depth of renal cortex without urinary extravasation |
| **III** | Laceration | > 1.0 cm parenchymal depth of renal cortex without collecting system rupture or urinary extravasation |
| **IV** | Laceration | Parenchymal laceration extending through renal cortex, medulla and collecting system |
| | Vascular | Main renal artery or vein injury with contained haemorrhage |
| **V** | Laceration | Completely shattered kidney |
| | Vascular | Avulsion of renal hilum that devascularises kidney |
| | | Advance one grade for bilateral injuries up to grade III |

* Tinkoff G, Esposito TJ, Reed J, et al. American association for the surgery of trauma organ injury scale I: spleen, liver, and kidney, validation based on the National Trauma Data Bank. J Am Coll Surg 2008; 207: 646-55

# Index